If I were a rich man could I buy a pancreas?

Medical Ethics series

David H. Smith and Robert M. Veatch, editors

If I were a rich man.../ could I buy a pancreas?

and other essays on the ethics of health care

by Arthur L. Caplan

Indiana University Press

Bloomington and Indianapolis

Library of Congress Cataloging-in-Publication Data
Caplan, Arthur L.
     If I were a rich man could I buy a pancreas? : and other essays on the ethics of health care / by Arthur L. Caplan.
         p.   cm. — (Medical ethics series)
     Includes index.
     ISBN 0-253-31307-4 (alk. paper)
     1. Medical ethics. 2. Bioethics.   I. Title. II. Series.
   R724.C34   1992
   174'.2—dc20
                                                                                       91-32112
   1 2 3 4 5 96 95 94 93 92

For Janet and Zachary

contents

Acknowledgments   x
Introduction   xii

Part I. The nature of applied ethics

1. Can applied ethics be effective in health care and should it strive to be?
    3

2. Moral experts and moral expertise: Does either exist?
                                        18

Part II. Ethical issues in animal and human experimentation

3. Beastly conduct: ethical issues in animal experimentation
                                        43

4 Moral community and the responsibility of scientists
                                        59

5. On privacy and confidentiality in social science research
                                        70

6. Is there a duty to serve as a subject in biomedical research?
                                        85

Part III. Advances in reproduction and genetics

7. New technologies in reproduction—new ethical problems
                                        103

8. Mapping morality: ethics and the human genome project
118

Part IV. Transplants and other unnatural acts

9. Requests, gifts, and obligations: the ethics of organ
procurement
145

10. If I were a rich man could I buy a pancreas? Problems in the
policies and criteria used to allocate organs for transplantation
in the United States
158

11. Ethical issues raised by research involving xenografts
178

Part V. Aging, chronic illness, and rehabilitation

12. Is aging a disease?
195

13. Let wisdom find a way: the concept of competency in the care
of the elderly
210

14. Is medical care the right prescription for chronic illness?
221

15. Informed consent and provider/patient relationships in
rehabilitation medicine
240

16. Can autonomy be saved?
256

Part VI. Money, medicine, and morality

17. The high cost of technological development: a caveat for
policymakers
285

18. Hard data is the only answer to hard choices in health care
302

· 19. Ethics, cost-containment, and the allocation of scarce resources
315

Index   337

Acknowledgments

The author gratefully acknowledges permission to reprint material previously published as follows:

Chapter 1 in *Ethics* 93 (Jan. 1983), pp. 311–19. Copyright © 1983 by the University of Chicago.

Chapter 2 in Benjamin Freedman, Barry Hoffmaster, and Gwen Fraser, eds., *The Nature of Clinical Ethics* (Clifton, NJ: Humana Press, 1989).

Chapter 3 in the *Annals of the New York Academy of Sciences* 406, pp. 159–69. Copyright © 1983 by New York Academy of Sciences.

Chapter 4 in *Acta Physiologica Scandinavia,* Blackwell Scientific Publications Limited.

Chapter 5 in Thomas L. Beauchamp, ed., *Ethical Issues in Social Science Research* (Baltimore: Johns Hopkins University Press, 1982).

Chapter 6 in *IRB: A Review of Human Subjects Research* 6, no. 5 (Sept.–Oct. 1984). Copyright © The Hastings Center.

Chapter 7 in *Annals of the New York Academy of Sciences* 530 (1988), pp. 73–82. Copyright © 1988 by New York Academy of Sciences.

Chapter 9 in *Transplantation Proceedings* 18, no. 3, suppl. 2 (June 1986), pp. 49–56. Copyright © 1986 by Grune & Stratton, Inc. Reprinted by permission of Appleton & Lange, Inc.

Chapter 10 was published in an earlier version as "Problems in the Policies and Criteria Used to Allocate Organs for Transplantation in the United States" in *Transplantation Proceedings* 21, no. 3 (June 1989), pp. 3381–87, copyright ©1989. Reprinted by permission of Appleton & Lange, Inc.

Chapter 11 in *Journal of the American Medical Association* 254, no. 23 (Dec. 20, 1985), pp. 3339–43. Copyright © 1985 by the American Medical Association.

Chapter 12 in S. F. Spicker and S. R. Ingam, eds., *Vitalizing Long-Term Care: The Teaching Nursing Home and Other Perspectives* (New York: Springer, 1984).

Chapter 13 previously published in *Generations* 10 (Winter 1985), pp. 10–14. Reprinted with permission from *Generations,* journal of the American Society on Aging, 833 Market St., Suite 516, San Francisco, CA 94103. Copyright ©1985 ASA.

Chapter 14 in S. Sullivan and M. E. Lewin, eds., *The Economics and Ethics of Long-Term Care and Disability* (Washington, D.C.: American Enterprise Institute for Public Policy Research, 1988). Reprinted with permission of the American Enterprise Institute for Public Policy Research.

Chapter 15 in *Archives of Physical Medicine and Rehabilitation* 69:312–17, 1988.

Chapter 17 in Anne S. Allen, ed., *New Options, New Dilemmas: An Interprofessional Approach to Life or Death Decisions* (Lexington, MA: Lexington, 1986).

Chapter 18 in *The Mount Sinai Journal of Medicine* 56, no. 3 (May 1989).

Chapter 19 is a revised version of an article originally written with Reinhard Priester and published in *Investigative Radiology* 24 (1989), pp. 918–26.

Introduction

An old friend of mine, a journalist not an academic, has for many years delighted in getting my goat by asking me what my philosophy is. Whenever we meet it is not long before he bellows, "You are supposed to be a philosopher, so what exactly is your philosophy? Have you figured one out yet?" I always find myself hemming and hawing. The best I can do is mount a half-hearted riposte along the lines that if I had a philosophy I would surely not reveal it to the likes of him.

The truth of the matter is that I do not have "a philosophy." The essays collected in this book do not represent the natural out-croppings of a rockbed moral theory. Such an admission is danger-ous, since the reader of a collection of essays on very different topics rightly expects some clue about what ties the elements together into a coherent whole.

While there is no overarching theory behind the papers included in this book, there are a variety of themes that may permit them to constitute an integrated whole. The articles address topics whose in-tellectual half-life seems to be more than a decade; the points made in them continue to appear to me to be valid. Another common bond is that many of these pieces previously appeared in journals or books remarkable for the degree to which their pages remain umblemished by the touch of a human hand.

Having said that no single moral theory or meta-ethical stance drives the analysis exhibited in these essays, I must also state that for me this is hardly a vice but is, rather, a virtue. I am deeply suspicious, as many of the papers reveal, of the still regnant view in ethics which seeks both unassailable foundations for normative statements and presumes that the same theory which is used to shed light in one domain of morality will work equally well when pointed in an en-tirely different direction. This is a view I like to refer to as "engineer-ing ethics," but it might more accurately be described as "universal foundationalism."

Foundationalists believe that one and only one moral theory must undergird a moral outlook. They also advance a one-theory-fits-all picture of moral analysis. Some foundationalists have not yet located the Holy Grail of the one true theory that is good for all moral seasons. In lieu of this discovery, they argue that anything having to do with applied ethics must remain on hold until philosophers (or, among exceedingly liberal-minded proponents of this view, theologians) figure out exactly which moral theory is true so that the requisite deductions of prescriptive statements with universal scope and psychic pull can be made.

Foundationalism in twentieth-century ethics cannot be understood without knowing how ethics has been kicked around by science for most of the century. One of the bitter ironies of twentieth-century moral philosophy is that those who do ethics have spent the bulk of the century trying to curry the favor of those most deeply suspicious that ethics is intellectually empty.

Early on in this century, in the years between the world wars, those who espoused logical positivism (the view that only the methods of science could provide warrant for beliefs about the world) dismissed ethics from the realm of serious intellectual subjects. Ethics was and could only be the study of subjective feelings and emotions, nothing more and probably a great deal less. Ethics was fit for only psychological or anthropological inquiry. Statements about right and wrong, good and bad were held to have about the same prospects for confirmation or disconfirmation as proclamations concerning the eating habits of fairies or the hobbies of those living in other galaxies. Ethical statements were meaningful but utterly unverifiable due to their immunity to validation or falsification by scientific methods. This outlook dominated philosophical thought in the Western world well into the 1950s and 1960s and had reverberations in the theological as well as the secular realms of ethics.

The bitter legacy of banishment from the kingdom of warranted knowledge was that those interested in ethics spent the better part of the century trying to return from intellectual diaspora. They believed their return to the philosophical promised land could be attained by beating the positivists, and those influenced by them, at their own game. The last bastion of ardent logical positivism in the English-speaking world is to be found in foundationalist normative ethics. Those interested in the theory of ethics have sought legitimacy and credibility by advancing theories whose structure and amenability to proof mimic, they hope, the theories and methods of the empirical sciences.

"Serious" moral philosophers spend their time trying to construct theories that are universal in their application to all moral quandaries, dilemmas and problems. Many mainstream moral philosophers believe that a moral theory, to be a good moral theory, must display an organization based on a core of axiomatic or unchallengeable truths. The principles and rules of the theory must be deducible from this core set of axioms. The refutation of the theory can be accomplished by finding moral phenomena which are inconsistent with one of the claims that has been deduced from the principles and axioms allowing for the conditions that prevail in a particular situation.

In other words, those who believe that ethics must be grounded upon a valid theory in order to make any contribution to the solution, resolution, or analysis of moral problems all too often believe that this theory must have all and only the attributes associated with well confirmed theories in the sciences—axioms, a deductive core of key principles, and a testable set of predictions or explanations. The only good prescriptive moral claims, according to foundationalist views of theory, are those that can be deduced from a single set of self-evident, universally accepted axioms.

The effort to out-science science in the quest for acceptance leads many moral philosophers to embrace what is commonly supposed to be the structure of scientific theories for their own theoretical constructions. But science mimicry does not stop here. The aping of science has extended through to the methodologies and tactics used to analyze moral problems.

One of the most popular stratagems in moral philosophy for the past few decades has been to construct theories using idealized assumptions about simple systems. As evidenced in their analyzing moral phenomena through a veil of ignorance or reconstructing a simple moral life in a virgin land with only a few "rational" beings to lay claim to the resources contained therein, the modus operandi popular among moral theorists is to climb into an armchair and imagine as hard as one can what human beings would choose to do with respect to the division of resources or the recognition of rights if they were put in a position of disinterested, disembodied, and disengaged existence.

The strategy of simplifying and idealizing as the route to discovering moral truth is a direct imitation of the most popular mode of inquiry in natural science—the scientific experiment. Scientists who want to understand a phenomenon try to isolate the variable that they are interested in from all other influences. By creating an artificial environment in the laboratory or in a mathematical model, one can see exactly how the variable of interest reacts to external changes and alterations.

To study behavior, psychologists will often expose pure-bred strains of mice or rats to a single stimulus in a highly controlled environment. The ecologist who wants to understand how organisms interact with one another in ponds or lakes may create a mathematical model which encompasses only a few species and a couple of critical variables to try and get a handle on their interactions.

Much of contemporary moral theorizing reflects the view that the only way to gain insight into morality is to isolate key variables in a simple system and then to vary certain parameters (mentally, not literally) in order to understand what the variables mean or do. Idealization and abstraction are the hallmarks of a great deal of contemporary moral theorizing. The discovery of the "true" moral theory can be accomplished only by escaping or at least negating the confusing moral cacophony of the real world in favor of an easier-to-understand, controlled, idealized, and simplified world.

The problem with this strategy is that there is little reason to presume that it will eventuate in a true moral theory. Not because a true moral theory cannot exist, although I very much doubt that one does. Nor is it for want of trying, since from Plato and Spinoza to Rawls and Nozick plenty of able thinkers have stepped up to the philosophical plate to take their swing at producing the big foundationalist theory. Rather, it is because the notion of theory structure and the modes of inquiry dominant among those in the foundationalist hunt for the correct moral theory are outdated caricatures of what scientists and students of the sciences have come to think constitutes theory structure and methodology within the sciences themselves.

Few students of the sciences believe that the only structure a theory in science may exhibit is an axiomatic-deductive hierarchy. Kuhn, Feyerabend, Lakatos, Bloor, Edge, and many others have debunked the notion that foundationalism is the only view—or even an appropriate view—of theories in the natural sciences. Few theories consist of logical axioms from which deductions are made to be compared against observations of the empirical world. Theories, to be blunt, are often a messy jumble of premises, crucial experiments, spin-off hypotheses, illustrative models, ideologies, and outlooks.

They are as much about ways of thinking as they are the logical structure of premises.

Nor is there any lack of critics for the position that idealization and simplification are the only roads to knowledge within the sciences. Among biologists, for example, every mathematical modeler has his or her counterpart in systematics, ethology, comparative psychology, or field studies of one sort or another. If anything, those in the life sciences seem to have moved toward the view that, for idealization, abstraction, and simplification to be valuable, they must be set against the claims and findings of those who try to observe and generalize from real-world events.

Those who do applied ethics need not and should not see themselves simply as servants to moral theoreticians. The engineer trying to figure out how to design a bridge to cross a river—or plotting a course for a spacecraft that will permit it to pass near enough to the sun to take pictures but not so close as to be turned into vapor—does not begin with string theory. The ethicist who wants to help decide whether a feeding tube should be removed from an elderly woman in a permanent coma or whether to defend the decision to attempt to use a baboon's heart to save the life of a dying infant need not await the ruminations of those engaged in meta-ethics concerning moral realism nor the announcement that a single valid moral theory has been discovered.

Sadly, the desire to link specific claims about bioethical issues to a single valid overarching moral theory has had a distorting effect on what problems in bioethics have drawn the greatest attention. The pursuit of the exception, the counter-example, or other equivalents of the "crucial experiment" that a belief in foundationalism inspires has led some of those doing bioethics to pursue the odd, the anomalous, and the rare in the hope of testing the limits of theory. This explains, in part, why there is a mountain of bioethical literature on baboon heart transplants and very little about the ordinary moral lives of those who live in nursing homes or receive their care in a doctor's office.

As I hope some of the essays in this collection show, there is as much of moral interest and importance in the mundane as there is in the extraordinary with respect to health care. The desire to see how fine a moral theory can grind can lead to fascinating nooks and crannies within health care, but it can also distort the recognition that these are only nooks and crannies.

If the organization, structure, and goals of bioethics and applied philosophy in general have much more in common with ethology and engineering than with the aims and organization of thermodynamics or cosmology, then it is quite probable that the equivalent of the unified field theory in bioethics will never be found. Not because there is no true moral theory but because the insights, skills, and knowledge that shed light on practical moral problems in health care cannot be derived from any single source. When the object of inquiry is not so much finding the right answer as trying to figure out the nature of the moral problem at hand, then many sorts of information—empirical, historical, sociological, economic, institutional, and ethical—will be needed.

It is fair to wonder whether the argument that bioethics can proceed in the absence of consensus about the validity of normative moral theory is nothing more than an exercise in transforming lemons into lemonade. This worry gains force in light of the fact that those who do bioethics, especially in clinical or policy settings, quickly learn that the subject commands respect among those outside the field. Gaining an audience is not always a difficult thing to do. There is a very real danger in such a climate that ideology and bias can masquerade as reasoned argumentation.

The ultimate test of claims in bioethics—as is true in other areas of applied activity, such as agriculture, engineering, or medicine—is not logical consistency with theory but pragmatic application. The good software engineer knows that the goal is to design a program that can be used by a variety of people to get a particular task done. So it is in bioethics. The aim of the enterprise is to determine the nature of the problem, to pinpoint the source, and to see if it is both possible and desirable to do anything about it. It is in the light of these goals that the following essays should be evaluated.

Part I

The nature of applied ethics

1.

Can applied ethics be effective in health care and should it strive to be?

I. Moral efficacy in medicine

A number of philosophers, theologians, and others with a major interest in ethics have, in recent times, found themselves plying their trades in the confines of a hospital or medical center. The extent of their involvement has grown to proportions which are sufficient to permit an inquiry into what exactly it is that these persons are supposed to be doing in such settings. This inquiry leads inevitably to a further and more significant question: are philosophers and others engaged in what has come to be called "applied ethics" in the "real world" of medicine able to do anything useful there? In mulling over such questions, it may be useful for the reader to ponder two examples which stand out in my own mind as the occasions upon which, through my involvement in a medical center, I felt I was most effective with reference to matters of applied ethics.

The first incident occurred in the course of teaching in the hospital of a large urban medical center. The elective was entitled "Ethics Rounds" and was team taught with a psychiatrist and an internist.

The course consisted of visiting various patients selected by students, interviewing the patients, and discussing some of the moral issues that the students and teachers felt were raised by the cases.

Early on in the course, the students had selected a 90-year-old woman with a fractured arm for an interview. She had no relatives, and the students were worried about what might happen to her upon discharge from the hospital. I came to the class fully prepared to discourse on theories of distributive justice at a moment's notice, since I rather naively believed the students might benefit greatly from a disquisition on Mill, Rawls, and Nozick in trying to figure out what to do with the old woman.

As soon as the medical instructors and students had gathered together, we hurriedly set off to find and interview the old woman. We all burst into her room just as she was in the process of defecating. To my surprise, no one was deterred by her behavior, and both the psychiatrist and the internist proceeded immediately to interview the woman about her life plans, goals, and personal aspirations. I remained uncharacteristically silent during this exchange, and it was only when the class had returned to the confines of the psychiatry lounge to discuss the case that I proffered the opinion that it might have been better to wait until the woman had finished her excretory functions before interviewing her. This observation was greeted with some consternation by both students and the other teachers. Of course I was correct, they conceded. Privacy was important to patients, as my comment showed, and physicians should not allow the press of their own busy schedules to override a patient's need for a certain amount of privacy. My insight was acknowledged with a great degree of gravity, and my esteem among the members of the course was assured for the duration of that particular clinical rotation.

The other paradigmatic example of my moral efficacy in a hospital setting resulted from a suggestion I made concerning a problem of scarce medical resources. Every summer the emergency room of the hospital filled up with persons suffering from emphysema and other respiratory ailments. The hot weather made it very difficult for such persons to breathe comfortably, and they came to the emergency room to receive oxygen. Unfortunately, there were only two oxygen units available, and there were often a dozen or more persons seeking to use them at various times during the day and night. The staff of the emergency room asked my help in developing a set of criteria for deciding what would be a fair and equitable allocation of their scarce medical resources.

My first response upon hearing their request was to consult the diverse anthologies in existence on medical ethics to see what various philosophers and theologians had to say about issues of micro-allocation and ethics. I found they had the predictable things to say about such matters—some defended a criterion of merit, some a criterion of need, some a criterion of social utility, and some a random lottery. I was fortunately bright enough to suspect that the medical staff could have gotten that far without me or the anthology. But, in thinking about the matter further, it occurred to me that it might be possible to solve the allocation problem by addressing the source of the scarcity. I asked some of the emergency room staff if Medicaid/Medicare covered the provision of air conditioners in the homes of persons suffering from respiratory ailments. It turned out, much to everyone's surprise, that the machines could be prescribed and the cost reimbursed. I ascended to the status of moral guru in the emergency room, famous as the man who had solved the oxygen machine crunch.

I mention these incidents not to impress anyone with my problem-solving skills. Indeed, I believe any person of reasonable intelligence possessing a bit of perspective on the behavior of the health-care professionals involved in both of these cases could have arrived at the exact same recommendations and solutions. It is interesting to note, however, that these two cases of efficacious moral action were hardly dependent on analytical rigor or theoretical moral sophistication for their genesis. Indeed, in both cases, ethical theory would have been the wrong place to turn for a solution to the issues under consideration.

II. What exactly is it that those in applied ethics do?

Of course it ought to be noted that philosophers and others working in medical settings engage in other activities besides behavioral reform. Philosophers with a background in ethics teach in various types of settings; attend rounds; serve on various kinds of committees, such as institutional review boards or hospital "ethics" committees; engage in health-policy formulation at the federal, state, and local levels; offer consultation and advice to interested parties in hospitals about a wide variety of ethical matters; and, on occasion, serve as moral fire fighters, rushing to various places within the hospital to help solve a moral dilemma or resolve a staff dispute. Not all philosophers working in medical centers do all of these things, but many of them have at one time or another been asked to serve as a teacher, lay representative, advisor, policymaker, or arbitrator. There are even media reports of philosophers and theologians prowling the floors of some hospitals armed with an electronic beeper and clad in a white coat, the better to respond efficaciously to moral crises and ethical emergencies.

"Beeper ethics" aside, it seems that philosophers and other persons with expertise in ethics believe that there are all sorts of contributions that they can and should make to the operation of medical centers and the well-being of staff and patients. What is less evident in considering these activities is exactly what skills and what expertise those in applied ethics think they possess that would make them effective in any way with regard to some or all of the various roles health professionals ask them to assume.

III. Philosophical qualifications for medical employment

One skill that philosophers seem to pride themselves on, in particular, is that of conceptual analysis. Oftentimes in the course of trying to explain to the uninitiated of health care what it is that philosophers do, those in philosophy and, in particular, applied ethics will mention such talents as being able to analyze the meanings of words, detect logical confusions and fallacies, and the ability to establish canons of sound and valid argumentation. Thus, one skill that someone expert in applied ethics can provide to those working in a medical setting is felt to be that of patrolling and policing logical malefactors.

Second, many persons working in applied ethics believe themselves to be in possession of a body or corpus of knowledge concerning ethical theories which can be brought to bear on moral problems arising in the practice of medicine. This knowledge includes both a mastery of ethical traditions within philosophy and, perhaps, theology, and an understanding of the ways in which moral beliefs and opinions can legitimately be justified through linking them to appropriate moral theories drawn from these traditions. Just as an engineer utilizes his or her understanding of the theories of physics to solve practical problems of transportation or heating of the sort which arise in everyday life, so the applied ethicist working in a medical setting can bring to bear the theoretical insights and lemmas of contemporary moral theory to solve the everyday moral quandaries of hospital life.

Third, some philosophers and ethical experts have noted that they bring an especially rare commodity into the health-care setting, the skill or ability to remain disinterested and neutral about moral events of the sort that arise in medicine. Philosophers who work in medical settings often view themselves as impartial observers of the medical scene. They are persons without a vested interest in the kinds of care that is delivered or the safety and efficacy of particular procedures, and they do not have a political need to align themselves with any individual or group within the medical settings. This perspective allows them, so they believe, to weigh alternatives and reflect upon policies in ways that those caught up in the system, either as providers or recipients of health care, cannot. Thus, as the two vignettes given earlier suggest, impartiality permits a person engaged in applied ethics to see the medical world in ways that are not available to those who are part of the scenery, often with beneficial consequences for all.

IV. The "engineering model" of applied ethics

This picture of ethics, emphasizing conceptual clarification, mastery of ethical theory, and impartiality, can usefully be referred to as the "engineering model" of applied ethics. It presumes that: (1) there is a body of knowledge concerning ethics that persons can be more or less knowledgeable about; (2) this knowledge becomes "applied" in medical settings by: (a) deducing conclusions from theories in light of relevant empirical facts and descriptions of circumstances and (b) analyzing properly the process of the deduction (i.e., watching for logical fallacies, ambiguities in the meaning of key terms, improper classifications of entities, misdescriptions, etc.); and (3) the process of applying ethical knowledge to moral problems in medicine can and must be carried out in an impartial, disinterested, value-free manner.

It is interesting to note that the engineering model is quite analogous to the model of nomological explanation regnant for so many years in the philosophy of the natural and social sciences. Explanation on the old N-D (nomological-deductive) model was held simply to be a matter of deduction from theory, the deduction being accomplished by the supplementation of laws and principles with the appropriate initial and boundary conditions, bridge principles, and empirical descriptions. The process of explanation was to be carried out in a value-free way by impartial souls dedicated solely to the advancement of human understanding and scientific progress.

In its applied-ethics reincarnation, moral justification has assumed the role of explanation. The process of explaining by subsuming data under a set of theoretical principles is directly mimicked by viewing the subsumption of moral "data" under a set of hierarchically ordered moral principles as the key to justification. Impartiality is the ethos held to pervade both undertakings. Why this model has taken hold in ethics when it has undergone such drastic revisions and modifications in the philosophy of science is surely an intellectual issue worthy of serious examination. But what is perhaps more interesting is the degree to which those who do applied work in ethics are wedded to the engineering model as a matter of self-perception, both of what they do and how they ought do it.

V. Have philosophers and others operating with the engineering model been effective in medicine?

There are numerous and obvious reasons for doubting whether it is possible to show if medical ethics, as practiced by on-site medical ethicists, has made any difference to the practice of medicine. Medicine is hardly an isolated system and, whatever one thinks of the appropriateness of doing beeper ethics, those philosophers in the trade have not been prowling hospital corridors for all that long a period of time.

Nevertheless, a few general observations about efficacy can be made. On the whole, those doing applied ethics have been far more effective in influencing the formulation of health policy at the federal level than at the bedside. Philosophers, both through arguments in the literature and through direct participation in the policy process, have had a hand in bringing about the creation and maintenance of committees, review procedures, regulations, and institutional controls pertaining to the practice of medicine and the delivery of health care. In large measure, for example, the continued existence of a system of institutional review boards at all medical centers receiving research monies from the National Institutes of Health can be traced directly to recent moral concerns about human experimentation and the attendant ethical issues this raises. These issues were and continue to be presented to a wide public audience by persons doing applied ethics.

Those in the applied ethics trade have been far less successful in some of the other roles and activities they have been asked or assigned, or have volunteered, to undertake. The teaching of medical ethics in the medical school curriculum has not been received with a great deal of enthusiasm by its intended audience. Students and faculty often find ethics courses boring and irrelevant. Many assign them low priority vis-à-vis other subjects. The ground swell of interest that surrounded the introduction of the subject in medical schools seems to have peaked, and there is some evidence that certain schools have, as often happens with rapid innovations in the medical curriculum, tired of this particular subject and may be moving on to newer and more lucrative ones.

Similarly, poor grades can be given in assessing the ability of philosophers and others in applied ethics to work well with medical personnel on matters of morality. Many in applied ethics simply find clinical work uncomfortable and do not choose to do it. When they do do it, however, health-care personnel often find themselves highly frustrated with the results. As one clinician acquaintance of mine observed about philosophers-in-residence in medical settings, "You guys like to talk about ethics, but you don't want to do any ethics." Health-care practitioners expect practical advice and counsel about actions they should take regarding specific patients. When such advice is not forthcoming, they become frustrated with the logic chopping of applied ethicists and turn to each other (or, rather, return to each other) for moral guidance and psychological support.

Few philosophers have been asked to help formulate sensitive hospital policies such as those governing admission to neonatal intensive care units or discharge from intensive care units. The issues of allocation and equity which arise on a daily basis in medical practice are usually resolved by senior medical personnel behind doors firmly closed to the wisdom of moral philosophers.

Those philosophers and theologians who are asked to "parachute" in to solve various crisis situations, such as when doctors and nurses are at odds about various hospital practices or when physical therapists, social workers, and occupational therapists are engaged in battles over turf, professional responsibility, or professional ego, do not last long. They usually meet the same fate as the psychiatrists who are likely to have preceded them—interest if they take sides, polite universal hostility if they do not.

Overall, the record of efficacy is a mixed bag. There have been some real policy triumphs at the national level; some schools have found philosophers to be useful in the classroom or on regulatory committees; and many health-care practitioners pay more attention to moral issues than they did before the applied ethicists appeared. On the other hand, most health practitioners find the writing and teaching of those in applied ethics hopelessly opaque and irrelevant, student interest in courses is weak, medical personnel find the skills of conceptual clarification and logical analysis to be of little use, and few philosophers have been asked to become involved in an active, ongoing way in hospital policy formulation on a day-to-day basis.

VI. Why has applied ethics enjoyed a mixed record of success in medicine?

If it is true that those doing applied ethics have not, to date, succeeded in carrying out the various kinds of tasks they find themselves engaged in within medical settings, then why might this be so? There is a temptation to turn, in light of the engineering model, to ethical theory as the causes of any failures that exist. Perhaps current moral theory is not adequate for solving the kinds of problems that exist in contemporary medicine. Ethics, like sociology and the other social sciences, must await its Newton, if those doing applied ethics are to be properly armed with theories that would enable them to work effectively with medical practitioners in solving the everyday moral puzzles of hospital life.

It may be true that some of the failures and disappointments arising in the course of recent work in applied ethics in medical centers can be blamed on inadequate theories in ethics proper. However, it may be that some of the difficulties have more to do with the uses to which such theories are put than with the adequacy or inadequacy of available moral theories, per se.

One difficulty confronting anyone attempting to utilize extant moral theories of justice, rights, or whatever to solve moral problems in hospital settings is that the problems are always complex and murky, particularly as a consequence of the dynamic nature of morality in medicine. Much of moral theory today presumes a static system whereby the abilities, interests, and needs of parties can be established and, once discerned, assumed to be constant. However, in the real world of medical morality, interests and needs constantly change and evolve. Patients learn to adjust to illness, nurses develop dislikes for particular patients, house staff grow eager to find an "interesting case" after dealing with a run of 20 alcoholics, and so on.

Not only do the phenomena of moral life constantly change and evolve in medicine, but it is not always clear how best to describe and individuate the moral data that appear in this constantly shifting context. Just as the N-D model of explanation in the philosophy of science foundered on the shoals of the observation/ theory distinction and the impossibility of locating a pure observation language, the engineering model of applied ethics shows signs of collapse when put to the test of locating pure moral "facts" whose descriptions are both intersubjectively verifiable and unbiased. Those in applied ethics have two difficulties in finding moral facts to submit to the test of moral theory. First, they do not always know enough about medicine to understand a situation adequately and describe it. And, second, even when they do, they come to the medical setting with a vast array of sophisticated preconceptions and theoretical biases that influence their moral perceptions and classifications. This view of ethical theory presumes it is possible simply to locate moral facts and test them against theory. But the process of observation, individuation, and description is no easier in the moral realm than it is in the scientific. So simpleminded a view of the relationship between fact and theory in ethics is certain to fail to be useful for purposes of problem solving.

But the failures of applied ethics to solve all the various problems that have been put before it cannot be attributed simply to an inadequate view of moral theory. The source of most problems for those involved in doing applied ethics is in great measure the engineering model of application which governs much of what is done with available moral theory in solving moral problems in medicine.

VII. The inadequacies of the engineering model of applied ethics

There are four important ways in which the engineering model of applied ethics both minimizes the efficacious use of moral theories and hinders the utility of applied ethicists in medical settings.

Problem selection and the definition of moral problems

On the engineering model of applied ethics, application is equated with deduction from a theory. Unfortunately, such a view presupposes that the analysis of what counts as a moral problem in medicine is either self-evident or predetermined by health professionals. On this model, the health professional presents a moral problem to a person trained in the fine points of ethics, who can then proceed to grind the problem through the available moral theories. While this kind of process sometimes works well in analyzing moral issues in medicine, more often than not those seeking advice or help in answering a moral problem are not in the best position to define the nature of the problem. By emphasizing deduction from theory as the main task of the applied ethicist, the engineering model obscures the fact that problem analysis and diagnosis are just as important in medical settings as is the solving of moral puzzles.

The situation confronting a person attempting to do ethics in the health-care setting is not all that dissimilar from that confronting a clinician in treating a patient with a medical complaint. Clinicians treat the complaints of patients as possible evidence of a medical problem. But they do not view what patients have to say as definitive with respect to identifying what the problem is, or even with respect to whether a problem actually exists.

Similarly, in analyzing a moral problem in medicine, it would be wrong to take the complaints of health-care professionals or patients simply at face value. Rather than attempt to solve problems within the framework of those who present them, as is encouraged on the engineering model, the applied ethicist must feel free to reinterpret complaints, disregard some issues, and, occasionally, move beyond the issues as initially framed by health-care professionals. Otherwise, applied ethics can become merely the palliative treatment of the symptomatology of ethical discontent.

Overemphasis on means rather than ends

Health-care professionals, like other busy people, place high value on the efficient solution of problems and quandaries. Those doing applied ethics along the lines indicated in the engineering model are highly susceptible to professional pressures on them to analyze and solve problems quickly. Efficiency becomes a prized value, while the analysis of the legitimacy of medical ends is easily discouraged. It is difficult to practice medicine and at the same time have someone around constantly questioning the value of the effort. However, after seeing case after case of 95-year-old women tied to their beds in intensive care units in order to permit the administration of drugs and fluids with a minimum amount of patient resistance, one may become convinced that there is a real need to resist the siren call of efficiency inherent in the engineering model in order to probe more deeply into the ultimate aims and goals of various medical endeavors.

Taking medical common sense seriously

There is a very strong tendency which the engineering model does nothing to discourage to view persons doing applied ethics as on a par with other consultants and experts who are present in medical settings. Just as the cardiologist and endocrinologist have their domains of expertise, so the philosopher or theologian is often thought expert in moral matters. Such a view discourages those doing applied ethics from taking seriously what health professionals have to say about moral issues in medicine. More important, it discourages close attention to the realities of illness and anxiety for patients and their families. By locating moral competence in the applied ethicist, the engineering model discounts the realities—of the sick role, of the inability to cope with fear, of the experience of pain, and so on—that are so important in understanding moral issues in medicine. All one need do is to take a casual glance through the literature on autonomy, paternalism, and personal responsibility in the journals of applied ethics to see how far moral expertise has wandered from moral reality.

Who wants moral expertise and who can pay for it?

Another problem inherent in the engineering model of applied ethics is that, by leaving problem definition in the hands of health professionals, the model tends to limit contacts between applied ethicists and health professionals to those health professionals who ask for help. For a variety of reasons, those likely to ask for help are physicians. This means that the tendency is to focus on moral dilemmas faced by physicians in clinical settings, and for those doing applied ethics to be identified with physicians. The fact that physicians are also the ones most often in the position of paying for the presence of persons doing applied ethics in medical settings does little to encourage attention to other parties. The engineering model not only skews ethics in the direction of technical competence, but also limits philosophical attention to those who seek and can pay for technical assistance.

VIII. When failure is not failure

There are a variety of reasons for suspecting that some of the difficulties encountered by those doing applied ethics in medical centers can be traced back to inadequacies in both current moral theories and in the model of application dominant in applied ethics today. But it ought to be noted that, while the engineering model assumes that those who ask for help or seek aid are sincere in doing so, this is not always the case. Sincerity is no more to be taken for granted in dealing with medical professionals than it is with persons claiming to want help in any walk of life.

There are a number of reasons health professionals may want to involve applied ethicists in their work that have nothing whatsoever to do with resolving problems or grounding moral beliefs on a firmer analytical foundation.

Moral theorizing as diversionary

There are all sorts of ways in which labeling a problem as a moral issue can be useful in diverting attention from other types of problems that arise in medical settings. Thus, for example, it is far better, from the point of view of the hospital administration, to have nurses discussing the morality of strikes than it is to have them engaging in such activities. If one must have a public participant on an institutional review board panel for reviewing human subjects research, it is much easier to deal with an academic than a real, live resident from the immediate hospital neighborhood. It is far easier to begin a moral discussion about the allocation of scarce resources, such as kidney dialysis units, than to ask health practitioners and patients to live with the fact that society has decided not to fund a sufficient number of machines to treat all who are in need.

Applied ethics as co-optative

Administrators and department chairs are frequently confronted with protests and complaints from underlings about the operation of a floor, unit, or ward. The usual response of medical administrators to such crisis situations is to find a way for staff to "let off some steam." People faced with a crisis are often quite prepared to utilize applied ethicists as harmless targets for the venting of anger and rage by hospital staff. However, often the complaints of the staff are legitimate and the invoking of ethics and moral analysis serves merely to sidetrack legitimate complaints and grievances that should be directed elsewhere.

Moral engineering as ceremony

Procrastination is a marvelous response to crises of all sorts, and this strategy has its proponents in health care as well. Oftentimes someone seeking the guidance of a moral guru is more interested in appearances than solutions. The time-consuming ethical meanderings of a verbose moral philosopher can provide a concrete and lengthy demonstration of concern over some thorny moral issue. Health-care professionals enjoy a performance as much as anyone else, and the virtuosity of moral engineers, while it is rarely taken seriously, can be at least temporarily entertaining for all concerned.

IX. The art of moral engineering

I have been fairly harsh on the engineering model of applied ethics in this essay. However, I am very much aware of the fact that engineering is a valuable and helpful activity even in a field such as ethics. But those who do applied ethics in any field must be aware of the limits and dangers inherent in the engineering model. In the rush to be efficacious, it would be a grave mistake to lose the freedom and independence requisite for sound prescriptive inquiry into any ethical issue.

Those who engage in applied ethics must decide for themselves exactly when and for whom ethical engineering is appropriate. In assessing the fruits of their labors, they must also remain aware that there are numerous reasons why efforts by applied ethicists in medical settings fail. Not all invitations to help are authentic, and there are many circumstances in which the process of doing ethics is more highly prized than the results of such a process. It is also true that certain moral dilemmas which chronically arise in medical settings serve various sorts of adaptive functions for health professionals. The prospect of finally resolving such dilemmas can be far more frightening to the persons involved than the need to accommodate their existence.

Ethical engineering like other forms of engineering is an art. It requires practical knowledge, theoretical understanding, and experience. It also requires a certain amount of independence and tolerance from those who engage the engineer. After all, moral efficacy is desirable only when the right questions are being addressed.

2.

Moral experts and moral expertise
Does either exist?

The growth in the utilization of moral experts

Recently a brochure was sent to a variety of health-care professionals and others interested in medical ethics announcing the existence of a new newsletter. "One bad ethical decision could destroy your career," the recipients were warned. In order to avoid this dire fate, prospective customers were encouraged to "get the answers and advice for your toughest medical ethics dilemmas." By subscribing to the newsletter, those with $148 to spare could, the brochure promised, avail themselves of expertise that might forestall costly lawsuits, avoid unnecessary conflicts with patients, and minimize the amount of time spent with various review committees. This is perhaps a flagrant example of a growing chorus of claims to moral expertise, but others, both implicit and explicit, are easy to find in the burgeoning field of applied ethics.

Claims about moral expertise are manifested not only in consulting roles for those who want to pay self-proclaimed moral experts for their advice. Philosophers now routinely sit on committees in medical and scientific settings and have full voting authority with respect to the resolution of problems and the determination of policies. They also have been active participants in commissions sponsored by both public and private organizations that have examined an array of moral issues in medicine. One reason that is sometimes given for allocating philosophers a seat at tables where decisions are made is that a philosopher can represent the interests and views of the lay public. I once sat on a human experimentation committee at Columbia University's Medical Center under the description of layman. In one sense this appellation was entirely apt. I had no idea what the researchers who were my fellow committee members were talking about much of the time. If ignorance is a necessary and sufficient condition of lay status, then, at least upon my initial appointment to the committee, I met that qualification.

But, of course, it is silly to think that philosophers are chosen for committees simply to represent lay interests of one sort or another. At least in the case of my own participation on a hospital human experimentation committee, I was in reality invited and treated as an "expert" in ethics. In general, the justification for according philosophers the privilege of participating in actual decision making seems to rest not on their ability to act as a sort of moral everyman or zealous advocate for the interests of patients and subjects, but rather upon the legitimacy of their claims to moral expertise.

It is not unusual for philosophers (and theologians doing work they describe as applied ethics) to be asked to present testimony before legislative bodies. It is reasonable to assume that the use of philosophers in this capacity results from a growing belief on the part of legislators that philosophers, or at least some philosophers, possess expertise about ethical matters. On the other hand, the explanation might be that philosophers, or at least some philosophers, have successfully hoodwinked others into believing that they possess expertise about ethical matters. In addition, a few philosophers, myself included on two occasions, have appeared in courtrooms as "expert" witnesses. Although such occurrences have been rare, it is interesting to note that some state and local courts have been willing to accept testimony from philosophers about various ethical matters on the grounds that they have expertise that might prove helpful in the resolution of legal conflicts.[1]

Although the use of moral experts in judicial, legislative, and practical decision-making settings does not yet rival the frequency with which social scientists, natural scientists, and various other professionals are utilized for their expertise, the activities of these philosophers merit serious discussion and reflection within and beyond the realm of philosophy. In fact, there has been surprisingly little written about the nature of experts or expertise in ethics. This paucity of discussion is difficult to understand given that claims of expertise and a willingness to adopt the role of moral expert appear to challenge some deeply rooted convictions about the undesirability of talk about ethical expertise and ethical experts. A good deal of the scholarship on Socrates sees him as having little positive to say about those who pretend to possess expertise in ethics.[2] And many modern scholars, such as Karl Popper,[3] have greeted with little more than scorn and derision Plato's attempt to defend a form of moral expertise and to create a caste of moral experts to run the state. Twentieth-century moral theorists have not exactly embraced the notion that their intellectual duties include a commitment to participate publicly in the resolution of either the controversial or the mundane problems of everyday moral life.

Despite the relative silence among philosophers and those in cognate fields about what some working in the area of applied ethics now do, or what is being done in their name by publishers, companies, and advertising agencies, the question of whether either moral experts or moral expertise exists is as germane today as it was in the time of Socrates and Plato. Is it appropriate for any philosopher under any circumstances to claim to be a moral expert? Should legislatures, courts, and other institutions of society seek out those with alleged moral expertise, or are such efforts incompatible with personal responsibility for one's actions and behavior as well as with any reasonable theory of democracy?

Quiet grumbling rather than written outrage

Statements about moral expertise or declarations of the status of moral expert have been greeted with more or less stony silence from the philosophers. Although one can find an occasional contemptuous dismissal of the notion that applied ethics rather than meta-ethics is the appropriate subject matter for ethics courses,[4] little written commentary has been offered by those within the field of ethics on the activities of those described either as moral experts or as possessing moral expertise.

On the other hand, the increasing frequency with which those doing applied ethics have described themselves or have been labeled either as experts or as possessing moral expertise has occasioned a great deal of behind-the-scenes sneering, derision, and contempt. Questions such as, "How does it feel to have to lower your standards of argument when you appear on television?"; "Why do you offer your philosophical services to the agents of repression within society?" (the reference here was to someone doing business ethics); and "Do you do any real philosophy besides medical ethics?" all capture the attitude of many philosophers toward claims of moral expertise, an attitude that suggests a somewhat less than ecstatic current of opinion about declarations of moral expertise.

Some philosophers, including former secretary of education William Bennett, see activities in applied ethics as no more than disguised political activism instigated by the upheavals surrounding Vietnam, Watergate, and the civil-rights movements for minorities and women.[5] Others view claims of moral expertise as nothing more than a dubious gimmick utilized by those unable to secure teaching positions.[6] Still others explain the growth of applied ethics as the co-opted response of those facing hard financial times in the humanities to the lure of power and easy money set out by the forces of power and repression in bourgeois capitalist states.[7]

It is true that some philosophers view applied ethics with enthusiasm, seeing the recent wave of applied work in philosophy as a refreshing break from the endless series of conceptual-thought experiments and artificial dilemmatic constructs that has passed for moral theorizing for a number of years.[8] However, it is doubtful that even this group is sympathetic either to self-proclamations of expertise or to calls for the creation of standards and certification requirements to protect the practices of a new guild of moral experts who aim to provide succor to the morally bereft and befuddled.

Claims of expertise are not unique to applied ethics, though. Those who teach moral philosophy in a university or professional school surely believe that they possess some sort of expertise that makes it appropriate for them, and not someone from a different discipline or profession, to teach such courses. However, the mores of academia do not encourage expressions of expertise as the basis for one's authority to hold forth in a classroom. Moreover, the subculture of the humanities within universities has little patience with, and no time for, those who would try to demean the profession of philosophy by making it a skill in need of a license, as is the case for psychologists, plumbers, and hairstylists. The expanding activities and influence of those doing applied ethics nevertheless demand that serious attention be paid to a question many moral philosophers would prefer to avoid or ignore—Is there such a thing as expertise in ethics, and if so, are there moral experts?

What have philosophers thought about moral expertise and attempts by moral philosophers to apply this expertise?

Though twentieth-century philosophers have written little about whether moral experts exist, most of what has appeared in print has been critical of both the possibility of expertise and claims to expert status. A. J. Ayer, for example, summarily rejects the notion of moral expertise in no uncertain terms:

> . . . it is silly, as well as presumptuous, for any one type of philosopher to pose as the champion of virtue. And it is also one reason why many people find moral philosophy an unsatisfying subject. For they mistakenly look to the moral philosopher for guidance.[9]

In the foreword to P. H. Nowell-Smith's widely read introductory text on ethics, Ayer is equally dismissive of moral expertise and experts:

> There is a distinction, which is not always sufficiently marked, between the activity of a moralist, who sets out to elaborate a moral code, or to encourage its observance, and that of a moral philosopher, whose concern is not primarily to make moral judgments but to analyze their nature.[10]

One might view Ayer's out-of-hand rejection of moral expertise as reflecting his general skepticism about objectivity in ethics. But other distinguished philosophers who have been far more sanguine about the prospects for objectivity in morals have had few kind words for those who would tout themselves as moral experts or advance claims about the privileged possession of moral expertise:

> . . . it is no part of the professional business of moral philosophers to tell people what they ought or ought not to do. . . . Moral philosophers, as such, have no special information, not available to the general public, about what is right and what is wrong; nor have they any call to undertake those hortatory functions which are so adequately performed by clergymen, politicians, leader-writers [editorialists]. . . .[11]

Philosophers have tended to confine their doubts about the possibility of moral expertise and moral experts either to concise dismissals or to private grousings to those with similar reservations. Those outside philosophy, who do not face the restrictions imposed by the norms of collegiality and professional tolerance that obtain within an academic field, have not felt similarly constrained, however, and have greeted such claims with scorn and derision.[12]

Are moral experts and moral expertise politically correct?

Claims about moral expertise have been subjected to rather vitriolic criticisms on political grounds. From the right, William Bennett, former secretary of education and then head of the National Endowment for the Humanities has written, "One of the most serious ethical problems of our time has become the fad of the new ethics and its defenders."[13] From the left, Cheryl Noble has written:

> To be amenable to these techniques [applying the expertise of the moral philosopher] moral problems must be abstracted from their social settings so that they appear purely moral. In fact, were moral questions more richly defined and conceived, the professional inability of philosophy to deal with them would be obvious.[14]

It is interesting that the political critics of moral expertise do not argue against the utilization of ethical theory in practical affairs or day-to-day matters on the grounds that moral expertise does not exist. None of those motivated by political concerns appears to doubt that, at least in principle, expertise in morals might be possible. What critics such as Bennett and Noble appear to believe is that:

1. Moral expertise might exist, but moral philosophers are no more likely to possess it than anybody else; and

2. Whether he or she has moral expertise or not, it is not the moral philosopher's job to utilize moral expertise to solve other people's moral problems, or to render judgments about moral matters in the professions or concerning practical affairs. Instead, the moral philosopher should be concerned with promulgating correct modes of thinking and reasoning about ethics to those in need of moral instruction.

Why are the philosophical critics skeptical?

It is difficult to know precisely what motivates the distaste many philosophers have felt, and many contemporary philosophers continue to feel, about claims of expertise or calls for the legitimation of moral experts. Most philosophers, at least in modern times, have been willing to identify and acknowledge all sorts of individuals as experts and to recognize many different kinds of claims concerning expertise. But there appears to be something unique to ethics that makes talk of moral experts and expertise grate on the ears of many philosophers.

A combination of factors seems to be responsible for the negative, skeptical reactions of academic philosophers to talk about experts and expertise in ethics.

A. *Moral expertise seems incompatible with the virtues of modesty and humility.* Socrates set the tone for philosophy's response to those who would hold themselves up as experts in ethics—skepticism combined with irony and cynicism.[15] Claims of expertise appear to violate the profession's own norms concerning the appropriateness of claims about knowledge, whether the subject is morality or something else.

B. *Moral expertise seems incompatible with democracy.* Moral expertise threatens the standard position on autonomy within liberal democratic theory because recognizing moral expertise seems to cast doubt on the ability of each individual to be his or her own best judge of values. Mill's highly influential arguments defending negative liberty against the inclination of persons and states toward crude paternalism—which he grounded in the right of each person, no matter how befuddled, to direct his or her own life—seem, particularly in the moral realm, incompatible with assertions of moral expertise by those who would call themselves or be called moral experts.

It is not accurate to argue, however, that Mill or a liberalism inspired by Mill has no tolerance for moral expertise. Mill was not concerned about the possibility that some individuals might possess more expertise than others in moral matters. Rather, he was disturbed by the prospect that persons, expert or not, might be allowed to force their judgments of right and wrong, good and bad on others.[16]

A more accurate characterization of the worry felt by some philosophers is that if moral expertise exists, its very existence undermines the possibility of democracy. Why should every citizen have a say in political and value issues if some are more expert than others at these matters? If there is moral expertise, then ought not experts guide society (as Plato suggested long ago) rather than the morally illiterate and backward?

C. *Moral expertise must be rejected because moral philosophers know they lack a warranted theory of ethics that can ground all moral beliefs and practices.* By vehemently denying the existence of moral expertise and contemptuously rejecting those who call themselves ethical experts, the dirty little secret of ethics—that in the absence of theological foundations all theories of morality appear to lack ultimate warrant—can be kept hidden. Ethics can remain part of the curriculum as long as those who teach it disavow any expertise in the subject. In this way no one can discern that the discipline has no epistemic clothes!

Skeptics, some old-fashioned Marxists, emotivists, and those who desperately wish to replace divine authority with some sort of irrefutable warrant for a comprehensive theory of ethics are prone to reject the possibility of either experts or expertise in ethics. Many in these groups doubt that an objective theory of ethics is possible, and as a result they dismiss claims to moral expertise out-of-hand.[17]

Many of those who believe in the possibility of objectivity in ethics, and who believe that a theory that can warrant moral beliefs and guide moral actions may yet be found, are skeptical of any attempt to do applied ethics in the absence of such a theory. Kai Nielsen, for example, complains that, without an epistemic Archimedean point, applied or practical ethics is meaningless, since the expertise required cannot be grounded in any defensible moral theory.[18]

Would-be experts would best be advised to delay their coronations until such time as meta-ethically minded philosophers produce a viable, comprehensive theory that can ground normative judgments about particular cases and problems.

D. *Moral expertise involves nothing more than being a moderately intelligent person who is adept at logical argumentation and who has the time and the inclination to learn about the history of ethics and to study the facts surrounding a particular moral issue.* In this view moral expertise might exist, but it is nothing more than a general set of intellectual skills. Anyone wanting public recognition on the basis of being generally intelligent thus seems to be nothing more than an intellectual fop—at best a person who is narrow-minded, elitist, and snobbish.

E. *Moral expertise is dangerous.* From the point of view of political and ideological commentators on the right, moral expertise reduces to nothing more than a journey through a boundless conceptual swamp of values clarification. "Real" expertise in ethics requires people to stand up for "good" values (usually meaning "American" values) such as patriotism, respect for life, civic virtue, obedience to proper authority, and so on. Philosophically disposed dispensers of moral expertise are seen as going on and on about the importance of clarifying moral arguments and the need to have good reasons for moral decisions, but such conceptual analysis is not the stuff of which "real" morality is made.

From the left, moral expertise is suspect because it appears to be entirely abstracted from social, economic, and class features of society. Moral expertise, at least as reflected in the writings of many who work in applied ethics, appears to isolate moral issues from the social contexts in which they arise in order to make conceptual analysis possible.[19] Moral expertise thus is bankrupt because it becomes nothing more than an apologia for the norms of the dominant class. Moral experts, as Hegel once warned, are doomed to be nothing more than conceptual handmaidens to the powerful and dominant within a society.

F. *Moral philosophers should not allow themselves to stoop to the practical level demanded in so many other intellectual arenas inside and outside the university.* Despite the fact that philosophers are usually courteous toward preachers and those giving advice in the newspapers on all manner of topics, most philosophers, following in the modern traditions of British and American philosophy, want to distinguish and distance themselves from the mundane labors of exhortation, character improvement, and positive thinking. Philosophy is seen to be the province of an intelligentsia, not a trade to be pursued in the manner of plumbing, automobile repair, or fishing. Moral experts, if such there be, are advised to hang their shingles out in some other discipline. Philosophy, properly understood as an intellectual's pursuit, has no room for those who would approach it as a trade, craft, or practical labor.[20]

Moral expertise is something that many philosophers seem to believe they possess, at least in terms of being qualified to teach the subject or edit journals devoted to ethics. But it is a skill that merits guilt, denial, and embarrassment when mentioned in public. According to this view of the role of philosophy, moral expertise certainly ought not to be seen as a license to present oneself as an expert practitioner outside university departments. Those who claim moral expertise may be quietly tolerated by the philosophical community, in the way that community tolerates self-proclaimed skeptics, solipsists, epistemological anarchists, and other philosophical deviants. But in many quarters it is a tolerance based on a mix of paternalism, pity, and superiority, not a product of respect for or credulousness about moral expertise.

Does expertise in ethics exist?

I believe that expertise does exist with respect to ethics. I think some moral philosophers have it and some do not. Moreover, I think it entirely possible for someone to acquire moral expertise without having any contact with moral philosophers or any training in moral philosophy. Neither is training in moral philosophy more likely to confer expertise about moral matters upon those who have had the benefit of such training as opposed to those who have not.

Some of the resistance by philosophers to public proclamations of moral expertise stems, as noted above, from a mix of views about the epistemic warrant, or lack thereof, for ethical theory. Others find expertise incompatible with commitments to autonomy, democracy, or the norms of humility and tolerance required for the practice of academic philosophy. It seems bizarre, however, to try to save moral philosophy from the sins of hubris or the psychic terror of living without a warranted foundational theory by simply pooh-poohing the notion of expertise in morality. If it is true that moral philosophers have no expertise about anything pertaining to ethics, that they know no more than anyone else about normative and prescriptive matters, then, as R. M. Hare has cogently observed, the time to "shut up shop" has long since passed.[21] If moral philosophy cannot in any way contribute to the resolution of normative and prescriptive matters, it is a field more akin to anthropology than anything else—interesting for the curiosities it reveals, but useless in terms of the logical support it can provide for normative practices and beliefs.

Before rushing out to hang "closed" signs over the doors of moral philosophers' offices, however, it might be useful to question: (a) whether the concept of expertise in ethics has been adequately analyzed; (b) whether there is any logical or epistemological connection between expertise and experts; (c) whether expertise is a status restricted to only a few or open to many and if so, by what means; and (d) whether expertise in ethics consists in anything more than the use of a moral theory to solve a moral problem. The answers that arise from considering these issues may not only shed light on some important questions about the relationship between theory and practice in any domain, but also will, or at least should, make academic philosophers feel less queasy about those who tout themselves as having expertise in moral matters.

What is expertise in ethics?

The question of what constitutes expertise in ethics is more complicated than the available analyses and comments on the subject reveal. One common strategy for trying to understand the nature of expertise in ethics is to see what those who call themselves experts in ethics know or do. But, as Socrates understood, this is not necessarily the best starting point for an examination of the concept.

One peculiar feature of moral experts is that anyone can claim to be one. Like psychics, water diviners, psychotherapists, and any number of other experts, moral experts need only the will and a public forum to claim the mantle of expertise. But this liberal admissions policy ought to cast doubt on the wisdom of drawing any logical connection between expertise and experts. The question of what to do about expertise is one that requires social, legal, ethical, and economic assessments that extend beyond the existence of people claiming to be experts.

It is an open question as to what ought to be done to or with moral expertise if some poor soul is believed to possess it vis-à-vis public policy, practical affairs, or politics. Our culture is enamored of and intimidated by experts of all sorts—revering specialization over generalization while at the same time admiring the flexibility of the generalist. But this should not blind us to the fact that, even if moral expertise exists and if moral experts who have expertise can be found, whether authority, autonomy, or privilege should be granted to these experts remains an open question. The late nineteenth century struggles between scientifically minded physicians and their other-minded rivals shows that the American public has not always known how to respond appropriately to expertise.[22]

As Mill pointed out in his discussion of paternalism, there may be sound reasons not to elevate anyone to the lofty status of moral expert with its concomitant authority to control and rule the lives of others. But this does not mean that expertise in matters moral does not exist, or that wise and prudent persons should not heed the advice of experts on a variety of subjects, including ethics, in deciding how to live or behave. It means only that the threat of abuse or error is so great that the social role assigned to moral experts or those with moral expertise must be confined to the tasks of exhortation and giving advice. Society should not create an elite of moral experts who have the authority to impose their judgments on others.[23]

What is expertise generally, and who are the experts?

Instead of analyzing who moral experts are and what it is that moral experts say and do, it is more useful to try to get some conceptual purchase on the concept of expertise itself. Ordinarily, expertise refers to the possession of a body of knowledge or a set of specialized skills. There is expertise concerning food and wines, French history, and mathematics, for example. There is also expertise concerning baking, detecting art forgeries, surgery, pole vaulting, and pottery making. In other words, expertise is possible, to use a famous distinction of Gilbert Ryle, with respect both to knowing how to do something and to knowing that some set of propositions is true or false.

What is striking about expertise is that, for many skills and areas of knowledge, it is difficult to obtain. People spend a lifetime studying signatures or examining watermarks in order to be able to claim expertise in narrow, restricted domains of inquiry. The years required to become a skilled pole vaulter or gymnast rival the degree of training required to become a physician or pharmacist.

Other forms of expertise are not, however, quite so demanding. The concept of expertise is associated in contemporary American culture with an exclusionary view of human knowledge—the only persons possessing expertise are experts. Expertise in our culture, to count as expertise, requires knowledge or skill that only a few persons can and actually do possess. It is often said that no one can be an expert in everything. By the same reasoning, if there are experts, they cannot be common. Pundits are prone to note that as the range of things to know and do expands, more and more experts will emerge.

One reason it seems odd to say that anyone can have expertise in ethics is that most moral philosophers and a great many psychologists[24] want to argue that each person has the capacity—perhaps a conscience or moral sense—to know and to do what is right. Part of the negative attitude toward the possibility of expertise in ethics is not that it is based upon the suspicion that some do not know more than others, but rather that it is a reaction to the exclusivity associated with moral expertise. If moral expertise exists, only a few of us can have it, and that seems strange and disturbing in a society committed to democratic liberalism, according to which everyone is capable of moral reasoning and moral points of view.[25]

But that our paradigmatic examples of expertise rely on specialized knowledge or the ability to perform certain skills at a high level of accomplishment ought not to obscure the possibility that expertise is not necessarily limited to only a few or a minority of especially gifted persons. Some forms of expertise may be more widely distributed among the population than others. Yet this possibility need not make the particular knowledge or skill any the less a matter of expertise. The existence of a body of knowledge about some subject or about how to perform some skill or activity is sufficient to create the potential for expertise. In many areas of life, lots of people have expertise about a variety of subjects and skills—how to use a telephone, drive a car, mail a letter, exhibit good manners, use a post office, play games, and so on. Other people may not possess expertise with respect to these activities, but most could probably acquire it if they were motivated and taught properly.

This last claim illustrates another ideological headache for those who subscribe to some form of liberal democracy. We like to think that all persons are equal, that drastic or important differences in intellectual ability or dexterity do not exist, and that everyone possesses the key attributes that really matter in life—free will, the ability to love, and so on. The best illustration of the importance of beliefs about human equality is the insistence by advocates on behalf of the elderly, women, and even children that these groups do not lack the skills and capacities possessed by those who control and dominate society, namely, white, middle-aged men.[26] Serious talk of expertise appears to threaten our commitments to both equality and equal opportunity, however. Moral expertise does so in a direct and obvious manner. But does the concept of expertise carry with it, inherently or analytically, the conceptual accoutrements of either exclusivity or inequity? Or are these worries that we project onto the concept for reasons that have more to do with our culture and ideology?

We normally do not think of ordinary skills such as using a telephone or simple forms of knowledge such as knowing the streets in one's neighborhood as representing expertise, partly because we often equate expertise with knowledge or skills that the possessor is self-consciously aware of possessing. But we ought not to allow familiarity to breed contempt with respect to descriptions of the vast areas of expertise each person possesses. One need only spend time with children or persons afflicted with mental diseases and disorders to appreciate how much expertise normal adults have. Nor do we have to accept the claim that expertise is by definition exclusionary. If all human beings knew how to cook Peking duck or were connoisseurs of fine wine, expertise in these matters would not disappear. Experts might not be possible in a world where many people knew a lot about a broad range of subjects or could perform a wide variety of skills and tasks, or in a society that demanded generalists rather than specialists for social or economic reasons—but expertise would still be possible.

Expert and expertise are concepts that have come to be used interchangeably in our increasingly complex, technologically oriented, specialized society. But this is not a conceptual necessity. Nor should we allow our ideological admiration of experts to blind us to the fact that universal expertise about lots of subjects and skills does not make that knowledge and those skills any the worse for wear as matters of expertise.

Singer and Wells's definition of moral expertise

Many of those who are embarrassed about proclamations of moral expertise or who are hostile to such claims on theoretical or political grounds have some basis for their unease. Often claims of moral expertise are highly abstract and not a little pretentious.

Among contemporary devotees of moral expertise, Peter Singer and Diane Wells are two of the few who have tried to give a serious analysis of the concept. But their analysis is unlikely to make skeptics, doubters, and critics go out and retain the services of a moral guru to guide their lives. In brief, their view is that moral expertise involves:

> (1) the ability to reason well and logically, to avoid errors in one's own arguments, and to detect fallacies when they occur in the arguments of others . . . ;
> (2) . . . an understanding of the nature of ethics and meanings of moral concepts. . . . A reasonable knowledge of the major ethical theories, such as utilitarianism, theories of justice and of rights, will also be useful . . . ; and
> (3) . . . being well informed about the facts of the matter under discussion. . . .[27]

I think Singer and Wells are right to claim that the concept of moral expertise makes sense. Moreover, it is surely valid to note, as they do later in their discussion, that moral expertise is not confined to moral philosophers, but can be acquired readily by any competent adult with a mind to do so.

Singer and Wells's explication of the concept nevertheless seems inadequate. Their first condition for moral expertise would apply to any type of expertise or, indeed, to any intellectual enterprise. If this were the only intellectual skill required, then logicians, not moral philosophers, ought to be encouraged to take up the field of ethics because they are, in this view of expertise, most suited for the field.

The second and third conditions show why logicians are not, on the other hand, especially suited to moral inquiry and the development of moral expertise. Singer and Wells are correct in noting that those engaged in moral inquiry or even moral problem-solving need to be acquainted with the "facts of the matter under discussion." But this phrase does not do justice to the level of acquaintance required for expertise in morals. Expertise, as noted earlier, can describe both knowledge about a subject and knowing how to perform a skill or activity well. In neither case would it do to say that expertise exists when one has simply a nodding acquaintance with the facts of a particular case or issue.

The application of moral expertise requires more than the facts

The notion that the use of moral expertise requires knowing the facts of a particular situation is closely related to a model of decision making that sees the application of moral theory as simply a matter of subsumption and deduction. The model that still predominates in many quarters is that moral theories are composed of axioms, laws, midlevel principles, and initial and boundary conditions. The "facts" are simply fed into this axiomatic hierarchy of rules and lemmas, so that a conclusion can be deductively arrived at by subsuming the facts under the relevant principles.[28] I have dubbed this model of how applied ethics proceeds "engineering ethics."[29] It presumes that:

1. Problems are presented to, not found by, philosophers.
2. Problem solving is the goal of applied ethics.
3. Problem solving is achieved by subsuming the "facts" relevant to a particular problem under a moral theory.

This model of what constitutes a theory in ethics seems to have been inherited from early and mid-twentieth century discussions in the philosophy of science concerning the nature of theory structure and explanation.[30] There are, however, serious problems with this view.

First, the notion of application utilized is closely wedded to a dubious view of theory. The most extensive analyses of the structure and content of theories have been advanced in philosophy of science.

Yet it is not clear that anyone currently working in philosophy of science, or in the history or sociology of science for that matter, believes that theories, to be theories, must be composed of axioms, laws, and principles arranged in an axiomatizable hierarchy. Powerful arguments have been given for the claim that such an account does not accurately describe all, or, in the eyes of some, even any theories in science. Among the most telling criticisms of the axiomatic-deductive view of theory structure and composition has been the point, made by Kuhn, Lakatos, Toulmin, and Laudan among many others, that theories, defined as axiomatic hierarchies of principles, are not the core units of inquiry in science. Often it is necessary to look at entire research programs, themata, or "strategies" to understand the evolution of scientific beliefs.[31]

Nor is there any reason to assume that theories, understood as deductive, axiomatic hierarchies, are or must be the basic units for understanding the evolution of ethical beliefs. Indeed, few, if any, philosophers who do applied ethics attempt to locate a single theory and apply it in the mode prescribed by the older, positivistic conception of theory. Rather, application often consists in drawing upon complementary moral theories or individual concepts to achieve clarification of points. On occasion, those professing expertise in ethics will invoke moral traditions such as rule utilitarianism or virtue-based approaches to morality that are not, at least in any obvious sense, compatible with one another. The expertise involved in this approach would seem to be knowing which tradition or research strategy in ethics is appropriate for a particular moral domain or problem. For example, it is entirely plausible to argue for a consequentialist moral view in thinking about the ethics of human experimentation. At the same time, one might adopt a Kantian perspective in response to questions about whether a market in organs from living donors ought to be permitted. The inconsistency would prove fatal to the arguments only if there were no significant differences between the two types of cases.

Utilizing a range of moral theories and traditions drives those committed to a univocal underpinning of all ethical knowledge batty. Yet expertise in both science and ethics appears to consist, in part, of knowing not only what theory or theories are defensible, or which moral traditions or paradigms are most defensible, but in how to pick and choose among theories and traditions to provide appropriate answers to specific problems or problematics.[32] It should go without saying that expertise also consists of knowing when theory and tradition have nothing to offer.

Unfortunately, moral philosophy, in its quest to replace God with a secure epistemic foundation for moral theory, has lost sight of the fact that very little of morality involves foundational questions. Rather, what is needed and what calls for expertise, and perhaps experts, is the knowledge necessary to individuate, identify, and classify moral issues and problems in order to bring existing moral perspectives—consistent or not—to bear.

It is not only the concept of theory that is suspect in the prevailing model of applied ethics, however. Telling criticisms have also been directed against the idea that "facts" can easily be separated from and identified independently of theories. The notion that a nodding acquaintance with the "facts" is sufficient to permit the exercise of expertise simply buys into a notion of moral facts that is highly suspect. Often expertise consists in recognizing that moral facts are problematic or identifying as relevant facts that are not recognized as such by those seeking help or advice.

Recently some philosophers have argued that analogical reasoning plays a crucial role in scientific theorizing, particularly in the biological and medical arenas. The use of paradigmatic cases seems to be a prominent feature of many such biological accounts.[33] The use of exemplary cases and analogical reasoning from clear-cut cases also seem to be important features of the logic of moral reasoning. Case examples and case studies play critical roles in many domains of moral inquiry. The axiomatic-deductive model of theory structure fails to capture this key attribute of theorizing in both science and ethics. The logical relationship of facts to theories, when paradigmatic exemplars are being used rather than deduction from theory, may require a different conception of the kinds of familiarity with the facts that is necessary than is suggested by the axiomatic-deductive model of theory structure.

More importantly, an analysis of expertise in terms of subsuming facts under theories to draw logically warranted conclusions is far too narrow an account of the various tasks and responsibilities of those who have moral expertise and of the way in which that expertise can be brought to bear to analyze moral problems.[34] Singer and Wells's account of expertise highlights the ability to solve problems as central to the possession of moral expertise. But problem solving is only one of many tasks that those with expertise are required to undertake to make a useful contribution to the solution of moral problems. Often, in the confused world of practical affairs, it is not clear exactly what the moral problems that require resolution are. Moral expertise is sought, not for problem resolution, but for problem individuation and identification. The kind of familiarity with the facts requisite for this task is much more complicated than that suggested by Singer and Wells's analysis. Occasionally, those involved in practical affairs are not even aware that a moral problem exists. The task of those with moral expertise may be to create moral perplexity where none existed. Again, the depth, comprehension, and degree of knowledge required to conduct moral diagnosis in a particular context is far more demanding than that suggested by Singer and Wells's requirement of general familiarity with the facts in a specific situation. The facts may not be as they appear even to those who request moral help. Those who offer their expertise must be sure that they allow themselves freedom not only in providing advice but, just as importantly, in defining the nature of the problem to be addressed.

Objections to expertise reconsidered

If the engineering model of applied ethics is allowed to go unchallenged, many of the criticisms that have been offered by prominent philosophers as well as the fears about moral expertise that are quietly espoused, at least orally if not in print, are impossible to defuse. But if one challenges the assumptions of the engineering model by pointing out that the model gives a false picture of what experts in ethics do, or at least ought to do, then it is possible to answer many of the criticisms that have been directed against both experts and expertise in ethics.

It is simply false to suggest that the professional virtues of modesty and humility are jeopardized by the possibility of moral expertise. If anything, it is those who lay claim to the mantle of expertise who best understand how little is known or understood with certainty about morality. The hubris inherent in contemporary efforts to locate a single foundational theory sufficient for warranting all moral beliefs is at least on a par with the hubris necessary to appear in public as an expert on matters moral. Expertise and experts are not, or need not be, co-optable to the forces of the left or right where ethics is concerned. This can happen only when moral experts allow themselves to operate as crude moral engineers, mindlessly funneling moral quandaries and dilemmas into the abstract apparatus of their favorite theories. Nor are expertise and its application any less worthy of intellectual respect than the activities of those who pursue meta-ethical investigations by means of thought experiments, hypothetical scenarios, or counterfactual case examples. Expertise in ethics demands a close, intimate understanding of the norms and values that prevail in a given institution or profession. It requires that those who wish to be perceived as experts know not only the theories and traditions of ethics, but also the nuances and complexities of the moral life as it is lived in a hospital, corporation, newsroom, court, or even legislative body.[35]

The engineering model makes it not only unlikely but impossible for those avowing expertise in ethics to contribute anything of use to those interested in the analysis of moral theory and meta-ethical questions. But if the assumptions of the engineering model are debunked, as they certainly ought to be, then a wide range of contributions can be seen to flow from practical experience and application to theory. To mention only a few such contributions, experts quickly learn that meta-ethics needs to reexamine the prevailing commitment to foundationalism rooted in a single theory that dominates so much discussion and debate within ethics. Similarly, the criteria used to identify and individuate moral "facts" and problems cry out for far more critical reflection than they have received to date. The role of modes of reasoning not built on deduction needs to be examined as well.

Most importantly, it must be appreciated that the recognition of expertise does not consign moral philosophers of either a theoretical or practical bent to the ranks of totalitarian elitists. One can admit the possibility of expertise in ethics without believing either that expertise is open to only an elite few or that society should create a social role that accords power and authority to moral experts. It is possible to live in a world where expertise abounds but there are no experts. Experts, oddly enough, are possible only when others decide to grant them status and authority.

Expertise, however, is a different matter. Expertise in ethics, or in any other area of knowledge or skill, is not, in itself, something to be feared or dreaded. Admittedly, there is no reason to believe that expertise exists merely because there are those who declare themselves to possess it. But that is hardly the problem in philosophy, where all claims of ethical expertise are regarded as suspect.

Expertise in ethics appears to consist in knowing moral traditions and theories. It also involves knowing how to apply those theories and traditions in ways that fruitfully contribute to the understanding of moral problems. But, most importantly, ethical expertise involves the ability to identify and recognize moral issues and problems, a skill that may be enhaced by training in ethics, but one that is not by any means restricted to those who have this training and that is not beyond the intellectual capacities of those who do not have this training. When the concepts of moral expertise and moral expert are understood in this way, we may be said to live in a world where moral expertise ought to be common but moral experts ought not.

References

1. Peter G. McAllen and Richard Delgado (1984) "Moral Experts in the Courtroom," *Hastings Center Report* 14, 27–34.

2. Gregory Vlastos (1971) "Introduction: The Paradox of Socrates," *The Philosophy of Socrates,* G. Vlastos, ed. (Doubleday, Garden City, NY), pp. 13–21.

3. Karl Popper (1963) *The Open Society and its Enemies,* vol. 1 (Harper & Row, New York, NY).

4. Gilbert Harman (1977) *The Nature of Morality* (Oxford University Press, New York, NY), pp. vii–ix.

5. William Bennett (1980) "Getting Ethics," *Commentary* (December), 62–65.

6. Samuel Gorovitz (1986) "Baiting and Bioethics," *Ethics* 96, 356–374.

7. Cheryl Noble (1982) "Ethics and Experts," *Hastings Center Report* 12, 7–9.

8. Stephen Toulmin (1982) "How Medicine Saved the Life of Ethics," *Perspectives in Biology and Medicine* 25, 736–750.

9. A. J. Ayer (1954) *Philosophical Essays* (Macmillan, London), p. 246.

10. A. J. Ayer (1954) "Editorial Foreword," *Ethics,* P. H. Nowell-Smith (Penguin, Baltimore, MD), p. iii.

11. C. D. Broad (1952) *Ethics and the History of Philosophy* (Routledge and Kegan Paul, London), p. 244.

12. Gorovitz, op. cit.

13. Bennett, op. cit.

14. Noble, op. cit.

15. Vlastos, op. cit.

16. John Stuart Mill (1961) "On Liberty," *The Philosophy of John Stuart Mill,* Marshall Cohen, ed. (Random House, New York, NY), pp. 185–319.

17. M. Lilla (1981) "Ethos, 'Ethics' and Public Service," *The Public Interest* 6, 3–17; P. Drucker (1981) "Ethical Chic," *Forbes* (September), 159–163; and J. P. Euben (1981) "Philosophy and the Professions," *Democracy,* 112–127.

18. Kai Neilsen (1982) "On Needing a Moral Theory," *Metaphilosophy* 13, 97–116.

19. R. Fox and J. Swazey (1984) "Medical Morality is Not Bioethics—Medical Ethics in China and the United States," *Perspectives in Biology and Medicine* 27, 336–360.

20. Daniel Callahan, Arthur Caplan, and Bruce Jennings, eds. (1985) *Applying the Humanities* (Plenum, New York, NY).

21. R. M. Hare (1977) "Medical Ethics: Can the Moral Philosopher Help?" *Philosophical Medical Ethics: Its Nature and Significance,* S. F. Spicker and H. T. Englehardt, Jr., eds. (Reidel, Dordrecht), pp. 47–61.

22. Paul Starr (1982) *The Social Transformation of American Medicine* (Basic, New York, NY).

23. Mill, op. cit., chapter IV.

24. See, for example, L. Kohlberg (1984) *The Psychology of Moral Development* (Harper & Row, New York, NY) and J. Rest (1979) *Development in Judging Moral Issues* (University of Minnesota Press, Minneapolis, MN).

25. Bruce Jennings (1986) "Applied Ethics and the Vocation of Social Science," *New Directions in Ethics,* J. P. DeMarco and R. M. Fox, eds. (Routledge and Kegan Paul, New York, NY), pp. 205–217.

26. See, for example, R. N. Butler (1975) *Why Survive?* (Harper & Row, New York, NY).

27. P. Singer and D. Wells (1984) *The Reproductive Revolution* (Oxford University Press, Oxford), p. 200.

28. Michael Bayles, "Moral Theory and Application," (1984) *Social Theory and Practice* 10, 47–70; R. M. Fox and J. P. DeMarco 1986) "The Challenge of Applied Ethics," *New Directions in Ethics,* J. P. DeMarco and R. M. Fox, eds. (Routledge and Kegan Paul, New York, NY), pp. 1–18.

29. Arthur Caplan (1980) "Ethical Engineers Need Not Apply," *Science, Technology and Human Values* 6, 24–32; and "Mechanics on Duty" (1983) *Canadian Journal of Philosophy* 8, 1–18.

30. F. Suppe, ed. (1977) *The Structure of Scientific Theories,* 2nd ed. (University of Illinois Press, Urbana, IL).

31. Arthur Caplan (1984) "Sociobiology as a Strategy in Science," *The Monist* 67, 143–160.

32. Abraham Edel (1986) "Ethical Theory and Moral Practice: On the Terms of Their Relation," *New Directions in Ethics,* J. P. DeMarco and R. M. Fox, eds. (Routledge and Kegan Paul, New York, NY), pp. 317–335.

33. K. F. Schaffner (1986) "Exemplary Reasoning about Biological Models and Diseases," *Journal of Medicine and Philosophy* 11, 63–80.

34. Tom Beauchamp (1984) "On Eliminating the Distinction between Applied Ethics and Ethical Theory," *The Monist* 67, 514–531.

35. Gorovitz, op. cit.

Part II

Ethical issues in animal and
human experimentation

3.

Beastly conduct
Ethical issues in animal
experimentation

The legitimacy of means and the legitimacy
of ends in animal experimentation

There has been a great deal of argument in recent years over the subject of animal experimentation. Few topics are able to elicit the degree of moral vehemence and passion that this topic does. Accusations of moral blindness fly back and forth between vivisectionists and antivivisectionists. Bills are submitted almost willy-nilly at both the federal and state level, lobbying efforts on both sides of the issue are best described as fierce, and the disputants seem to delight in holding meetings and conferences at which their opponents are persona non grata—on both sides opponents are rarely invited, and, if they somehow manage to appear, they are made the object of calumny usually reserved only for criminals or even politicians.[12]

Despite the political and sociological vortex surrounding the issue of animal experimentation, it would be wrong for those on either side to underestimate the sincerity and thoughtfulness that can underlie much of the noise and rhetoric characteristic of current public debates over the issue. In recent years a rather rich philosophical literature[10,11] has developed on the subject of the moral responsibilities of human beings toward animals, and this literature surely must be reckoned with by all parties to the debate. Just as it is wrong to suppose that all vivisectionists are callous brutes, unconcerned about the effects of their work on their animal subjects, it is also wrong to assume that all antivivisectionists are misanthropic kooks who are too emotionally unstable to recognize the benefits that derive from research involving animals.

Before considering some of the moral questions that arise in the context of the practice of experimentation involving animals, it is important to make a distinction between two issues that are often conflated by parties on both sides of the issue. Oftentimes scientists go to great lengths to demonstrate to each other and the general public that they take every possible precaution to assure the humane treatment of any animals that may be used for experimental purposes. Scientists often note with pride that they have, through their own voluntary efforts, established clear codes of conduct about the care and handling of laboratory animals. Moreover, most reputable scientists in America and other nations go to great lengths to minimize, through the use of anesthetics, anesthesia, and other means, the pain or suffering that animals endure as a result of the process of experimentation.

The many efforts now made to reduce animal suffering and to ensure the proper care and handling of animals used for research purposes are often brought forward in response to criticisms leveled by antivivisectionists concerning the enterprise of animal research. Unfortunately, persons who question the moral legitimacy of animal experimentation are not likely to be dissuaded from their view by demonstrations of the care and concern shown by those engaged in the practice.

There are really two issues involved in thinking about research involving animals, and questions of humane care are pertinent to only one of them—(1) Is it morally legitimate to conduct research upon animals? (2) If it is morally permissible to utilize animals for research purposes, what moral responsibilities must be discharged by those engaged in such research? Questions on what conduct constitutes humane care, guidelines on the handling and transport of animal subjects, and efforts to teach students and professionals techniques that will minimize animal suffering and pain consequent to research interventions are all only relevant to the question of professional duty within the research context. However, before these issues can be usefully discussed, it is necessary to examine the prior question of whether it is morally justifiable to conduct any research on animals. For if the answer to this question is no, then no amount of guidelines, restraint, educational effort, or codified standards will suffice in response to criticisms of the activity.

The major areas of contention concerning the moral legitimacy of animal research

If one reviews various public pronouncements[1,3,6,7,10,12] made about the issue of animal experimentation by parties on both sides of the issue, it quickly becomes evident that there exist three major areas of dispute. First, there is a good deal of disagreement about the need to conduct any research upon animals. Second, there is much disagreement about the moral value to be assigned to animals. Much of the attention to issues of animal sentience and consciousness in debates about the ethics of animal research are spin-offs from this issue, since the more animals are felt to possess mental powers equivalent to or closely resembling those possessed by humans, the more various people feel disposed to assign moral worth to such creatures. Third, there is a good deal of tacit or between-the-lines argument about the moral priority that ought be accorded the whole issue of the ethics of animal experimentation. Many persons admit that the question of the legitimacy of animal experimentation is a vexing one, but there is no agreement over whether the topic is one that ought to command wide public attention and legislative concern. Other issues, such as human starvation, malnutrition, war, crime, poverty, and the like are felt, oftentimes, to deserve precedence over the fates of animals in research laboratories.[12]

It is interesting to compare and contrast the positions taken by the pro- and antivisection camps on these three major issues. To some degree some of the stereotyping and caterwauling so characteristic of disputes over this issue can be defused by a little reflection over the stances adopted by the parties to the debate on the major question surrounding the legitimacy of the research enterprise.

The provivisection point of view

Need

Provivisectionists argue that it is ludicrous to talk at the present time about the complete elimination of animals from the context of experimentation. If human health and well-being are to be improved, if human safety is to be assured in both medical and nonmedical contexts, and if human knowledge is to advance, then some amount of animal experimentation must be conducted. It is simply not possible, given our present knowledge, to utilize alternatives to animals and simultaneously maintain publicly acceptable levels of human health and well-being. In part, this is due to the fact that testing chemicals or pharmaceutical substances on cells or other limited organic systems fails to capture the complexities involved in the processing of such substances by whole organisms. The pursuit of such universally recognized human goods as health, safety, and knowledge requires that some animals be utilized in research contexts.

Moral equality

Most provivisectionists do not accept the equation of animals and humans as entities deserving of equal moral consideration and concern. Some believe that animals do not suffer or feel pain in ways analogous to that experienced by human beings, and, thus, do not deserve the same sort of protections and considerations as human beings do in experimental settings. Others favoring vivisection simply see human beings and their goals and purposes as more worthy of moral respect than the goals and purposes of members of the animal kingdom. Thus, the general health of human beings or the welfare of any specific individual human being counts for far more, in their view, than the well-being or health of any single animal or group of animals. This view is reflected in the fact that scientists will often comment to each other in private that they have actually heard some antivivisectionists say that they would rather one baby be used for experimental purposes than one thousand rats. Such statements are held up as exemplifying the moral blindness of those who would equate animal welfare with human welfare.

Priority

Many persons involved with or supportive of the use of animals in experimental studies find it hard to believe that so much energy, money, and time are devoted to this issue by opponents of such practices. They note that there is plenty of misery about in both the human and animal kingdoms and that antivivisectionists might better devote their frenetic energies to obviating the many other clear injustices that exist in the world. Why, it is sometimes asked, don't antivivisectionists attempt to stop such practices as pet abuse, hunting, or meat-eating rather than focus as they do on animal research? The numbers of animals who suffer at the hands of humans are surely greater in these other contexts, and these would therefore seem to be more appropriate places for political and legislative intervention by those concerned with animal welfare.

The antivivisectionist point of view

Need

Antivivisectionists believe that while it may be true that not all animal experimentation can be abolished (some believe that all could), it is nevertheless true that far more could be eliminated than is presently the case. They argue that there exist many techniques for replacing animals in experiments, including cellular studies, computer simulations, and careful field studies upon animals in natural settings. Moreover, they argue, even more could be done in the way of replacement and reduction in the number of animals used in scientific research but for the pernicious influence of the animal-breeding industry, which has no obvious interest in seeing animal experimentation curbed or in developing suitable substitutes for whole live animals. Antivivisectionists see the continued and ongoing reliance of scientists upon animal studies as the natural outcome of an economic and political situation in which various parties have powerful vested interests in assuring the continuance of the status quo with regard to animal research.

It should also be noted that while most opponents of animal

research do not challenge the legitimacy of such goals as the assurance of human health and safety or the advancement of human knowledge, they find defenses of animal research couched in terms of these broad social goals inadequate. First, they argue, it is not clear that human knowledge is likely to be advanced by the kinds of studies and experiments to which animals are currently put by scientists. There is simply too much waste, replication, and redundancy in scientific experimentation to justify the toll imposed on animals in the name of advancing scientific knowledge. Second, it is not clear that human health is always advanced by animal research since ultimately all drugs and procedures must be tried on humans anyway.

More importantly, they note, a good deal of animal experimentation is conducted in order to assure the American consumer a suitable range of cosmetics, toiletries, and other aesthetic paraphernalia. These are hardly indispensible aspects of human existence, and the antivivisectionists have been quick to note that safety with regard to perfumes and underarm deodorants is hardly an awe-inspiring moral imperative when assessing the legitimacy of the animal sacrifices involved in order to attain safety with regard to these frivolous ends.

Moral equality

Sophisticated critics of the entire enterprise of animal research argue that science itself is in many ways responsible for skepticism about the acceptability of animal research. While there have existed strong traditions within both science and religion committed to the view that animals are nothing more than dumb brutes or automata, the fact is that scientific research has, over the years, revealed essential similarities between humans and animals with respect to many physical and mental properties. Surely, such critics note, we know enough about the physiology, neurology, and behavioral capacities of higher vertebrates to make us realize that these creatures can feel pain, can suffer, and that they ought not to be treated any differently than we would treat any human being endowed with such capacities and traits. There is an implicit demand for consistency behind much of the antivivisectionist opposition to research on animals—what we would not dream of doing to a child, a fetus, a newborn, a demented person, a retarded person, a senile person, a comatose person, or a dead person, we ought not dream of doing to a sentient animal.

The argument from consistency does not commit the antivivisectionist to the equation of animals and humans in terms of their moral worth. Rather, the view held by most antivivisectionists is that animals have the minimal properties capable of conferring moral standing upon an entity—sentience, consciousness, or the capacity to feel pain. These properties, or some one of them, seem sufficient for according moral status to animals. Animals and humans both possess, on this view, minimally sufficient attributes for becoming the objects of moral concern. Both kinds of organisms satisfy minimal requirements for being valued, and in this sense they ought be viewed as of equal moral worth.

Priority

While antivivisectionists argue that animals and humans are equal in terms of capacities that qualify them for moral concern and respect, antivivisectionists give a higher priority to the need to attend to animal suffering than do many proponents of research. The primary reason that seems to motivate the view that animal suffering deserves our legislative and regulatory attention is that animals are not in a position to avoid the types of suffering they encounter in the laboratory. While it is true that animals cause each other harm in nature, the fact remains that the sorts of suffering they often encounter in research settings is entirely due to the activities of human beings. Human beings, thus, are responsible for inflicting an additional measure of pain and suffering upon creatures who are unable to protect themselves against these evils. While human beings can, presumably, avoid at least some of the pain and misery they inflict on their fellows in various situations, animals in laboratories cannot and thus possess a special claim to human moral attention because they are so utterly dependent on humans for alleviating the suffering they encounter.

The issue of moral equality

Having presented the basic outlines of the dispute about animal experimentation, the rest of this essay will focus on the thorny question of the moral worth of animals and humans. For, if it is true that at least some partisans on both sides of the issue are in basic agreement that human health, well-being, and safety are desirable goods, and, that the production of human knowledge that promotes these ends is also good, then it would seem that the real issue dividing pro- and antivivisectionists is the degree to which sacrifices and concessions have to be made with regard to these goods in order to promote animal well-being and decrease animal suffering. Both the level of priority accorded the enterprise of animal experimentation as a moral question and the zeal with which alternatives to animal use are pursued pivot around the degree to which animals are seen as worthy of moral concern. The moral equality of animals and humans is thus the crucial issue dividing the two sides in current disputes, and it is this question which merits close, critical scrutiny if any progress is to be made toward settling the issue.

Much of the basis for the belief that animals and humans have an equal claim to moral consideration arises from an awareness of recent history in the discipline of ethics.[11] During the past two hundred years or so, many human beings have come to realize that differences in sex, race, ethnic group, or sexual preference are not relevant properties for excluding individuals from the moral realm. The popularity of the story of the Elephant Man in the movies and on Broadway derives in part from the message conveyed by the leading character of the play, John Merrick, that despite his deformed and even ghastly appearance, he is still a person worthy of moral concern and respect. Physical form and appearance are not in themselves reasons for excluding someone or even something from the sphere of our moral concern. Thus, while animals are certainly different in their shape, form, and physical appearance from human beings, these differences are not in themselves sufficient for establishing a relevant moral difference between animals and humans any more than are the various shapes, colors, and sizes of human beings.

Some persons have turned to criteria other than physical differences for distinguishing between the moral worth of animals and humans. Reason, language, intentionality, self-awareness, and a sense of personal identity have all been suggested as properties possessed by humans which distinguish them from animals with respect to their moral worth.[2] But there are problems in using these properties as a basis for distinguishing animals from humans concerning moral worth. Many human beings lack some or all of the aforementioned properties. Certainly fetuses, comatose persons, and dead persons can be said to lack all of them. Yet, we do not feel free to do as we please with individuals who are in one of these categories of humanhood. It is also the case that the mental powers of many humans are, at various times, severely impaired or entirely absent (when they are asleep, under the influence of drugs, etc.), and yet we do not believe that the moral worth of such persons evaporates with the temporary disappearance of their mental powers.

Nor is it evident that animals lack the capacities and abilities to manifest some or all of the mental properties often held to distinguish man and beast. There is a voluminous literature in ethology and comparative psychology that indicates that at least some animals are capable of primitive forms of reasoning, intentionality, language, and self-awareness.[1,3,5] Certainly enough evidence has accumulated in the behavioral and biological sciences to cast suspicions on claims for the complete absence of higher mental states and abilities in the animal world. Given the uncertainty surrounding the question of animal awareness, it seems reasonable, in light of what we know about other similarities and commonalities between humans and animals, to err in the direction of commonality when in doubt until definitive evidence can be produced—that what has proven true with regard to genetic, morphological, physiological, biochemical, and anatomical properties is not true with respect to mental properties.

Given the fact that not all humans always possess fully developed mental powers and the likely circumstance that at least some animals do, there would appear to be no basis for drawing a hard and fast line between animals and humans in terms of physical or mental properties. What is important about this claim is that the moral worth of entities does seem linked in important ways to abilities and capacities to suffer, feel pain, or have their goals and purposes frustrated. While it is evident that bodily form or physical appearance are unimportant in deciding whether one ought to be concerned about the welfare of another creature, it is true that certain properties must be presumed if talk about welfare is to make any sense. The ability to feel pain, to suffer anxiety or stress, and the capacity to have one's desires, purposes, or intentions frustrated, all seem to be grounds for speaking meaningfully about the welfare of something. If a creature can experience pain, then, other things being equal, it certainly seems wrong to inflict pain on that creature. Similarly, if an organism, be it human or animal, seeks to fulfill some purpose or end—to drink some water, return home, to rest—it seems wrong (again, other things being equal) to frustrate such desires or purposes.

Sentience and purposiveness seem to be the kinds of properties that confer moral worth on creatures. Any entity, human or non-human, terrestrial or non-terrestrial, that could reasonably be said to possess sentience or purpose seems to be the sort of thing to which it is reasonable to attribute moral worth.[4,6] Unless some reason can be given for interfering with or hindering a creature so endowed, it seems inherently wrong to inflict pain on a sentient entity or to frustrate the purposes and goals of such a creature.

It is with respect to the properties of sentience or purposiveness that humans and animals can be said to be of equal moral worth. Most humans and many animals seem to possess some degree of sentience. They are alert to stimuli and will seek those they find pleasant and attempt to avoid those they find noxious. Many animals and most humans seem to harbor any number of desires, aspirations, intentions, and purposes as can be inferred from the efforts they will make to attain certain goals or to overcome certain obstacles that may stand between them and the objects of their desires. While the issue of sentience and purposiveness is in part a scientific question, at least with regard to the distribution and degree of such properties in the biological world, there would seem to be good reasons for thinking that these properties represent excellent candidates for conferring moral worth upon entities.[4]

It should be noted that in arguing that sentience and purposiveness are sufficient properties for attributing moral worth to an entity, this does not mean that both or either property is necessary for having moral worth. Creatures may someday be found on this or other planets that lack these traits, but possess still others that might make them objects of our moral respect. Moreover, the fact that an entity possesses sentience or purposiveness only satisfies the minimal conditions requisite for having moral worth. It may be possible to distinguish further among various creatures as to which ones have more or higher degrees of these salient features. It would surely be a logical error to infer from the fact that animals meet minimal conditions for having moral worth that there are no relevant differences with respect to these properties that distinguish humans and animals—for example, few animals will modify their behavior toward other animals as a result of reading this book, while it is possible that some human beings may do so.

If it is true that the existence of sentience and/or purposiveness are sufficient traits for imputing moral worth to someone/something, then it would seem there exist what philosophers term *prima facie* duties[2,9] that ought be exercised toward such creatures. Unless one can justify the behavior by an appeal to some higher moral reason or purpose, it would be wrong to harm or frustrate any creature, including an animal, for no reason. Perhaps the cruelest or meanest activity that humans can engage in is the harming or frustrating of others, human and animal, for no reason other than simple meanness of spirit. In some ways human beings are actually in a better position than minimally endowed animals to cope with the frustration and pain of being deceived, fooled, hindered, tricked, or duped since humans are at least bright enough to occasionally figure out what is going on and take steps to avoid or end their suffering. Animals, confronted with malevolent owners or mischievous children, are competent enough to serve as the objects of malevolent intentions (as the pet owners or children know all too well), but are not competent enough to avoid or evade their plight.

It is important to distinguish between an entity's having moral worth, a status I have argued derives from the properties of sentience and purposiveness, and an entity's being a moral agent. Or, in other words, to distinguish between being a moral object and being a moral agent. It is true that many animals and some humans lack all of the properties of mentation we commonly associate with *Homo sapiens.* It would be ludicrous to think that we could hold all animals and humans morally responsible for their actions or that we should expect moral reciprocity from any creature capable of sentience and purpose. What is sufficient in terms of properties that concern moral worth or standing is hardly sufficient in terms of properties that confer moral agency and moral responsibility. We need not determine the nature of the properties that would be sufficient for establishing moral competence among creatures (although it is interesting to note that historically not a few animals have been punished by their owners and even by courts as liable for the untoward outcomes of their behavior!). All that need be noted is that the class of moral agents is far smaller than the class of moral objects, and that arguments about the moral equality of animals and humans concern the latter status and not the former.

Sentience and purposiveness as criteria of moral worth

I have argued thus far that both sentience and purposiveness seem to me to be properties sufficient for conferring moral worth on entities who possess them. However, I have not faced the question of whether both of these properties must be present, or whether either one of them is sufficient by itself for establishing moral worth. Since moral considerableness entails a number of responsibilities for human agents in terms of their not harming or interfering with creatures that have moral worth, it is important to look carefully at these two properties to see whether they are independent and individually adequate for conferring moral worth.

In arguments about the ethics of animal experimentation, some philosophers,[10,11] notably and most vocally Peter Singer in his book *Animal Liberation,* have argued for the sufficiency of sentience as a property for conferring moral worth upon entities. Singer presents a four-part argument in this book that runs as follows: (1) Any creature that is sentient has an interest in not suffering and not feeling pain; (2) all interests must be taken into account in deciding how we ought to behave; (3) equal interests in not suffering or experiencing pain must be counted equally; (4) we should act to bring about the greatest amount of good and to minimize suffering and pain. Thus, if animals can suffer and feel pain as a result of being sentient, Singer argues we must treat them impartially in assessing the practice of animal experimentation. What counts is not only the degree to which human safety is assured and human health promoted, but the degree to which animal suffering is exacerbated by experimental procedures. We should not engage in any particular experiment where the degree of suffering or pain produced in sentient creatures is not outweighed by the amount of benefit to be produced for other sentient creatures, animal and human.

Singer's position is one of classical utilitarianism—the costs and benefits of every action must be computed as best as possible, and decisions about the acceptability or non-acceptability of any action or practice turn on the beliefs we have about the overall effects of the action or practice in terms of goods versus suffering produced. In most cases, Singer argues,[11] animal experiments fail to be justifiable

since, given animal sentience, the degree of suffering involved cannot, with certainty, be predicted to be outweighed by the goods to be
obtained by engaging in any given case of animal experimentation.
Since we should be impartial as to the source of suffering when it
occurs, animals and humans being equally deserving of moral consideration when they are capable of suffering or feeling pain, we ought to
modify our current experimental practices accordingly and drastically decrease the use of animals in research.

The difficulties confronting Singer's criterion of sentience and
his four-part argument are many.[9,10] For example, it is not clear that
most scientists would disagree with the claim that human benefit
ought to outweigh animal suffering if animal experimentation is to be
morally legitimated.[2] Indeed, as critics of Singer's view point out, the
issue of how much suffering is caused by animal experiments is an
empirical question, and it is not clear that the benefits do out outweigh the harms in assessing most cases of animal research.

More seriously, Singer's argument against animal experimentation founders on two other issues. First, his position would seem to
permit experimentation on any creatures which cannot, for whatever
reason, suffer or feel pain. Thus, if we made animal experimentation,
or human experimentation for that matter, pain free, we would appear to be justified in conducting research that would produce benefits in terms of health, well-being, safety, or knowledge. Also, if we
could produce vast benefits to animals or humans by utilizing only a
few animals or humans in painful experiments, this practice would
also escape moral condemnation since, on Singer's construction of
the argument, it is only the net outcome of experimentation that
legitimates the activity.

I suspect that sentience and the corresponding ability it confers
upon animals to suffer or feel pain is a bit too lofty a standard to
invoke in thinking about the question of moral worth. It seems wrong
to treat humans or animals who are incapable of suffering or feeling
pain as undeserving of moral respect and consideration. For example,
even if—by surgical intervention or through the use of drugs—a human being were rendered unable to feel pain or to suffer, I doubt
whether members of our society would want to say that such persons
could then be used in any way scientists deemed useful in the process
of research.

It is interesting to note that Singer's view, while popular in antivivisectionist circles these days, does not lead to the view that all

animal experimentation is wrong. Nor does it lead to the view that animals have rights—a concept that is antithetical to a utilitarian analysis of moral worth. However, if we look to purposiveness and intentionality rather than sentience and the ability to suffer as the standard of moral worth, I think we come closer to locating the kind of criterion that motivates much of the moral concern about animal experimentation.

If animals and humans are so organized as to be purposive creatures with various desires, drives, intentions, and aspirations, it seems wrong to cavalierly frustrate these purposes. It might be argued that if animals and humans are biologically constituted so as to pursue their own existence, which is a fact quite consistent with current thinking in evolutionary theory, then it is morally wrong to interfere or to deprive animals of the opportunity to fulfill this basic drive. In other words, animals and humans, endowed by nature with a will to survive, have a right to survive—rights being consequent upon the purposiveness and teleological orientation of living things.[9] If all creatures who possess purposiveness have a right to be left alone to pursue their ends, then the basic moral repugnance felt by many people about animal experimentation can be easily understood—most experimentation deprives animals of the right to exist, or, at minimum, frustrates certain basic drives and intentions they manifest. While human beings are under no moral obligation to aid their fellows or animals in the pursuit of their basic purposes, they do appear to be under some constraint not to interfere uncaringly with other organisms.

I believe that purposiveness rather than sentience is a property that suffices for conferring moral worth upon entities. When organisms have sufficient organization to have basic drives, desires, and intentions, be they amoebas, bees, birds, or retarded humans, it is wrong to interfere with their efforts to fulfill these desires. It needs to be quickly added that such interference is wrong unless there exists some other reason or justification for doing so. The fact is that—mirroring attitudes in the abortion debate—most persons erroneously believe that once animal rights are established, the issue of animal experimentation will be settled.[2] If it is wrong to interfere with purposive creatures, then no animal research could ever be morally legitimate. But such a view confuses the question of how moral worth and moral rights arise with the question of what to do when rights conflict—a common, ordinary, and unavoidable consequence of the nature of the world we live in.

No animals or humans capable of purposiveness should be interfered with by others, other things being equal. But other things are rarely equal. If humans are to survive, they must eat, and animals may have to suffer the consequences. If human beings are to fulfill their desires to have medicines, then some creatures will have to suffer in the course of our determining whether different substances have therapeutic value. While it is true that we ought not to interfere with or hinder the bringing to fruition of the desires and purposes of others, animals and humans, in a world of limited resources and conflicting purposes, some creatures will, of necessity, have their basic rights overridden.

The legitimacy of animal experimentation reconsidered

It should be evident from the preceding discussion that science has no one to blame but itself for the existence of worries about the ethics of animal experimentation. Science has shown the degree to which sentience and purposiveness permeate the animal kingdom, and thus has raised doubts about the validity of causing harm to or interfering with creatures who may not differ all that much from human beings in the properties that count from a moral point of view. If sentience or, minimally, purposiveness are sufficient for conferring moral worth on things, and if we are to be consistent in our moral practices and beliefs, then we may have to rethink our ordinary attitudes about the legitimacy of animal experimentation.

Perhaps the strongest caveat to emerge from an analysis of the morality of animal research is that the burden of proof always rests upon the experimenter to justify the use of animals in experimental contexts. The antivivisectionist has nothing to prove; many animals used in experiments are sentient and purposive, and thus have *prima facie* rights to live and be left alone. Those who would override or abrogate these rights must provide compelling reasons for doing so. Humility and sensitivity, not arrogance and hubris, must be the hallmarks of animal research, since it is only out of ignorance and expediency that we put members of the animal kingdom to our purposes rather than theirs.

The other conclusion that follows from the analysis of the moral legitimacy of animal experimentation is that such activity is always morally tragic. No matter what goods are promoted by the process, some creatures who are unable to alter their circumstances will have their basic rights to life and fulfillment infringed. Since this is so, it would seem imperative that steps be taken to reduce waste and duplication in the use of animals for research purposes, put more funds toward the development of alternatives to animal testing, and make the public aware of the moral trade-offs that must be faced in deciding how best to achieve human well-being, health, safety, and knowledge at the expense of animal suffering. Ultimately, the public will have to decide what sorts of trade-offs are morally acceptable when animal and human interests conflict.

1. Bowd, A. D. 1980. "Ethical reservations about psychological research with animals." *Psychol. Rec.* 30(Spring): 201–210.

2. Caplan, A. L. 1978. "Rights language and the ethical treatment of animals." In *Implications of History and Ethics to Medicine—Veterinary and Human.* L. McCullough & J. P. Morris, eds.: 126–135. Texas A&M University Press. College Station, Tex.

3. Fox, M. S. 1981. "Experimental psychology, animal rights, welfare and ethics." *Psychopharm. Bull.* 17(2): 80–84.

4. Goodpaster, K. E. 1978. "On being morally considerable." *J. Phil.* 76(6): 308–324.

5. Griffin, D. R. 1976. *The Question of Animal Awareness.* Rockefeller University Press. New York.

6. Hoff, C. 1980. "Immoral and moral uses of animals." *N. Eng. J. Med.* 302(2): 115–118.

7. Morris, R. K. & M. W. Fox, eds. 1978. *On the Fifth Day: Animal Rights and Human Ethics.* Acropolis Books. Washington, D.C.

8. Passmore, J. 1976. *Man's Responsibility for Nature.* Scribner's. New York.

9. Regan, T. 1980. "Animal rights, human wrongs." Environ. Ethics 2(2): 99–120.

10. Regan, T. & P. Singer, eds. 1976. *Animal Rights and Human Obligations.* Prentice-Hall. Englewood Cliffs, N.J.

11. Singer, P. 1975. *Animal Liberation.* Avon Books. New York.

12. Visscher, M. B. 1979. "Animal rights and alternative methods." *The Pharos* (Fall): 11–19.

4.

Moral community and the responsibility of scientists

Why is there such interest in animal experimentation today?

During the past decade, the debate over the use of animals in scientific research, educational demonstrations, and toxicological testing has commanded increasing attention. Many scientists believe that contemporary concerns about animal welfare are based upon nothing more than sentimentality about animals and perhaps nothing less than misanthropy.

This interpretation of the animal welfare movement is simply wrong. The movement that has evolved during the past fifteen years is rooted in the insights of philosophers and the belief of some scientists that what we now know about the abilities and capacities of animals may force us to rethink our traditional understanding of their moral status. In fact, contemporary concerns about the moral status of animals are closely linked to debates about the moral standing that ought be assigned to various categories of human beings. Debates about the moral propriety of using fetuses, the mentally retarded, the comatose, and the dead for various scientific purposes have led directly to a concern about the morality of using animals in research, education, and testing.

Many of those in the animal welfare movement have noted that if it is wrong to experiment on human beings with severely limited or underdeveloped mental abilities then consistency demands that we reexamine our practices with respect to animals—at least those animals that have the same abilities and capacities as the weakest and most vulnerable members of our species. For unless some significant difference can be shown to exist between embryos, fetuses, children, the retarded, the comatose, and animals, what we view as ethically proscribed in terms of educational, testing, and research practices for these creatures ought to be equally proscribed for animals.

Do animals have rights?

In recent years the most vocal proponents of animal rights have been the Australian philosopher Peter Singer and the American philosopher Tom Regan.

Singer (1976) argues that consistency concerning the moral status of such organisms as fetuses, children, and the comatose demands a revision in our attitudes about animals. He believes that mere membership in a particular species is not a morally relevant distinction in thinking about whether a creature has moral worth. Rather, he utilizes a rather concise argument to show why it is wrong to harm or hurt animals in research or testing:

> All sentient creatures have an interest in not suffering.
> All interests must be considered in ethically evaluating an action or policy.
> Equal interests count equally.
> We should always act to maximize goods and minimize suffering.

Singer argues that, unless we are speciesists, animal interests and human interests in avoiding suffering must be counted equally. If they are, then few animal experiments pass the test of maximizing good and minimizing suffering given the large number of animals that must be used to produce benefits either for other animals or for humans.

Regan (1983) argues that Singer's brand of utilitarianism is flawed in that it allows individual animals or humans to be used as a means to benefit others whenever a sufficiently large number of other animals or humans may benefit. Regan presents an important and elegant argument for according rights to animals. His argument is, roughly, as follows:

All organisms which can be said to be "subjects-of-a-life" have inherent value.

Any organism can be said to be the subject-of-a-life if it has beliefs and desires, perception, memory, a sense of the future, a sense of identity over time, and can be benefitted or harmed.

Those individuals who have inherent value ought be treated in ways that respect their value.

Inherent value is a sufficient basis for according respect.

We fail to respect the inherent value of creatures when we do anything that harms them.

I think there are flaws in both Singer's and Regan's positions, which I shall return to at the end of this paper. But regardless of my own views, those scientists who favor using animals for scientific purposes must take such arguments seriously.

Should scientists involved in animal research take their critics seriously?

Some scientists have argued that the best response to all the talk these days about animal rights and about legislating animal experimentation out of existence is to say and do nothing. Many scientists believe that anti-vivisectionism should not be lent credibility by showing it serious consideration. In their view the best response is no response, particularly when the advocates on the other side of the issue seem so strident and entrenched in their views. Proponents of what might be termed the "ostrich approach" believe that it is ethically and tactically wrong to spend valuable time arguing with individuals who do not understand the methods and aims of scientific research and who do not represent the mainstream of public opinion on the matter of animal experimentation.

Other scientists believe that the best response is to make the strongest possible case for animal research to both legislators and the general public. Those committed to the value of research believe that the issue of whether animal research should be done is not open for debate—it is being done, and the general public wants research to continue. This "let it all hang out" strategy suggests that the research community carefully explain what is being done to animals (and why it is being done) and highlight the steps being taken now—and that might be taken in the future—to assure that the interests of animals are being protected in the course of scientific research and testing.

It is easy to understand why scientists conducting research with animals often become exasperated by the critics of animal experimentation. Time and again scientists note that the only way progress can be made is by using animals in education, testing, and research. It seems that there is no real choice between using human subjects and using animal subjects—animals must be utilized.

The benefits that have accrued to humankind as a result of animal experimentation are real and indisputable. Many scientists therefore believe that any moral argument that animal experimentation is wrong and ought be stopped *must* be invalid. No intellectual gymnastics can obscure the fact that animal experimentation has and continues to provide humankind with safe, efficacious, and needed drugs, therapies, and products. The exasperation of the scientific community with respect to the more strident critics of animal experimentation raises an interesting (although somewhat abstract) methodological issue concerning all moral arguments. How should we evaluate moral claims that conflict with our moral common sense?

Intuition and common sense in ethics

Advocates of particular moral views often reach conclusions that directly conflict with ordinary commonsensical intuitions about what is right and what is wrong. When such a situation arises, two choices are available to those who do not agree with such a conclusion—to modify what are sometimes deeply held moral convictions, or to dismiss the argument on the ground that it reaches a patently absurd conclusion.

The problem with the latter strategy is that many ordinary or everyday moral intuitions about right and wrong have ultimately been recognized as being false. Perhaps the most obvious and familiar such instance was the ordinary and quite common moral view—current for thousands of years—that slavery is morally acceptable.

The moral acceptability of slavery was a view that had currency in Greek and Roman society, as well as in broad segments of American and British society during the eighteenth and nineteenth centuries. Nevertheless, few today would disagree that, despite the ordinary intuition of the resident of the Greek polis or the early settlers of the United States, slavery was as morally wrong then as it is understood to be now.

The example of slavery shows that not all moral arguments that reach counterintuitive conclusions can be simply dismissed out of hand. If every counterintuitive or oddball moral claim were dismissed on this basis, then some of the most basic advances in the history of ethics—advances concerning the treatment of slaves, blacks, women, ethnic and religious minorities—would never have been made.

This having been said, it is also true that some moral arguments arrive at conclusions that, for all their apparent elegance and sophistication, can only be described as goofy. Any number of philosophers and theologians through history have argued that the only reasonable response to life on this planet is suicide. While such arguments can make for some interesting after-dinner conversation, they are—by the very nature of the conclusion they advance—at least highly suspect and in all probability wrong. Any healthy soul who proceeded to dispatch him- or herself on the basis of some ornate bit of philosophical sophistry which adduced suicide as the only answer to life's problems would be making a grave and deeply regrettable mistake.

The problem in ethics is that, when facing an apparently bizarre or threatening moral claim, it is difficult to know whether it falls into the category of arguments against slavery (counterintuitive to the majority of those who first entertained the idea but correct in an important and basic way) or into the category of arguments favoring universal suicide (counterintuitive to those who entertain the claim and rightly so).

There is no doubt that claims to the effect that animal experimentation is wrong and must be stopped strike most scientists and indeed most ordinary citizens as *prima facie* wrong. Such claims appear to have much more in common with arguments about the moral desirability of suicide than they do with arguments about the moral perniciousness of slavery. There is a strong temptation to simply ignore them.

I believe such a response is wrong. It is wrong since a persuasive case can be made that animal research is both necessary and beneficial for both humans and animals. But more importantly it is wrong because it is not consistent with the responsibilities borne by any scientist conducting research at public expense in a democratic society.

The responsibilities of scientists in a democracy

Science in most nations is a public enterprise. It is public in the sense that the funds for scientific research are obtained through taxation, either directly from the citizenry or indirectly by allowing exemptions to foundations and companies that devote monies to basic research. Those who are the beneficiaries of pubic money incur a responsibility to the members of the society which supports their work. They must be prepared to justify their work to the public either directly through the media or indirectly through appearances before legislators and governmental bodies.

If it is true that scientists who use public funds have an obligation to be publicly accountable for their work, then it is wrong for scientists to fail to take their critics in the animal welfare movement seriously. For the critics are surely among the members of the general public who help foot the bill for scientific research through their tax dollars.

Democracy, moral uncertainty, and controversy

One of the most valuable features of democratic societies is that they try to treat odd or counterintuitive moral views in a serious fashion. Not only do all citizens have the basic right to express their views and opinions, but the government has an obligation to listen to all such views and incorporate them into its deliberations. While the number of ethical "false positives" produced in such a system may be high in terms of the amount of time and newsprint given over to silly, banal, or even malicious views, democratic theory is committed to the assumption that the cost of allowing "false negatives" in ethical matters is so great as to be intolerable.

Is the conclusion to be drawn from this argument that animal experimentation is morally wrong because a few citizens say it is? Or ought we to conclude that the moral views of a small minority should be allowed free reign over those of the majority whenever a conflict arises? Or is it the case that the only way of evaluating the moral claims of any interest group within a democratic society is by public meetings followed by referenda? None of these conclusions is valid.

What does follow from the arguments concerning the unreliability of intuition in ethical matters and the moral responsibilities of scientists in democracies is that all opinions concerning matters of public policy be treated seriously, courteously, and respectfully. It does not matter one bit that the militant critics of any and all forms of animal experimentation may be wrong. What matters is that researchers realize that they cannot and should not dismiss the claims and arguments of their critics as so much benighted hot air or as nothing more than the visible manifestation of some grave psycho-pathological condition.

The greatest enemy of scientific research is not militant animal welfarism but scientific arrogance. The most convincing arguments against allowing researchers to conduct experiments involving animals have nothing to do with talk of "animal rights" or photographs of gruesome animal experiments. The argument that the public is likely to find most persuasive against animal research is the argument that researchers are so morally arrogant that they will not deign to take their critics seriously.

What are the issues in animal experimentation?

If it is true that scientists have an obligation to address themselves to the concerns of those with objections to animal experimentation, what then should the nature of their response be? Must scientists justify the entire enterprise of animal experimentation every time someone raises an objection to this practice?

All but the most zealous critics concede the fact that some experimentation and testing is useful and that there are as yet no viable alternatives to the use of at least some animals. Certain issues merit serious consideration by the scientific community: (1) At what price in terms of safety and scientific progress can fewer animals be used in research? (2) Are current regulatory guidelines and practices concerning animal welfare adequate and, if they are not, what ought be done to modify them? (3) Do greater efforts need to be made to educate the research community about their responsibilities in using animals for research purposes? (4) Are there new techniques or practices which can reduce the suffering of those animals that are used as subjects in research, education, and testing?

I said at the beginning of this essay that I have reservations about the adequacy of the arguments of both Singer and Regan. These reservations are relevant in thinking about all four of these questions.

Very simply, my reason for not being persuaded by Singer's argument is that the claim that animal interests and human interests ought to count equally appears to me to be false.

I think Singer is correct in observing that both animals and humans are capable of suffering and that this capacity gives both kinds of creature an interest in avoiding this state. However, it is a big step from the observation that both animals and humans can suffer to the conclusion that their interests in avoiding suffering ought to be counted equally.

Most humans can do far more than suffer. They can plan, hope, desire, intend, fear, doubt, blame, know, and engage in a variety of other complex mental activities. Most animals cannot. These differences in mental and cognitive abilities seem quite relevant in thinking about the weights that ought be assigned to animal and human interests in thinking about whether it is morally acceptable to use them in scientific testing and research.

Singer seems to make a basic conceptual mistake in arguing that, since animals have some of the capacities and abilities necessary for having ethical standing, they must be counted as the equals of humans, who also have such properties. But he fails to show that equal consideration is appropriate or deserved since there are other traits that make a moral difference and most animals appear to lack these.

Regan's view is far more compelling than Singer's in terms of assigning rights to animals. Regan explicitly grounds his view of animal rights in a commitment to the inherent equal worth of animals and humans. Moreover, he argues for a principle of respect for the inherent value of all creatures that would not allow some animals to be used to benefit others regardless of the degree of benefit involved.

I believe Regan is correct in arguing that those creatures which can satisfy what he terms the "subject-of-a-life" criterion qualify for moral standing (Caplan, 1983). I doubt whether many species of animals can reasonably be said to be capable of the various conditions necessary for fulfilling this standard. But some animals such as the primates and perhaps other mammals come very close.

My difficulty with Regan's argument is that it is not sufficiently sensitive to the reasons we have for using animals rather than human beings for scientific research and testing. I agree that some animals may have inherent value. I also agree that this value is due respect and that it may make sense to signify this in the language of rights. However, I do not agree that having inherent value is sufficient to make one immune from harm or the violation of right in any and all contexts. Nor do I agree that inherent value itself is simply an all-or-nothing proposition. Most importantly, I do not believe that the only thing that matters in deciding what to do with animals in scientific contexts is to determine whether or not they have inherent value.

A single example may help to illustrate the differences between most animals and human beings that lead me to assign more weight to human rights than animal rights. If you kill the baby of a baboon the mother may spend many weeks looking for her baby. This behavior soon passes and the baboon will go on to resume her normal life. But, if you kill the baby of a human being, the mother will spend the rest of her life grieving over the loss of her baby. Hardly a day will go by when the mother does not think about and grieve over the loss of the child.

The morally relevant difference between the two cases is that, while animals may be the "subjects-of-a-life," they lead lives that are more independent and far less interconnected than the intertwined lives of human beings. Human beings have a level of interdependence that would seem far to exceed anything that prevails in the animal kingdom.

Our notions of family, parenting, friendship, kinship, community, and patriotism bind us to one another in ways that do not appear to be true of the animal kingdom. While respect for families, communities, and country can and have been taken to extremes, these relationships appear to be morally important and worthy of respect. If we do not experiment upon fetuses, conduct toxicology testing upon embryos, or farm the comatose for useful medical products, it is surely out of respect for the feelings and values of families and friends—not (as Singer and Regan appear to suggest) simply out of an obligation to respect the value which inheres in the lives of these individuals.

Respect for the inherent value of life demands that we not harm, hurt, or frustrate the aims and interests of those creatures capable of commanding respect. Uniquely human mental capacities and abilities to relate to one another differentiate humans from animals in morally significant ways. If one aim of morality is to foster and maintain such interrelationships, then we may have to assign greater moral weight to the moral status of humans (and of any animals capable of these interrelationships) than we do to creatures which are capable of having only inherent value.

If this argument is valid, it may be possible to defend the use of animals in research, testing, and education when no alternatives exist and when their use will lead to the preservation of morally important relationships among human beings. It may be necessary to violate the rights of animals for scientific purposes when no alternative exists and when such uses advance the bonds of social cohesion and interconnectedness that ought to prevail among human beings. We should not equate the moral worth of baboon babies and human babies if in so doing we would lead human parents to care less about the welfare and interests of their children. We might choose to experiment on rats rather than retarded children if such a choice promotes essential values such as family, community, and mutuality.

Nonetheless, it seems to me that scientists would still be under strong obligations to minimize the use of animals in scientific contexts. If situations do exist in which animal research is poorly designed, in which researchers are unnecessarily duplicating the efforts of other researchers, in which alternative techniques are available but not utilized, then procedures must be created to detect and remedy these situations.

The scientific community is making many efforts to achieve these ends by means of revising existing guidelines on animal welfare, by introducing the subject of animal welfare at professional society meetings, by introducing the subject of animal welfare into undergraduate and graduate training programs, and by strengthening the committee review process for animal research. All these efforts are laudable and ought be continued.

It is important that scientists working for animal welfare realize any change must come, not in response to outside public pressures, but because certain moral responsibilities inhere in the role of scientist. It is equally important that scientists engaged in animal research not become defensive or arrogant about animal welfare. The public is right to demand thoroughness and concern on the part of scientists, and scientists are right to demand these virtues from one another. At least to this degree, agreement should be possible among all of the parties concerned about animal welfare.

References

Caplan, A. 1983. "Beastly conduct," *Ann. N.Y. Acad. Sci.*, 406: 159–169. (Reprinted in this volume.)

Regan, T. 1983. *The case for animal rights.* Berkeley: University of California Press.

Singer, P. 1976. "Are all animals equal?" In *Animal rights and human obligations*, eds. T. Regan and P. Singer. Englewood Cliffs, N.J.: Prentice-Hall.

5.

On privacy and confidentiality in social science research

Why worry about privacy?

Worries about privacy play a key role in arguments for the regulation of inquiry in the social sciences, Many social scientists have argued that the amount of physical or mental suffering caused by social science research is so small as to make the need for regulation, both internal and external, nonexistent.[1] Physical harm, when it occurs in social scientific inquiry, is almost always a matter of malpractice, misconduct, or error. Psychological harm is difficult to assess and often transient in duration. Violations of privacy, confidentiality, or dignity, by contrast, are often felt to be at the heart of moral concern about the activities of social scientists.

Social scientists often *do* seem to infringe upon persons' privacy. Covert observation, random surveys, and the analysis of information pertaining to identifiable individuals or groups are all examples of common activities in social science that can jeopardize privacy. This is particularly apparent when behaviors such as drug use, sexual activity, or criminal activity are the topics of social scientific inquiry.

Social scientists are interested in studying a wide variety of human activities which many consider private and personal. It is a concern over the intrusive and invasive nature of the activities and methods of social science research that fuels much of the interest in, and discussion of, ethical issues about such research.

If this is so, then it becomes important in discussions of ethical issues in social science research to know exactly what is meant by the concept of privacy, and to discuss the status of this concept relative to other moral goods and evils present in everyday life. If worries about privacy and its violations are the source of most moral musings about research in the social sciences, the analysis of the meaning and weight of this concept becomes pivotal.

At first glance, this claim might appear to be only an instance of the typical philosopher's refrain—"Before we can decide what to do about x, in this case the regulation and promotion of social scientific inquiry, we must come to a clear understanding of concepts such as y, in this case privacy. Such concepts are loosely bandied about in all the extant ethical and legal discussions of this topic." This refrain is solemnly intoned by philosophers at the outset of nearly every discussion of an ethical matter, the solemnity displayed for nonphilosophers being balanced by a certain amount of internal glee. The philosopher's glee issues from the anticipation of yet another exciting ethical safari during which numerous thorny cases will be slashed clear, many dangerous conceptual pitfalls avoided, and terrifying counterexamples wrestled into logically consistent submission. The nonphilosopher, or at least the nonphilosopher with some prior travel experience in the company of philosophers, is likely to pale at the prospect of another gloomy and endless journey through the conceptual moral bush. These trips consume time and often result in undersized or worthless conceptual trophies.

I mention this safari metaphor because I fear that many persons may have come away from Terry Pinkard's essay "Invasions of Privacy in Social Science Research" with a keen sense of disappointment. For the meager quarry flushed out of his conceptual analysis seems to be that privacy has no clear meaning. It is a concept, Pinkard suggests, that is "essentially contested." Its meaning is to be understood in terms of what is deemed appropriate behavior in various social roles, and the contestable nature of the concept "appropriate" breeds a relativistic morass from which no clear-cut definition of privacy can ever be culled.

It must be noted that Pinkard is not alone in his view of the slapdash nature of the concept of privacy. As he himself points out, the concept of privacy in the law is a jerry-built affair that includes activities having to do with disclosure, misrepresentation, intrusion, and restrictions of personal liberty. Frederick Davis provides a useful summary of this view of privacy when he states: "Invasion of privacy is, in reality, a complex of more fundamental wrongs. . . . The individual's interest in privacy itself, however real, is derivative and a state better vouchsafed by protecting more immediate rights."[2]

Philosophers have also found themselves puzzled by the notion of a *right* to privacy. Judith Thomson notes that

> Nobody seems to have any very clear idea what the right to privacy is. . . . The right to privacy is "derivative" in this sense: it is possible to explain in the case of each right in the cluster how we have it without ever once mentioning the right to privacy. Indeed, the wrongness of every violation of the right to privacy can be explained without ever once mentioning it.[3]

For Thomson, the concept of privacy is useful only as a placeholder to capture a complex set of concepts concerning ownership, liberty, freedom, and harm.

In a recent review of the literature on privacy, H. J. McCloskey comes to a similar conclusion about the derivative nature of privacy. He writes:

> Any right to privacy will be a derivative one from other rights and other goods. This means that it will be a conditional right, and not always a right. Whether or not it will be a derivative right . . . will depend on practical considerations as to whether respect for privacy is necessary for the enjoyment of these [other] rights.[4]

McCloskey realizes that if privacy is a placeholder concept or a derivative right useful only as a means for achieving justice, freedom, or autonomy, then privacy becomes a topic of derivative or secondary moral concern. He notes:

> Each restriction of privacy for the sake of liberty must be weighed against the loss of liberty involved in the legal protection of privacy and in the light of the liberty that is protected. A blanket protection of privacy is not justified by this argument from liberty. Much liberty, more importantly, the liberty to inquire and to gain knowledge, more particularly about man and men, the liberty to engage in

psychological, historical, biographical inquiries, and to publish and share with other scientists, historians, thinkers, the world, what one has discovered is a basic liberty, one that is the very core of the structure of our liberal society. So to protect privacy that this liberty, and similar kinds of liberties, are curtailed or lost, is to threaten the very life of our society as a liberal society.[5]

McCloskey, Thomson, Davis, and others[6] who think of privacy as a derivative or instrumental right raise a central problem for those concerned to defend the right of privacy as a legitimate area of central concern in assessing social inquiry. If privacy is a derivative moral concept, either reducible to more basic moral notions or a convenient placeholder for a diverse range of relatively minor worries and concerns, much of the starch goes out of the view that respect for privacy ought to be a dominant concern in conducting social inquiry. On these suppositions, concerns about liberty, autonomy, justice, and benefits (a) will be most appropriate to discussions of the ethics of social research and (b) will always trump worries about privacy. Privacy will often wind up taking a back seat to social benefits when inquirer and subject meet.

Since Pinkard believes not only that the concept of privacy is derivative but also that it is essentially contestable, his arguments deserve careful scrutiny. If he is right and privacy is ultimately in the eye of the beholder, there will be little point in going to great lengths to protect it.

Is privacy an essentially contested concept?

Pinkard argues for two significant attributes of the concept of privacy—that it is "essentially contestable," and that it is derivative from the principle of respect for persons. He appeals to these features to adduce a definition of an invasion of privacy, and uses this definition in turn to formulate a right to privacy which there can be no "utilitarian or knowledge-based justification for overriding."[7] I think his arguments are flawed on a number of points. Since, however, Pinkard and I both agree that privacy is worth taking seriously as a matter of moral concern in performing and evaluating social research, these flaws must be exposed and repaired.

Pinkard notes that a number of senses of privacy float around in the legal, philosophical, and scientific literature. These senses—plus the facts that privacy is appraisive in character, internally complex, admits of different worths, and is relative to changing circumstances—lead him straight to the essential contestability of the concept. One obvious problem with these points is the ease with which they can be applied to any and every concept in ethics, aesthetics, and large chunks of the sciences. Consider the notion of "width." It is appraisive, complex, admits of different descriptions, and varies with changing circumstances. Does this make "width" an essentially contestable concept? If so, then every normative term will be essentially contestable. This may be so, but it will not help much in the analysis of privacy and of its importance to know that the essentially contestable concept of privacy must be balanced against the essentially contestable concepts of justice, rights, dignity, autonomy, freedom, liberty, etc. We already know that much.

Pinkard has been deceived by the multiplicity of meanings available for privacy and by its diverse cultural and social manifestations into thinking that privacy is essentially a relativistic morass. This is a conclusion unwarranted by either definition or cultural pluralism. It is surely erroneous to conclude that since different people have different standards of privacy, the concept has no core meaning. This is simply ethical relativism in miniature.

Pinkard is undaunted by his own assessment, for he takes the messy notion of privacy developed in the first part of his essay and refines it substantially in order to demonstrate that a right to privacy exists. He writes:

> It is surely a truism that control over one's life entails control (to some degree) over what is known by others about oneself and control over some set of crucial (private) areas of one's life. From the general moral principle of respect for persons an abstract right to privacy thus follows.[8]

There are some puzzling features in this passage. First, all the alleged vagaries of meaning about privacy have evaporated. Control over what is known about one's life becomes Pinkard's "unattainable" definition. This mysterious attainment of the impossible—a definition of privacy—can best be explained in two ways. Pinkard tacitly realizes that there is another option besides essential contestability when faced with a multiplicity of definitions and assessments of a concept: trim the excess. Some things lumped together in legal definitions of privacy—say, freedom of choice regarding abortions—merit culling, and Pinkard's definition reflects this need.

Moreover, the fact that people disagree over what counts as privacy or how much privacy is enough does not mean that they disagree about what privacy is. It may be that they disagree about the scope or applicability of the definition. Contestability, after all, can be a product both of definitions *and* of the criteria for satisfying them.

Somewhat more puzzling than the appearance of a definition for a notion that is essentially contestable is the argument in this same passage that privacy is derivable from the principle of respect for persons. In Pinkard's view, privacy is a subset of personal autonomy; the principle of respect for persons demands that we respect autonomy and, thus, privacy. The problems with this argument for a right to privacy are numerous. Pinkard gives no defense of the principle of respect for persons. Without such a defense, it is unclear whether this principle is one that any rational agent must follow, or what type of rights would be contingent on such a principle. Neither is it clear that respect for a person's autonomy demands a respect for personal privacy. One might watch or study various forms of behavior without affecting autonomy. Simply knowing or learning something about persons does not necessarily impair their capability for "forming conceptions of their own good and how they should lead their lives" or their ability to "act according to those conceptions."[9] Knowing things about others does not in itself affect their ability to act freely or autonomously. A social scientist who knows something about my personal habits in my bedroom or bathroom can threaten my autonomy only by acting on such knowledge in some way. Knowing is not sufficient.

Pinkard has not given us sufficient reasons for his view that there are no utilitarian or knowledge-based justifications for overriding privacy. It is not clear that privacy is a part of autonomy, for it is not clear that free and informed action licenses control over the access of information concerning such action. Neither is it clear that a right to autonomy could not be overridden by a right to liberty or certain goods, such as knowledge or health. Moreover, it is not at all clear that we cannot know precisely what we are talking about when we invoke the concept of privacy.

What is privacy and how important is it?

In writing about the characteristics of total institutions, Erving Goffman remarks upon the phenomenon he calls "mortification of self." In many prisons, hospitals, religious orders, and schools, there is an interest in changing or remaking the person who enters. One of the central ways in which this is done is to invade or destroy the privacy of the person. Goffman writes:

> Beginning with admission, a kind of contaminative exposure occurs. On the outside, the individual can hold objects of self-feeling—such as his body, his immediate actions, his thoughts, and some of his possessions—clear of contact with alien and contaminating things. But in total institutions these territories of the self are violated; the boundary that the individual places between his being and the environment is invaded and the embodiments of self profaned.[10]

Goffman's perceptive remarks indicate that privacy plays a key role in self-identity and personhood.[11] The ability to control access to thoughts or actions is closely tied to our notions of personhood, personal identity, and selfhood. Those who run political prisons or concentration camps realize that the key to destroying personal identity and selfhood is to remove any sense or possibility of privacy. Political prisoners often report that during imprisonment they found it necessary to create a sense of mental isolation or seclusion in such environments in order to maintain their sanity and identity as persons.

Anthropologists have noted that all cultures, even the most open and highly exposed, make some provision for the privacy of their members. The Mehinacu Indians of Brazil, who live in an almost totally nonprivate society—lacking doors, barriers, and many natural obstructions such as hills—still have some provisions for seclusion. Even in this community where individual behavior can quickly become a matter of public knowledge (and comment), individuals "have a number of ways of establishing a measure of privacy for themselves even though they are often hard-pressed to do so."[12] These include various taboos, social conventions, ceremonies, affinal avoidances, and the practice of civil inattention whereby certain public events are consciously and studiously ignored.

The universality of at least some cultural practices for attaining privacy[13] is paralleled in other areas of social life in both humans and animals. Territoriality and conventions as to social distance and social spacing are well known among various animal species and human cultures. The deleterious effects of crowding, of constant violations of cultural norms as to territory and spacing, and the negative effects of prolonged residential density on health and behavior are amply documented in the literature of biology and psychology.[14]

The importance of space seclusion and territory in animal and human behavior, and the deleterious effects of many practices within total institutions on personal identity, reveal what is at the core of the concept of privacy. Privacy refers to the human need for voluntary access to an exclusive space or environment. Human beings, if they are to be well-functioning persons, require noninvaded personal control over some part of their environment if that environment is publicly accessible to others.

Privacy is a basic human need. Without privacy, it is not possible to develop or maintain a sense of self or personhood. In deriving privacy from autonomy, Pinkard has the cart before the proverbial horse. Autonomy and self-determination are concepts that can be predicated only of persons. But to be a person and to remain a person, human beings require a modicum of privacy. Although questions as to exactly how much space, or what degree of spatial exclusivity, remain unsettled, the findings of social scientists and biologists clearly show that some measure of privacy is requisite for personhood. Without privacy self-governance or autonomy becomes impossible because there are no selves or persons to govern or be governed.

The claim that privacy is a basic human need on a par with needs for food, shelter, liberty, etc., is borne out by the deleterious consequences which result from the denial of privacy. If privacy is a basic human need, then negative consequences should accompany its absence. This is precisely what the literature in psychology and medicine reveals. In the absence of privacy, cognitive functioning is impaired, physical and mental disorders occur, the individual's sense of well-being is harmed, and the sense of personhood and of self is injured.[15]

Ironically, science provides the best available answer to the question of how important privacy is relative to other human goods. If the core notion of privacy concerns the control of personal space, then privacy is as basic and as fundamental a need as any other basic human need. Indeed, respecting the rights persons have to privacy is as basic a requirement as there can be in ethics; in the absence of privacy, there are no persons to serve as either the subjects or the agents of moral action and moral description.

The buying power of privacy in the moral marketplace

Privacy is not a derivative or secondary right. It stands as a basic human need and as such is on a par with rights rooted in other basic human needs. If this analysis is correct, it means that we must take the right to privacy seriously when it collides with the rights of other humans or with social practices. While Pinkard and I disagree about why it is so, we both agree that good reasons must be given for overriding so fundamental a right as the right to privacy.

Wallace agrees that the right to privacy is a serious and basic right. But he maintains that utilitarian considerations of the social or common good may sometimes justify violations of an individual's right to privacy. The main problem with this view is a pragmatic one—the calculation of utility may not often produce the kind of disciplinary privacy waiver that Wallace seeks. Wallace is particularly concerned with providing a justification for the violation of privacy rights by epidemiologists. He notes that the driving forces behind social inquiry in epidemiological research are the prevention and control of disease—both widely accepted social goods. If these goals are to be obtained, Wallace maintains, certain conditions have to be met in epidemiological research. These conditions can be reconstructed from his discussion as follows:

1. Individually identifiable medical and vital information must be available to researchers.
2. The rerelease of identifiable health information should be permitted.
3. Most medical records should be retained.
4. Researchers should be granted immunity from the subpoena power of the state.

What is the likely response to the suggestion that people must give up some freedom and privacy for the general good of the public?

Note that this request issues from the public health community and not from the police or duly elected legislators. It is easy to imagine one sort of response coming from certain libertarian circles—peals of laughter, followed by "not one iota of freedom, not one infringement or invasion of privacy." In this view, no one can or should be compelled to help, aid, or abet the good of another, much less the *general* public—whoever that unwashed mass might be—at a cost of individual rights.

This claim obviously arises in response to Wallace's overtly utilitarian argument that more benefits will accrue to the public if a policy of leniency is adopted toward privacy concerns vis-à-vis the health benefits of vigorous epidemiological research. A large group of persons is unlikely to be moved by this logic. Their freedom and privacy are not barterable. No one, for any reason, can infringe on basic rights and feel morally justified about the infringement. For this crowd, a utilitarian argument for infringing on privacy is entirely wrongheaded. The concern with privacy, as I have tried to suggest, is rooted in basic human needs. Defenders of individual rights are not likely to be assuaged by appeals to greater public goods. In fact, it is just this impassioned defense of privacy that is behind some of the current pleas of social scientists against any form of regulation.[16] Why not argue that scientists qua scientists have basic rights to freedom and privacy, too, and let the libertarians hash out how the various and inevitable rights conflicts will be resolved? One does not have to resort to utilitarianism to justify one person's invasion of another's privacy.

Another objection to public-spirited arguments for allowing some transgression of privacy in the name of public health is based on the claim that epidemiology can provide the promised public goods even if all of Wallace's conditions for research are not fulfilled. One might argue, following Robert Boruch, that Wallace overstates the case for the need for identifiable health information. Clever statistical maneuvering may suffice to protect privacy while allowing the promotion of public health. Similarly, one might say that making medical records available to researchers is necessary, but that a law providing for a ten-year shield before release might permit roughly the same degree of prophylaxis and cure at a lower cost to privacy.

Wallace's plan for utilitarian exemptions for epidemiology can be challenged even on his own utilitarian grounds by questioning the accuracy of his moral calculations. He argues that disease prevention and health are worth the cost of some confidentiality and privacy. But his calculations are not complete. A few well-placed subpoenas may provide social utility far in excess of the cost of the privacy of a few individuals, the autonomy of a few epidemiologists, or a few days in jail for the overprotective public health officer. Or perhaps there are other, more efficient paths to health than the long route of epidemiological detective work. Imposing strict pollution controls and modifying personal behavior in light of present knowledge may go further toward prevention and cure at less cost to privacy than further epidemiological research. Once one's foot is firmly planted on the utilitarian path, it may be hard to avoid all that lies in this road.

Finally, one could critique the ordering of goods found in the utilitarian calculus. Health may be nice, but a maximization of liberty—or sexual pleasure, or the thrills of risk and danger—may be just as desirable, if not more so. This line of criticism is compelling when one realizes that determinations of public good will, in Wallace's view, be made by small groups of health professionals in institutional review boards (IRBs). Wallace's utilitarianism and concern for the public weal thus may not take him where he wants to go. Even on utilitarian grounds, it is far from clear that the cost–benefit calculation will come out the way he thinks it will. The IRBs upon which Wallace depends may require research practices drastically different from those anticipated by the author. I am willing to walk down the utilitarian primrose path quite a way in thinking about reasons for overriding privacy. But danger lurks down this road—there are libertarian muggers all about, and the road may lead elsewhere if epidemiology cannot really deliver on its promise of concrete improvements in public health.

Protecting privacy can be good for scientific health

I have few criticisms to offer about Boruch's views. While I make no claims to competency in assessing the adequacy of the various statistical stratagems and techniques Boruch describes, I applaud his attempts to protect privacy in the course of social research. His goal of maximization of research opportunity and minimization of privacy risks is laudable. Sometimes humanists rebel at the suggestion that technical solutions might be available for solving ethical worries. This intolerance is silly. If Boruch and his colleagues can devise clever modes of protecting privacy and confidentiality while retaining an acceptable basis for scientific inquiry, then hurrah for them!

One of the delicious ironies of Boruch's essay is that it illustrates how moral concerns have fueled imaginative advances in statistical research methodology. If moral worries were at least responsible for the evolution of some of the techniques Boruch reports, this would give the lie to the old chestnut that moralists are only concerned with restraining or prohibiting free scientific inquiry. Boruch provides an example of the way moral worries about science can lead to better, or at least richer, science. Perhaps by putting ethics courses into the graduate curriculum of schools of social science, we might further advance scientific methodology and technique! Unlike many of his colleagues in the social sciences, Boruch has responded to moral concern with cleverness and respect rather than whining and pleading.

This being so, let us consider some criticisms, quibbles, and whinings of my own. One might reasonably ask, "How widely applicable are the techniques and methods Boruch discusses?" I pose this question with a number of senses of applicability in mind. First, what is the realistic scope of techniques involving the aggregation of data or the avoidance of identifiers through linkage for all areas of social inquiry? What are participant observers to do about their privacy and confidentiality problems? Second, how widely known are these techniques? Has the profession devoted sufficient time in training and continuing education to make the utilization of these methods a reality? Third, how feasible are these methods? Boruch is at a large university where he is the director of a program explicitly devoted to methodology and evaluation research. The facilities and staff available at his institution may simply not be available to other persons at other places. What is the poor survey researcher at Green Acres State to do, given his or her limited resources?

Next, consider the possible moral problems posed by the availability of nonidentifiable statistical information that can be used or linked with other bits of data. Social research on identifiable social groups sometimes poses examples of what Herbert C. Kelman calls risks of social harms.[17] When people sign on for an experiment or agree to be in a survey, they have consented to these procedures and to nothing else. But when eager researchers begin to search for anonymous data with which to do other studies, different sorts of problems may appear. Minority groups, for example, may see their social or economic status as contingent upon various scientific findings in the social sciences. People who agree to participate in one sort of study (say reading ability) may be shocked to see anonymous data about them used in other studies (say busing) whose results may pose serious harms to them. Personal privacy is no guarantee of group privacy. The protection of an individual's privacy may not be sufficient for preventing harm to the individual if the individual is a member of an easily identifiable social group.

This sort of moral problem can elicit some odd complaints from scientists. Some charge that worries about the social implications of publicly available social knowledge are reflective of ideological biases or blind political commitments. But the issue involved is one of control over information. It seems morally suspicious not to inform potential research subjects that data they provide may be pooled, aggregated, linked, or reused (in anonymous form) by others. If this seems to be an excessive restriction on social science—medical researchers and natural scientists rarely worry about the social impact of their work—the excess nonetheless seems justified. This is an area where social science is different in a morally relevant way from other modes of scientific inquiry. Policies are made, money distributed, and interests met on the basis of social science findings. The keen interest of government in social science research is legitimate, but also legitimates special protections for those who might become subject to government programs based upon the work of social science researchers.

This point brings me to my last comment. Boruch sometimes writes as if the empirical demonstration of a lack of concern about privacy or disclosure on the part of subjects is evidence of, or constitutes a rationale for, a diminshed concern in social science about confidentiality and privacy. Politically speaking, he is probably right. Ethically speaking, he is probably wrong. Surveys in certain U.S. communities in the 1920s would have revealed a significant number of persons (perhaps a majority) who thought that blacks should sit at the rear of public buses. But the common citizen's opinion is far from binding on moral inquiry. It is of interest, but hardly definitive, whether research shows that most people do not consciously care about privacy. This, in itself, would not constitute proof that we ought to loosen regulatory policies governing privacy. Majority opinion does not, as a matter of course, override minority concerns in all moral matters. Protecting the rights of the uninformed, the uninterested, or the incompetent may be paternalistic, but it is still morally important. As I have tried to argue, social science itself reveals a fact which we ignore at our peril: privacy is a basic human need and, thus, a basic human right.

Notes

1. See E. L. Pattullo, "Modesty Is the Best Policy: The Federal Role in Social Research," in T. L. Beauchamp, R. R. Faden, R. J. Wallace, L. Waters, eds., *Ethical Issues in Social Science Research* (Baltimore: The Johns Hopkins University Press, 1982): 373–90; also Ithiel de Sola Pool, "The New Censorship of Social Research," *Public Interest* 57 (1980): 57–66.

2. Frederick Davis, "What Do We Mean by 'Right' to Privacy?" *South Dakota Law Review* (1959): 20.

3. Judith J. Thomson, "The Right to Privacy," *Philosophy and Public Affairs* 4 (1975): 331–32.

4. H. J. McCloskey, "Privacy and the Right to Privacy," *Philosophy* 55 (1980): 37.

5. Ibid., p. 35.

6. S. I. Benn, "Privacy, Freedom and Respect for Persons," *Nomos 13* (1971): 1–26.

7. Terry Pinkard, "Invasions of Privacy in Social Science Research," in T. L. Beauchamp, R. R. Faden, R. J. Wallace, L. Waters, eds., *Ethical Issues in Social Science Research,* p. 272.

8. Ibid., p. 264.

9. Ibid.

10. Erving Goffman, "The Mortification of Self," in R. Flacks, ed., *Conformity, Resistance and Self-Determination* (Boston: Little, Brown & Co., 1973), p. 178.

11. See also J. H. Reiman, "Privacy, Intimacy and Personhood," *Philosophy and Public Affairs* 6 (1976): 26–44.

12. J. M. Roberts and T. Gregor, "Privacy: A Cultural View," *Nomos 13* (1971): 209.

13. Margaret Mead, "Neighborhoods and Human Needs," *Ekistics 123* (1966): 124–26; K. Greenawalt, "Privacy," *Encyclopedia of Bioethics,* ed. W. Reich (New York: Free Press, 1978), vol. 3, pp. 1356–64.

14. J. Rodin, "Density, Perceived Choice, and Responses to Controllable and Uncontrollable Outcomes," *Journal of Experimental Social Psychology* 12 (1976): 564–78; D. Stokols, "Environmental Psychology," *Annual Review of Psychology* 29 (1978): 253–95; D. P. Barash, *Sociobiology and Behavior* (New York: Elsevier, 1977).

15. J. B. Calhoun, "Population Density and Social Pathology," *Scien-*

tific American 206 (1962): 139–48; P. B. Paulus et al., "Density Does Affect Task Performance," *Journal of Personality and Social Psychology* 34 (1976): 248–53; S. D. Webb, "Privacy and Psychosomatic Stress: An Empirical Analysis," *Social Behavior and Personality* 8 (1978): 227–33; L. M. Dean et al., "Spatial and Perceptual Components of Crowding: Effects on Health and Satisfaction," *Environment and Behavior* 7 (1975): 225–36; J. W. Chapman, "Personality and Privacy," *Nomos* 13 (1971): 236–55; and P. M. Insel and H. C. Lindgren, *Too Close for Comfort* (Englewood Cliffs, NJ.: Prentice-Hall, 1978).

16. Lauren H. Seiler and J. M. Murtha, "Federal Regulations of Social Research Using 'Human Subjects': A Critical Assessment," *American Sociologist* 15 (1980): 146–57.

17. Herbert C. Kelman, *A Time to Speak: On Human Values and Social Research* (San Francisco: Jossey-Bass, 1968). Kelman's later and more elaborate reflections on these problems are found earlier in T. L. Beauchamp, R. R. Faden, R. J. Wallace, L. Waters, eds., op. cit., chapter 2.

6.

Is there a duty to serve as a subject in biomedical research?

Most contemporary discussions of the ethics of human subjects research focus on the adequacies and inadequacies of informed consent in combination with peer review by institutional review boards (IRBs) for protecting subject welfare. Little has been written about the moral reasons that ought to lead someone to participate in research in the first place.

The strong impression conveyed by all the scholarly attention to consent and committee review is that the main problem in the area of human experimentation is the prevention of the practice of murder or mayhem against those poor unfortunates who fall into the maw of biomedicine. While it is true that one does occasionally encounter the grousings of a researcher or two concerning the possible negative effects ethical concerns have had on the pace of biomedical research, the major preoccupation of those writing about the ethics of research appears to be the protection of subjects who wind up in research settings solely as a consequence of infirmity, insanity, or inanity.

I do not mean to suggest that research subjects would be better off without the dual protections of informed consent and IRB review.

While there are many reasons for doubting the sufficiency of these mechanisms for protecting the interests of those who serve as subjects, there can be little doubt that the current regulatory provisions in the United States have done much to eliminate the more egregious examples of moral atrocity from the domain of human experimentation. Nevertheless, the frequent claims that the current system of regulations and protections is a success because it has prevented the recurrence of the flagrant moral abuses of the past is a telling comment about the nature of the moral concerns that originally fueled the establishment of these protections.

Moral scandals and their prevention

A review of the articles and books written during the 1960s reveals the importance of examples of subject abuse by biomedical researchers in setting the tone of ethical discussion. The Nuremberg trials of the physicians and scientists involved in barbarous medical experimentation during World War II played an especially central role in determining the direction of subsequent discussion concerning the ethics of experimentation. Nazi medical experiments exemplified what crass utilitarian concerns and total disregard of subjects' rights and welfare could lead to if followed faithfully and systematically.[1] The airing of research abuses in the landmark studies of Henry K. Beecher, Paul Freund, Jay Katz,[2] and many others drew public and academic attention to the serious problem of subject abuse in our own research settings.

The tradition of motivating concern about the ethics of human subject research by focusing on the serious harms that have befallen subjects continues today in both the anthologies and textbooks of bioethics.[3] It is easy to understand the current emphasis on the protections of informed consent and peer review in the light of the role played by moral scandals in focusing public attention on the ethics of human experimentation.

The desire to protect individuals against blatant abuses of medical authority and power led many scholars and physicians to emphasize the central role of autonomy in human experimentation. Lawyers, philosophers, and physicians agreed that voluntary choice, as evidenced by written informed consent, was the best protection against abuse in medical contexts.[4]

The desire to assure the welfare of research subjects eventually resulted in the complex array of state and federal regulations that now govern human subjects research in the United States. However, the provision of these safeguards does not in any way address the basic issues raised by the need to involve human beings in research: Who will serve and why?

What is known about subjects?

Unfortunately, very little is known about the composition of the pool of persons who actually participate in biomedical research in the United States. The available data shed little light on the way in which subject participation is obtained, and, more important, on the specifics of how the benefits and burdens of biomedical research are distributed in our population as a whole.

There is some reason for concern about the makeup of the subject pool. One of the few available studies of subject participation suggests that

> . . . studies involving greater therapeutic benefit for the subjects are more likely than those of lesser benefit to be done using subjects the majority of whom are private patients, whereas studies with minor or no benefit for subjects are most likely to involve mostly ward or clinic patients.[5]

While it is difficult to obtain hard data on the socioeconomic background of those currently participating in research there is at least some reason for concern that the poor and disadvantaged bear a disproportionate share of the research burden.

A number of authors have also noted that the underrepresentation of females of reproductive age in research trials may have a deleterious effect upon the health and welfare of the members of this group. Similar concerns have been voiced about the relative absence of elderly subjects, children, and even fetuses in research trials of new drugs and procedures.[6]

There is little reason to doubt that the brunt of contemporary research in biomedicine is borne by those who are ill, institutionalized, or both. The benefits enjoyed by the public as a whole of improved medical care, better drugs, and increasingly powerful technological therapies have been acquired at a cost that has not been shared equitably among all the members of our society.

If it is true that some individuals or groups never or rarely participate in medical research, and if many Americans behave as "free riders" when it comes to obtaining the benefits of medical research, then discussions of the ethics of research should not be limited to considerations of the adequacy of current protections of subject safety and welfare. While it is morally laudable that our society has instituted these protections, their moral value is greatly diminished if some groups within our society are far more likely to need to avail themselves of them than are others.

Bad science and skewed subject pools

Justice is not the only reason that compels attention to this question. Important methodological reasons also point toward the need for the broadest possible public participation in biomedical experimentation.

The biases introduced into research findings by the selective use of volunteers or nonrandomized subjects are poorly understood but much discussed by those designing research protocols. A number of recent studies have shown that unblinded randomization and non-random assignment can have a deleterious impact on the adequacy of controlled clinical trials.[7] If double-blind randomization is the method of choice in clinical trials, then it is surely of the utmost importance that such trials draw their subjects from a statistically representative sample of the general population. A system that relies primarily on the recruitment of subjects from among those who are sick, institutionalized in one way or another, or who volunteer, cannot rest easy about the reliability and soundness of its research conclusions.

It is not even clear that participation in most blinded randomized clinical trials is ethical. There are few trials where the researcher can believe with certainty that there is no difference among the treatment arms of the trial. In such cases it may not be ethical for the physician to solicit volunteers if there is reason to think that one form of treatment might be preferable to another.[8] Yet the need to conduct randomized clinical trials even on widely disseminated and accepted procedures in medicine is well known. In such cases informed consent does not appear to be consistent with the requirements of therapeutic ethics since it is often difficult to ethically justify entering patients randomly in one arm of a clinical trial knowing that one treatment appears preferable to another but with less certainty than is required to satisfy the traditional canons of statistical significance.[9]

Can a duty to be a subject be generated?

There have been a few attempts in the past decade to locate a moral basis for participation in biomedical research. The arguments for participation have taken two forms: (1) There is an obligation to participate, which is incurred because the benefits of biomedical research are available to all; and (2) there is a tacit "cross-generational" social contract that compels each person to participate.

Physicians such as Walsh McDermott, Louis Lasagna, and Leon Eisenberg have argued eloquently the view that participation is justified by the fact that the results of biomedical research are public goods. None argues that the state has a right to force participation in research in the name of the social good. Rather, they argue that health, safety, and knowledge constitute public goods—goods that accrue not to a majority of the members of a society, but to all members of society.[10] The duty to participate in research, in this view, derives from the fact that the production of public goods requires public participation.

The counterarguments have been persuasively made by, among others, Hans Jonas and Charles Fried.[11] These authors note that (1) it is not self-evident that health, safety, and knowledge are public goods, and (2) the moral pull exerted by the desire to have public goods is counterbalanced by the far more powerful moral force of respect for individual autonomy.

Certainly in our society it would be difficult to argue that the benefits of biomedical research are equally available or even desired by all citizens. Nor is it evident that anyone need feel an obligation to produce any and every public good no matter how valuable that good might be.

But even if one were to grant that health and safety were public goods, it is not clear what the relationship is between biomedical research and these goods. As Jonas correctly notes, research aims at improving or advancing health and knowledge and, while one might be obligated to engage in activities that maintain public goods, it is hard to see why such an obligation would extend to the improvement or advancement of such goods.

The other means of generating a duty to participate in research is by positing some version of a "social contract."[12] Since those now living have benefited from the participation of previous generations in biomedical research, we owe our own participation in research to future members of society, born and unborn, as a way of discharging this debt. By accepting the benefits of scientific and medical knowledge in the form of better therapy, diet, lifestyle, and so on, we affirm, obliquely but overtly, our duty to those individuals whose past sacrifices made these benefits possible. We incur a powerful moral obligation of reciprocity to bear additional burdens so that future generations may reap similar benefits.

But it is not at all clear that those persons who participated in research in the past did so believing that they were creating a debt that had to be discharged by those who reaped the benefits of their participation. Indeed, such a view diminishes the sacrifice of previous generations of research subjects by stripping their actions of any suggestion of altruism.

Many of those who participated in dangerous and deadly experiments in the past did so out of a desire to benefit humankind. It is simply a conceptual mistake to think that a duty to reciprocate is the obligatory response that must be made to a gift that was freely given—at most, we are obliged to be grateful for a gift.[13]

It would, of course, be naive to think that those who participated in biomedical research in the past all did so out of pure altruism. Many subjects were compensated for their participation; some others were coerced or tricked into participating. However, it is hard to see how any obligation is generated among the existing members of a society who have obtained the benefits of research produced as a result of either compensation or duplicity.

Furthermore, it is not clear that a contract exists unless someone has directly benefited from the actions of those involved in previous forms of biomedical research. The only persons with a contractual claim on the living would be the members of the past generations who gave of themselves with the thought that such giving had to be reciprocal. Unless these claims are cashed in, it seems mistaken to speak in a general way about abstract duties to society or to past generations and simply wrong to generate duties to participate in research on the basis of hypothetical claims by future generations.

The counterarguments against a duty to serve as a subject in biomedical research seem to have been so persuasive as to have made the topic otiose. While there have been discussions in recent years of the moral acceptability of involving prisoners, children, retarded people, and other classes of so-called "vulnerable" subjects in research, these discussions have hinged almost exclusively upon the reliability of the informed consent mechanism for protecting these classes of persons from abuse rather than over the issue of an individual's duty to serve in research.[14] However, if inequities exist in the ways in which the benefits of human subjects research in the biomedical sciences are allocated, and if some research requires involvement that cannot be justified on the grounds of immediate personal benefit, then other grounds should be sought in support of a duty to participate in research.

One way of generating a moral duty to participate in biomedical research is to acknowledge that the public status of the goods or benefits of research—knowledge, health, and safety—is questionable, but another approach is to insist that those individuals who actually accept the benefits of such research incur certain obligations, central among them a duty to participate in research. H. L. A. Hart describes such obligations as arising

> . . . when a number of persons conduct any joint enterprise according to rules and restrict their liberty, those who have submitted to these restrictions when required have a right to similar submission from those who have benefitted by their submission.[15]

John Rawls[16] has coined the term "fair play" to describe this type of obligation. He argues that those who benefit from participation in various cooperative social schemes—for example, the creation of a food co-op, a block patrol, or even a political state—have obligations to each other when called upon to bear the risks or burdens that involvement in cooperative endeavors often entails. The members of a cooperative group can legitimately expect each group member to accept the burdens and risks of participation in such enterprises if the members have profited from the activities of the group. The members of cooperative enterprises are on sound moral footing in chastising and excluding any "free riders" that are discovered taking benefits but shirking responsibilities.

The notion of fair play, which properly governs the actions and ethical evaluations of the members of voluntary associations and organizations, requires that a distinction be drawn between those who derive benefits from various social enterprises as knowing participants, and those who simply have such benefits forced upon them without their consent. For example, Robert Nozick[17] has persuasively argued that no obligations can be said to be incurred by persons who inadvertently or unavoidably derive benefits from social schemes and cooperative endeavors that they neither approve of nor consent to.

Nozick argues that even if I am lucky enough to benefit from the security afforded me by the existence of a block patrol in my neighborhood, I incur no obligation to pay for or serve in such a patrol merely because I happen to live in the locale where this group is active. I incur no obligations or duties to the members of social groups merely because they choose to make me the beneficiary of their group largesse. Nozick maintains that the principle of fair play is binding only upon those who explicitly consent to participate in cooperative enterprises and social schemes.

This principle of fair play can, however, be restricted in a way that avoid the kinds of difficulties Nozick raises. No doubt it is true that innocent beneficiaries of group activities incur no obligations toward other group members. But one need not give explicit consent to be recognized as a full-fledged participant in a group activity or enterprise.

If someone is constantly, continuously, and knowingly receiving benefits as a result of some cooperative social activity and if such a person also makes no effort to avoid receiving such benefits when it is possible to do so with little inconvenience, then it seems reasonable to argue that this person has tacitly consented to membership in the group's activities.[18] If, for example, I set up a receiving dish on top of my house in order to obtain the broadcasts from my neighborhood cooperative television satellite, it will hardly suffice as a reason not to pay the required monthly charge for me to argue that I am an innocent and unwilling beneficiary of the group's largesse. My conscious and purposeful efforts to get the benefits of television broadcasts would seem to obligate me to pay the fees that the group has agreed to levy upon all of its members even if I never actually consent to membership in the cooperative. Those who knowingly seek out and obtain benefits from social enterprises appear to bear a general obligation to share in the costs, if any, of creating these benefits.[19]

The teaching hospital as a social cooperative

One way of viewing the institutions and organizations of biomedical science is as social cooperatives—often vast ones, but, nonetheless, enterprises that depend upon the voluntary cooperative efforts of many individuals to produce specified benefits. They also generate burdens and costs that have to be shared according to some fair scheme. Consider the example of a relatively small biomedical cooperative—the teaching hospital.

Physicians often state that patients who receive care in such institutions have an obligation to serve as subjects for teaching and demonstration purposes. If patients do fully understand the nature of the institution, I believe that these physicians are correct.

Those who freely choose to receive care in the context of a teaching hospital do incur an obligation to serve as the subjects in various teaching activities. The teaching hospital is one form of a scientific social cooperative—physicians, scientists, and patients organize themselves into a social unit to promote certain ends and to obtain certain benefits. Those who receive the benefits of such a scheme can legitimately be said to incur certain duties as a result. Fair play requires that those who *knowingly* and *willingly* seek out and accept the benefits of better care, closer attention, and the higher levels of medical skill that are often available in a teaching hospital incur a general obligation to serve as the subjects of medical teaching.

Of course the distribution of the burden of service as a teaching subject must be fair and equitable. But as long as this is so, those who willingly accept care in such settings fall under the requirements of fair play that govern all forms of voluntary social cooperation.

Of course, it should be quickly added that a sense of fair play among the participants in this kind of hospital setting requires that some burdens not be assignable. For example, no one is obligated to serve as an illustration of the effects of lethal drugs on human beings. Because those who knowingly receive the benefits of care in a teaching hospital incur a duty to serve does not mean that such a duty abrogates their other rights, including the basic rights not to be seriously harmed or killed.

Most of those who work in teaching hospitals do not believe that they have the right to demand participation in teaching activities whenever they see fit. Despite their belief that patients have a duty to make themselves available for teaching purposes, physicians will often exempt certain patients for both physical and psychological reasons from such activities. Patient consent is usually obtained, as it should be, with respect to both the specific teaching activity and the convenience of the patient. Those who choose to receive their care in teaching hospitals incur a duty that can be discharged in a manner most consistent with their wishes and their convenience as long as, at some point, the duty is discharged.

The obligation to serve as a subject

Is it not the case that those who benefit from or receive care in hospitals and health-care facilities that openly identify themselves as research institutions incur an analogous duty to participate in research? Fair play seems to require that those who reap the benefits of greater therapeutic knowledge and skill that are derived from biomedical research should be called upon to bear the burdens and costs of pursuing such activities. There is no more reason for tolerating free riders in research contexts than there would be in any other voluntary social cooperative. As long as all patients freely and voluntarily choose to receive care in research settings, and as long as the burdens of being a subject are fairly allocated among all who benefit, a general obligation to be a subject appears to exist.

There are important restrictions on those who demand the discharge of this duty. They must (1) openly disclose the nature of the institution; (2) recruit among all those who are sufficiently competent to have chosen to receive care in a research context; (3) not compel participation in studies that pose significant risks to health or well-being; (4) obtain consent from all individuals who are asked to participate, since the determination of significant risk requires the involvement of each individual; (5) assure that all subjects have a fair chance of obtaining the benefits derived from research; and (6) ensure that all potential subjects have freely chosen to receive the benefits of better health care.

If it is accurate to say that biomedical research and its constitutive hospitals, organizations, and practitioners constitute voluntary social cooperatives, then a number of interesting ethical consequences can be drawn. First, biomedical scientists must recognize the distinctive nature of their enterprise and fully inform those persons who have an interest in reaping its benefits about the choices they have and the burdens and costs they are likely to incur. Second, as members of such social cooperatives, biomedical scientists must also be considered eligible for bearing the costs and reaping the benefits of the enterprise—the duty to serve in research is one that is owed both by patients and researchers. Finally, the existence of duties generated by the principle of fair play should not abrogate the obligations of researchers to respect the basic rights of those who choose to be in such settings.

A duty to participate in research does not void the rights of subjects to choose and consent to specific research protocols. Nor does the existence of a duty to serve as a research subject diminish in any way the need for prior peer review of research protocols. Just as the proposition that a fetus has a right to life does not settle the question of what to do when rights conflict, so also the demonstration of an obligation to serve as a research subject does not settle the question of how conflicting obligations in this context are to be resolved. But the fact that conflicts between subjects' duties and rights can arise does not weaken the case for positing a duty to discharge the burdens incurred by freely accepting the benefits of a particular social activity.

There is a strong case for arguing that biomedical research constitutes a form of voluntary social cooperation. The hospitals and institutions in which research usually occurs are quite analogous to other forms of social cooperation where the obligations generated by fair play demand equal participation in sharing the benefits and burdens of voluntary social activity. Any competent person who voluntarily seeks out and takes the benefits of care resulting from biomedical research can legitimately be said to be a consenting participant in the enterprise and, thus, the bearer of a duty to share in the costs of producing the desired goods.

Possible objections to the argument

There are a number of possible objections to this claim. It is not always clear that those who benefit from biomedical research voluntarily choose to do so. Nor is it clear exactly what level of participation in research will suffice to discharge the general obligation.

Some people may have no choice about whether they will or will not avail themselves of the services of any given biomedical institution or practitioner. Since, as Nozick and other critics of the concept of fair play have been at some pains to point out, those who receive the benefits of cooperative social activity without choosing to do so incur no obligations as a result of being benefited, such people are not under any general obligation to serve as subjects.

It is sometimes difficult to ascertain whether those who utilize research hospitals or receive care from physicians who are engaged in biomedical research knowingly choose to do so. Some patients come to research institutions not by choice but simply because no other facilities are available to care for them. Others become sick suddenly and have little say in who will treat them or in what setting. People who receive care in such circumstances do not appear to be under any general obligation to serve as subjects in biomedical research since they cannot be said to have either had or made a choice about receiving the benefits of such research.

But these situations are relatively rare. For the most part those who seek health care consciously and often conscientiously seek out the "best" or "most advanced" hospitals and clinics. In fact most consumers of health care attempt to locate those practitioners who are the most up-to-date and those institutions with the most up-to-date equipment and facilities. This sort of medical consumer, surely the majority of those receiving medical care in this country, can hardly be described either as having no choice or as not intending to choose the benefits of biomedical research in seeking care when they receive care in institutions that have research as one of their primary goals.

Implications of the argument

If it is true that those who knowingly and consciously seek out the benefits of care in research institutions incur, as a consequence of being bound by the principle of fair play, a general obligation to participate in biomedical research, then there are strong moral arguments against complacency about the composition of the current research subject pool at many institutions. If it is true that the sick, the poor, or the young are bearing a large portion of the burden of biomedical research, then measures should be taken by IRBs and researchers to redress these imbalances by making every effort to include as subjects all of those who freely choose to receive the benefits of research.[20]

Admittedly, there are many persons, both healthy and ill, who do not seek care from physicians or institutions that avowedly identify themselves as committed to biomedical research. Nonetheless, it is surely true that many hospitals, nursing homes, and private physicians make regular use of the knowledge that is gained as a result of biomedical research. Does the general obligation to participate in research extend to these persons?

Furthermore, many patients in research institutions must pay for their care. If a general obligation to participate in research can be said to exist, what behaviors suffice to meet or discharge such an obligation—payment, participation as a subject in a controlled clinical trial of a new drug, having one's blood drawn for tests?

If cash payments are to be allowed as a method for discharging the general obligation to serve as a subject in research contexts, then surely policies about this option must be discussed and debated by all the members of the research enterprise—subjects as well as researchers. And if the scope of the general obligation to participate in research is to extend to all persons who receive any sort of health care, then patients will have to be much more informed about the various costs and burdens of having health care available.

These are provocative and important issues but they should not be allowed to distract the reader's attention from the main point of this article: in identified research settings, the knowing beneficiaries of care incur a general obligation to participate in research. How, when, and in what manner this obligation ought to be discharged are all subjects for future debate and deliberation. But, if my arguments are valid, they are questions that those who design or participate in research ignore at their own moral peril.

Notes

1. Alexander, Leo. "Medical science under dictatorship," *NEJM*, 241: 39–47, 1949.

2. Beecher, H.K., "Ethics and clinical research," *NEJM*, 274: 1354–60, 1966; Freund, P.A., ed., *Experimentation with Human Subjects*, New York: George Braziller, 1970; Katz, J. *Experimentation with Human Beings*. New York: Russell Sage, 1972.

3. See for example the selections in chapter three of Gorovitz, S., et al., eds., *Moral Problems in Medicine*. 2nd ed. Englewood Cliffs, N.J.: Prentice Hall, 1983.

4. Ramsey, P. *The Patient as Person*, New Haven: Yale University Press, 1970; Rutstein, D.D., "The ethical design of human experiments," *Daedalus*, 98; 523–41, Spring, 1969; and Jonas, H., "Philosophical reflections on experimenting with human subjects," *Daedalus*, 98: 219–47, Spring, 1969.

5. Barber, B., et al., *Research on Human Subjects*. New York: Russell Sage Foundation, 1973, p. 55.

6. See the papers by Lawton, M.P., and Ostfeld, A.M., in "Do elderly research subjects need special protection?" *IRB: A Review of Human Subjects Research* 2: 5–9, October, 1980.

7. Schafer, A., "The ethics of the randomized clinical trial," *NEJM*, 307: 719–24, 1982.

8. Taylor, K. et al., "Physicians' reasons for not entering eligible patients in a randomized clinical trial of surgery for breast cancer," *NEJM*, 310; 1363–1367, 1984.

9. Marquis, D., "Leaving therapy to chance," *Hastings Center Report*, 13; 40–77, 1983, and Angell, M., "Patients' preferences in randomized clinical trials," *NEJM*, 310: 1385–1388, 1984.

10. See, for example, McDermott, W., Opening comments to colloquium: The changing mores of biomedical research, *Annals of Internal Medicine*, 67: 39–42, 1967.

11. See Jonas, op. cit., note 4; Fried, C., *Medical Experimentation*, New York: Elsevier, 1974; and Donagan, A., "Informed consent in therapy and experimentation," *Journal of Medicine and Philosophy*, 2; 310–27, 1977.

12. See Jonas, op. cit., note 4.

13. Simmons, A. John, *Moral Principles and Political Obligations*. Princeton: Princeton University Press, 1979.

14. One interesting exception is McCormick, R., "Proxy consent in the experimental situation," *Perspectives in Biology and Medicine*, 18: 2–20,

1974, which attempts to justify the participation of children in research by arguing that parents have an obligation to cultivate virtue in their offspring.

15. Hart, H.L.A., "Are there any natural rights?," *Philosophical Review,* 64, 1955; reprinted in Melden, A., ed., *Human Rights.* Belmont, CA: Wadsworth, 1977, p. 70.

16. Rawls, J., *A Theory of Justice.* Cambridge: Harvard University Press, 1971.

17. Nozick, R., *Anarchy, State and Utopia.* New York: Basic Books, 1974, pp. 90–97.

18. Arneson, R., "The principle of fairness and freerider problems," *Ethics,* 92: 616–33, 1982.

19. A useful summary of other efforts to generate an obligation to participate in biomedical research is provided in Levine, R.J., *Ethics and the Regulation of Clinical Research.* Baltimore: Urban and Schwarzenberg, 1981, pp. 85–87.

20. This would mean that IRBs ought to take far more seriously than they often do the requirements of 45 CFR 46.111a (3) which charges IRBs with ensuring that the "selection of subjects is equitable."

Part III

Advances in reproduction
and genetics

7.

New technologies in reproduction— new ethical problems

Framing the issues: standard IVF in the United States

To discuss the ethical problems raised by the development and dissemination of new technologies for assisting reproduction in the space of a chapter, I will have to somewhat arbitrarily narrow the scope of my discussion. Rather than addressing the broad spectrum of techniques that have evolved to assist those who find themselves to be infertile, my comments will be directed solely to *in vitro* fertilization (IVF). Indeed, nearly all of my examples will be drawn from what I have elsewhere termed "standard" IVF[1] and what others have called "simple" IVF.[2]

Standard IVF refers to those situations in which the woman who contributes the egg to be fertilized *in vitro* is also the woman who will bear any conceptus that may result and who fully expects to act as the social parent to any child who is born. In standard IVF, the man who contributes the sperm to be used in fertilization is either married to or has maintained a long-standing, stable relationship with this same woman. He too fully expects to assume parental responsibilities toward any child who may be born as a result of the use of the technique.

There are obvious and indeed notorious variations from standard IVF which raise a host of important ethical problems, including the acceptability of using either paid or voluntary surrogates, the selection of sperm donors and gestational mothers for eugenic purposes (as is done at the so-called "Nobel Prize" sperm bank in California), and the utilization of IVF techniques by homosexuals or single parents. These non-standard forms of IVF raise so many fascinating issues, however, that there is a danger of losing sight both of the legacy of earlier debates about IVF upon contemporary ethical discussions and of the continuing need to come to terms with the ethical issues raised by even the most mundane form of IVF.

The first phase of the ethical debate: do no harm

Philosophers, theologians, physicians, and lawyers on both sides of the Atlantic have been debating the morality of IVF for decades. With the scientific reports of Menkin and Rock in the late 1940s of the fertilization of human eggs *in vitro* and the suggestion by Shettles in 1955 that IVF might be applied in the treatment of infertile women,[3] a heated debate arose in the United States—and, to a lesser extent, in the United Kingdom—about the morality of undertaking IVF in human beings with the intent of creating a baby.

At the heart of this debate was the issue of whether or not IVF techniques could be used without causing harm to any infants that might be born. Those involved in extending IVF techniques from animals to humans worried well into the late 1960s and early 1970s that "the normality of embryonic development and the efficiency of embryo transfer cannot yet be assessed."[4]

Critics of IVF such as Paul Ramsey and Leon Kass argued that if there were risks associated with IVF, then IVF "constituted unethical medical experimentation on possible future human beings" and as such ought be ". . . subject to absolute moral prohibition."[5] The possibility of doing irreparable damage to a potential child, a child incapable of giving consent to serving as an experimental subject, was held by such critics to be a sufficient moral basis for prohibiting all forms of IVF involving human gametes.

Persuasive arguments have been made against the view that any and all forms of risky research upon nonconsenting subjects are morally illicit.[6] But, whether the rebuttals of the prohibition against research on children and other subjects incapable of consent are persuasive or not, the fact remains that objections to the use of IVF in human beings were highly influential throughout the late 1950s and 1960s.

Phase two of the debate: nature knows best

The birth of Louise Brown in 1978 had an enormous impact on ethical debate concerning the use of IVF. Earlier ethical arguments presumed that the use of IVF to treat infertile women was clearly experimental. While one might condemn the decision to try IVF, the birth of Louise Brown, and a few thousand more like her in Australia, the United States, the United Kingdom, and other Western European countries, ended all arguments about the safety and, therefore, the experimental nature of IVF.

For the most part, recent (meaning after Louise Brown) ethical and legal debates concerning reproduction by means of IVF have been concerned with examining the morality of procreation and conception outside the surroundings normally associated with heterosexual intercourse. The March 1987 Vatican pronouncement on assisted reproduction spends little time expressing concerns about the experimental nature of IVF. Instead, the unnaturalness of separating sexual intercourse and procreation, and the adverse impact of IVF-based techniques on the nuclear family are the basis for the condemnation of IVF as morally illicit.

Similar, albeit secularly grounded, criticisms are in evidence in the more recent ruminations of Leon Kass. He notes in the course of a discussion of the ethics of ectogenesis that it is "incompatible with the kind of respect owed to its [the embryo's] humanity that is grounded in the bonds of lineage and the nature of parenthood."[7]

The problem with ethical arguments that locate the moral illicitness of IVF in the unnaturalness of the procedure is that they are impossible to take seriously on anything other than religious grounds without rejecting most elements of modern obstetrics. No evidence exists that the use of glass rather than protein as the medium to facilitate conception has any adverse impact on either the children who have been conceived in this way or their parents. And there is no reason to expect that it would any more than the discovery that one's entry into the world was assisted by forceps or a caesarean section.

Natural origins are of ethical interest only to the extent to which societies attach stigma or opprobrium to other methods of procreation. If society views medically assisted conception as morally irrelevant to the dignity and worth of human beings in the same way that no opprobium is attached to being born in a hospital rather than a home, there is no reason to presume that there is anything morally illicit about extracorporeal fertilization.

The transformation of IVF from experimentation to therapy

It is extremely interesting to note that the appearance of Louise Brown and many hundreds of other healthy infants was seized upon by proponents of the use of IVF to remove the labels of experimentation and research. The desire of the medical community to quickly shed the label of experimentation has interesting analogues in other areas of moral dispute concerning medical interventions within the American context.

Those involved in the first artificial heart implant and the first xenograft of a heart to an infant were quick to declare their efforts therapeutic and non-experimental.[8] The therapeutic status of these interventions was seen as established by the demonstration of the mere feasibility of the undertaking.

There are many reasons why those involved in the development of new medical interventions wish to dispose of the label "experimental" as soon as they can. "Experimental" carries with it connotations of the unknown, the risky, and the especially dangerous, dimensions of medical innovation which make it harder to recruit willing participants. Such connotations are unfortunate and unfair, since there are many experiments which are relatively safe and risk free, and many therapies which are precisely the opposite.

Another reason for the desire to transmute experiments into

therapies instantaneously involves the psychological needs of those who are sick and of those who care for them. For those seeking to offer hope to those who are desperately ill or beset by a severe disability, therapy seems far more conducive to optimism than does experiment.[9] Those involved in the development of new drugs to treat terminal cancers and AIDS find it much easier to offer comfort and solace to the dying under the banner of therapy than research.

Therapy also serves to establish a kind of priority of discovery for a research team which is not associated with the language of research. If the first artificial heart implant is still experimental, or the first baby born as a result of IVF represents the outcome of research, then it will fall to others to lay claim to the first truly "successful" application of a new technology or technique. Priority is no small matter in a scientific world of fierce competition for grants, fame, and recognition for one's institution and even country.

The pervasiveness of competition in the world of medical research even extends into the realm of medical ethics. Western European ethicists have been known to complain about the imperious attitude American ethicists display in commenting on developments at the frontiers of medical research. The source of hubris appears to be nothing more than the fact that American researchers have been involved in many such pioneering developments.

IVF is, of course, an exception to American medical hegemony over medical innovation. As a result British and Australian ethicists can be quite insistent about their authority regarding the ethics of IVF. When the influence of competition can be seen even in the attitudes expressed by those interested in the ethical implications of medical developments, there can be little doubt that the desire to be first plays a powerful role in decisions to drop the language of experimentation in favor of the language of therapy.

Fiscal motivations are especially important in understanding the desire to shed the label of research. In the American context, disposing of the label of experimentation allows researchers and their subjects to seek access to reimbursement for their undertakings. Until liver transplants were declared therapies by various federal agencies there was no way for American hospitals or recipients to pay for them except through personal income insofar as that could be augmented through personal or family begging through media appeals, bake sales, and car washes.

Currently in the United States, most third-party payors, public and private, will not cover the costs of IVF. This has led to an increased stridency in the frequency and solemnity with which the label "therapy" is brought to bear in descriptions of IVF at federal and state legislative hearings.

Most importantly, from the point of view of IVF, the association between IVF and experimentation gave critics of the intervention their strongest argument. It is a compelling point to argue that experimentation ought to be permitted only on those capable of understanding and consenting to it. Children, therefore, and certainly embryos, so the argument went, cannot legitimately serve as research subjects in any form of human experimentation. The ethical argument based on viewing IVF as research seemed ironclad—as long as the possibility of harm existed, no one could ethically undertake IVF with human gametes in order to ascertain whether harm really would befall the embryo.

Once Louise Brown appeared, was photographed, hoisted about and otherwise exhibited as a paragon of pediatric normality, the thrust of the ethical worry about IVF could be deflected by putting to rest the sticky matter of the acceptability of undertaking risky research on the unconsenting. Therapy upon the unconsenting seems far less morally vexing.

Technology or technique?

The shift away from discussion of IVF under the rubric of research to that of therapy is not the only major shift to characterize ethical discussions of IVF in the United States and the United Kingdom since the 1950s. Contemporary ethical analyses of IVF are usually conducted under the aegis of labels such as the "new reproductive technologies" or "test tube" babies. This has the effect of grouping IVF with such high-falutin and somewhat awe-inspiring medical technologies as artificial hearts, organ transplants, and neonatal intensive units.

But, the reality of the matter is that there is not a great deal of complicated technology involved in attempts to assist reproduction using standard IVF techniques. Whatever complexities there are have far more to do with scientific ignorance of the natural processes of ovulation, fertilization, development, and implantation, than anything having to do with especially complex gadgets, machines, or gizmos.

Indeed, calling IVF a technology is misleading precisely because much of what goes on under this rubric is actually more a matter of technique than technology. Some centers are very good at getting babies via IVF while others are not.[10] I doubt that many of these centers would attribute such differences to differences in their technologies. Rather there is something about the techniques employed in one center that leads to success more often than do those employed at others.

It is interesting to note that many centers have had no success in producing babies whereas others have enjoyed quite a bit of success. Why these differences exist is not well understood. However, the language of technology may serve to deflect attention away from another pertinent fact about standard IVF. Standard IVF in both the United States and the United Kingdom, despite all the babies produced by this technique, does not work very well.

The efficacy of IVF

It is often observed that more than 2,000 babies were born in England alone in the first ten years after the appearance of Louise Brown in 1978. Optimism and declarations of success attend many public and even private scientific discussions of IVF. Moreover, the proliferation of American clinics and hospitals offering standard IVF since 1980, when the Norfolk Clinic first opened its doors, has been rapid enough to persuade even a casual observer that IVF is a technique that works regardless of the moral reservations some may feel about it.

But these facts do not convey the whole story with respect to IVF. Even if one looks to the most charitable presentations of the success rates associated with standard IVF, the figures are not impressive. For example, the Ethics Committee of the American Fertility Society (1986) states that:

> Success rates with human IVF techniques have steadily improved since the first birth in 1978. Currently, the success rates vary but have been reported to be up to 25% per cycle of treatment.

The twenty-five percent figure in and of itself might seem impressive, since it can be interpreted as showing that all persons who use IVF techniques can expect to have a baby at the end of four attempts.

But matters are hardly that simple or that efficient. Success rates in IVF are often measured not in terms of babies but in terms of successful implantations following upon the reinsertion of an embryo back into the mother. But few couples want to undergo the hormonal treatments and psychosocial rigors of IVF simply to produce an implantation or even a longer pregnancy. Babies are and must be the final standard by which the technique is assessed.

It might be objected that it is not kosher to criticize IVF on the grounds that even at the most experienced centers it succeeds in producing babies only ten to fifteen percent of the time.[11] After all, engaging in reproduction in the old fashion way results in babies only about ten to fifteen percent of the time. IVF specialists are doing at least as well as the birds and the bees in producing future generations of humankind. But such an argument misses crucial differences between having babies as a result of sexual intercourse and having them whipped up in a dish.

The costs of IVF are not small. Per cycle charges in American fertility clinics are usually around $5,000. Nor is the process of egg retrieval, drug treatments, and intensive monitoring by various specialists a matter of indifference to the couples who receive IVF.[12] Most importantly, expressions of satisfaction with a twenty-five percent implantation rate obscure the fact that relatively little is known yet about the techniques involved in standard IVF.

There are still basic components of IVF techniques which are not at all well understood. The proper components of the media in which sperm and egg are joined, the dosage levels for various hormones to produce superovulation, the best temperatures and environmental circumstances for storing and reimplanting embryos, which embryos are most likely to implant, and many other basic questions are still shrouded in a fair degree of mystery. Not only are the rates of success of standard IVF low, but the understanding of why this is so is quite high. At best, even standard IVF is still more empirical than scientific. There is more trial and error than systematic inquiry present in the manner in which IVF is carried out.

It might also be argued that since there are no generally accepted standards of the level of efficacy that demarcates experiment from therapy, it is not fair to pick on IVF because it is poorly understood and has a relatively low rate of success. After all, the "therapies" used to treat lung cancer or AIDS have even lower rates of efficacy.

But, surely more is involved in identifying medical interventions as research than safety or risk. Outcome would seem to matter. If one takes the rule of thumb applied by American insurance agencies, then a fifty percent success record of achievement over a five year span based on the performance of all providers seems reasonable. Even on a generous view of efficacy, success rates of twenty or twenty-five percent at the most experienced centers would not seem to be sufficient warrant, in itself, for bestowing the label of therapy on IVF.

Furthermore, the moral case for undertaking more research is undercut by the elevation of IVF to the status of a therapy on the basis of a ten to twenty percent success rate. Calling IVF therapy fuels false hope on the part of those beset by infertility.

The failure to view IVF as experimental or at least highly innovative on the grounds of poor efficacy, leads many in the field to a regrettable indifference toward the formulation of adequate and comprehensive international data bases, the tolerance of less than high quality performance by some practitioners and clinics, and the inability to engage the public in a rational inquiry into the question of whether the time has yet arrived for public funds to be allocated for reimbursing the costs of IVF. In the short run, the talk of therapy may have served to deflect moral criticism of early IVF programs. In the long run, it deflects public policy away from the hard choices that need to be addressed in order to refine and perfect the technique.

Reproductive rights and liberties

One possible explanation for the relative indifference that most commentators display to the question of where standard IVF ought be placed on the experiment/therapy continuum is to be found in the widely expressed view that such questions are irrelevant, since the government has no proper business attempting to restrict access to IVF, whatever its scientific status.[13] Some commentators believe that all human beings enjoy an unrestricted and fundamental right to procreative liberty. They find support for such a claim in such documents as the United States Constitution, the Universal Declaration of Human Rights of the United Nations, and declarations concerning human rights issued by various other national and international organizations. For example, the United Nations Declaration holds that every person "of full age" has the right "to marry and found a family."[14]

American courts have been concerned to protect procreation from outside interference by third parties. The Supreme Court held in the Eisenstadt vs. Baird case that

> if the right of privacy means anything, it is the right of the individual, married or single, to be free of unwarranted governmental intrusion into matters so fundamentally affecting a person as the decision whether to bear or beget a child (405 US 438, 453 [1972]).

The report of the Ethics Committee of the American Fertility Society, "Ethical Considerations of the New Reproductive Technologies" (1986), cites this case in arguing that the right of privacy vis-à-vis reproduction implies that IVF and related methods for assisting reproduction ". . . may not risk sufficient tangible harm to the parties or the offspring to warrant state interference with the constitutional right to procreate."[15] The report concludes that:

> Intangible religious, moral or societal concerns about the nature of reproduction, family, the reproductive roles of women, and the power of science would not ordinarily justify interference with procreative liberty. . . . Moral, religious, or symbolic concerns that do not have direct, tangible effects on others are not sufficient constitutional grounds for interfering with fundamental rights of persons. . . .[16]

Such arguments are not, however, persuasive if it is granted that the state of knowledge and efficacy associated with IVF and related methods for assisting reproduction is so low as to justify its continued classification as experimental rather than therapeutic. Certainly the parties seeking IVF as well as any children that might result have a right to state protection from the risks, uncertainties, and harms associated with human experimentation.

Moreover, even if one acknowledges a right to procreate or a right to reproductive freedom for every man and woman, this does not mean that the state has no legitimate interest in monitoring or regulating the practice of IVF. It is true that competent individuals have a right to be free from governmental or state interference with their procreative activities under the interpretation that American courts have given of cases involving access to contraception and abortion. However, the acknowledgment of a negative right, the right to be free from interference with one's sexual and reproductive actions, does not thereby entail the existence of a positive right to be aided or assisted by the state or any other third parties in fulfilling one's procreative desires.[17]

The government is under no obligation to assure the availability of IVF to any person who might desire to have an offspring any more than it is obligated to help find willing mates for the unmarried. While there may exist a negative right to be free from interference with respect to sexual activities between consenting adults there is no reason to think that there is a complementary right which entitles anyone to services for the treatment of infertility by any means available, especially if those means are probably still best viewed as experimental.

Matters of respect

If it is true that IVF is properly viewed as experimental then the need to address the issue of the moral acceptability of research aimed at improving the efficacy of the technique needs to be addressed. If it is further true that those seeking help for infertility require the protection of the state in utilizing procedures that are still experimental, then there is a need to understand the values that might guide legislators and bureaucrats in regulating research in the area of IVF.

One of the benefits of acknowledging that low rates of efficacy are a sufficient basis for classifying the technique as research is that it helps answer the question of what purposes ought to govern research in this area. The sole reason individuals seek access to IVF is for the purpose of creating babies. Some may seek IVF treatment because they are known to be incapable of having a child in any other way. Others may desire IVF because of concerns about the health risks posed to them by a pregnancy or even for reasons of convenience.

Since IVF is still experimental and since access to IVF is still relatively difficult, it would be hard to justify making it available at the present time to anyone other than those who cannot have children in any other fashion or for whom a pregnancy is known to be life-threatening. Research ought be undertaken on those whose need for benefits are the greatest, not upon those who seek to be subjects for convenience or for the other reasons.

Research at this point in the evolution of IVF should concentrate on those studies most likely to lead to the improvement of the efficacy of the technique. To some extent this will require the creation of registries and systematic means of reporting results so that IVF clinics can learn from one another about success and failure with various approaches to IVF. Third-party payors, both public and private, surely have an interest in insisting that such basic epidemiological research be undertaken as a precondition of eligibility for reimbursement.

To some extent, research will also be required on sperm, ova, and upon embryos to ascertain methods by which the technique can be refined so as to produce more babies at less cost and with less risk, physical and psychological, to prospective parents. It makes no sense in light of the shortage of reproductive materials for research and the low efficacy of IVF to use embryos or gametes from those seeking assistance for infertility for any purpose other than improvements in the rate at which IVF produces babies.

It is often said that whatever other moral rules ought to govern the treatment of gametes or embryos these biological materials ought to be "treated with respect."[18] One major difficulty with such prescriptions is that it is not self-evident what a commitment to respecting human biological materials entails. Can one espouse a commitment to research upon embryos, for example, while still adhering to a norm of respect for them?

Ironically, if it is true that more research is needed to help advance IVF to the status of a full-fledged therapy, and if research upon techniques aimed at increasing the efficacy of IVF for the infertile ought to have the first priority among other research goals that might be undertaken, then the moral question of the acceptability of research on the unconsenting must still be addressed. If it is true that research that carries risk or danger cannot ethically be done, as an earlier generation of critics of IVF maintained, then it is hard to see how a norm of respect can be compatible with experimentation involving human reproductive materials.

It seems clear that whatever else is entailed by a norm of respect, it is difficult to insist upon respectfullness solely on the basis of the intrinsic properties possessed by gametes or embryos. While an ovum or an embryo is clearly human material, and while there may be the potential present for the development of a human being from such materials, the potential is not inherent solely in gametes or embryos themselves. A woman must be willing to carry these materials in her body under somewhat restricted circumstances for a significant period of time for that potential to be fulfilled.

What we must respect about human reproductive materials then is not their potential personhood but the fact that they are human materials. The attitudes, practices, and interventions we will tolerate with such materials ought to be no more liberal or lackadaisical then those we would tolerate where other human materials (such as tissues, organs, and cadavers) are concerned.

This may mean that we ought not, as a matter of respect, to allow sperm, ova, or embryos to be bought and sold. It may also require that certain routines and customs govern the procurement and manipulation of such materials. It may further require that those who wish to utilize such materials for any purpose obtain the permission of those from whose bodies they came and from committees or other groups that society may deem appropriate to insure that the goals undertaken and the benefits to be produced by using such materials are consistent with public sensibilities.

There is a long history in Western law and morality which establishes the nonproperty status of persons and their bodies as a sign of special respect for what is human. It would seem imperative in order to remain consistent with this tradition to extend the same nonproperty, noncommercial status to human reproductive materials. Moreover, if we are to respect not only the humanity of the materials involved but also the humanity of those persons from whom such materials are obtained then there would seem to be an obligation to obtain informed consent at all times from those who provide such materials for each and every use of such materials.

If it is the case that those seeking IVF are at a special disadvantage in that they are especially vulnerable to the requests of researchers for access to a form of intervention that they desperately seek, it may make sense to insist upon independent committee review for each and every case of procurement of human reproductive materials. If it is the case that we are confident that those seeking IVF can still make intelligent, informed, and free choices about the fate of their reproductive materials then their consent may form a sufficient basis for procuring such materials.

Whatever else is entailed by the notion of respect it certainly must be interpreted to include both the donors of reproductive materials and the materials themselves. These individuals ought to have the right to determine the uses to which gametes and embryos are put.

But consent is not the sole determinant of the acceptability of research on human reproductive materials. It might be argued that the potentiality inherent in such materials forces the question upon us of whether research that might damage or destroy such materials is morally licit.

If the aim of such research is to improve the efficacy of IVF then it would seem possible to justify the use and even the destruction of these materials. The reason is quite simple—unless such research is done, the potential inherent in human reproductive materials is likely to remain only that—potential. If the goal of allowing the potential of a sperm, ovum, or embryo to be expressed in the form of a baby is a morally justifiable one, then it would seem morally acceptable to allow the routine fulfillment of that goal.

Those who wish to see IVF accepted as a routine element of medical practice have thought it best to use the language of therapy in describing the technique. However, while it is true that IVF seems to entail no harms for those children who are created in this manner, it is also true that medical science is not yet capable of making the technique work in a reliable way without imposing significant burdens on those involved. The only way to modify this situation is to come to terms with the moral reality that it is only by encouraging further research on human reproductive materials that respect for human life can be exemplified.

References

1. Caplan, A. L. 1986. "The Ethics of In Vitro Fertilization." *Primary Care* 13(2): 241–254.

2. Waller, L. 1983. Report on Donor Gametes and In Vitro Fertilization. Victoria, Australia (unpublished document).

3. Fishel, S. 1986. "IVF—historical perspective." In *In Vitro Fertilization.* S. Fishel & E. Symonds, Eds. 1–16. IRL Press, Oxford.

4. Edwards, R. G., P. C. Steptoe & J. M. Purdy. 1970. "Fertilization and cleavage in vitro of preovulator human oocytes." *Nature* 227: 1307–1309.

5. Ramsey, P. 1972. "Shall we reproduce?" *J. Am. Med. Assoc.* 220(10): 1346–1350.

6. Gorovitz, S. 1982. *Doctors' Dilemmas.* Macmillan, New York, NY.

7. Kass, L. 1979. "Making babies revisited." *The Public Interest* 54(Winter): 32–60.

8. Caplan, A. L. 1985. "Ethical issues raised by research involving xenografts." *J. Am. Med. Assoc.* 254(23): 3339–3343.

9. Katz, J. 1985. *The Silent World of Doctor and Patient.* Free Press. New York, NY.

10. Feichtinger, W. & P. Kemeter. 1986. "Variations in current ivf programmes—the in-patient versus out-patient treatment." In *In Vitro Fertilization.* S. Fishel & Symonds, Eds. 147–154. IRL Press, Oxford.

11. Rowland, R. 1987. "Making women visible in the embryo experimentation debate." *Bioethics* 1(2): 179–188.

12. Ibid.

13. Ethics Committee of the American Fertility Society. 1986. "Ethical considerations of the new reproductive technologies." September.

14. Ibid.

15. Ibid.

16. Ibid.

17. Warnock, M. 1987. "The good of the child." *Bioethics* 1(2): 141–155.

18. Kass, L. 1979 & L. Andrews. 1986. "Legal and ethical aspects of new reproductive technologies." *Clin. Obstet. Gynecol.* 29(1): 190–204: Ethics Committee, 1986.

8.

Mapping morality
Ethics and the human
genome project

I. What is the project to map the human genome?

During the past few years, much attention and discussion has focused on the wisdom of launching a project to map and sequence the human genome. Many expert groups and organizations have studied the feasibility, cost, and desirability of such a project (National Academy of Science, 1986; National Research Council, 1988; Office of Technology Assessment, 1988; American Association for the Advancement of Science, 1988; McKusick, 1989). While there are some experts within the scientific community who doubt the soundness of the project (Office of Technology Assessment, 1988; McKusick, 1989), the National Institutes of Health, in consultation with the Department of Energy and the Congress, decided in 1989 to make funds available for the project.

The estimated cost for mapping and sequencing the human genome is three billion dollars. The project, or more accurately, the set of interrelated activities at various universities and companies that the

NIH and the Department of Energy intend to support under the general rubric of the genome project, is expected to be finished in about fifteen years.

The general tasks which must be performed in mapping and sequencing the human genome are

(1) the creation of a high resolution genetic linkage map
(2) the creation of a collection of ordered DNA clones
(3) the creation of a high resolution (nucleotide sequence) physical map

(National Research Council, 1988)

Genetic linkage maps are created by studying families to measure the frequency with which two different traits are inherited together, or linked, over generations. This information can then be used to create maps which exhibit the relative positions of genes for these traits on various chromosomes.

Ordered DNA clones are genetically engineered replicas of known DNA sequences. They are used in conjunction with various recombinant techniques to reveal the positions of individual genes on chromosomes.

Low resolution physical maps—banding patterns of the kind visible under a microscope and formed by staining different pairs of chromosomes—are currently in wide use in many areas of the biological and agricultural sciences. A high-resolution physical map would show the actual sequence of nucleotides, the smallest unit of genetic information in a segment of DNA drawn from a chromosome. The resolution of such a map is so precise that distances are measured in terms of the number of linked pairs of nucleotides that separate one site from another on a particular DNA segment.

As of January 10, 1989, 4,584 genes had been identified in the human genome (McKusick, 1989). About 1,500 of these have been mapped to specific sites or regions on a specific chromosome, and 600 of these have been cloned and sequenced. It is estimated that somewhere between 50,000 and 100,000 genes will have to be mapped in order to complete the map of the human genome (McKusick, 1989).

Mapping the genome is not the same as understanding how the human genome works. Even if scientists had the complete set of nucleotide sequences possible for each chromosome of a human being, they would still be faced with the daunting project of trying to understand how this information is transformed and translated into the traits that we ordinarily recognize as constitutive of human beings. But mapping and sequencing the genome is a first step toward such understanding.

II. Why map the human genome?

The debate about whether the federal government ought to fund a systematic, centrally planned effort to map and sequence the human genome was won by persuasive arguments concerning the possible applications of this information. Those who favored funding the genome project argued that mapping and sequencing the genome would permit a much greater understanding of human growth and development, greatly increase the possibility of offering early diagnoses of many diseases and disabilities, and provide new avenues for therapy against some. Proponents also argued that mapping the human genome, in conjunction with similar ongoing efforts to map the genomes of other species, would be important in the development of techniques to accomplish molecular farming of a broad spectrum of biological products with both therapeutic and industrial value. A brief review of the promises contained in the various reports and studies which supported undertaking the genome project is fascinating for the range and degree of benefits that are supposed to be generated by funding the genome project.

A. Benefits for understanding fundamental questions in the human and life sciences

By mapping and sequencing the human genome it should be possible, proponents say, to rapidly accelerate scientific understanding of how various genes function in mediating the processes of normal development and growth. The processes of mutation and sexual recombination would be amenable to careful description and analysis. Scientists could use high-resolution genome maps in constructing evolutionary trees which would aid efforts to understand both human and animal phylogeny (Cann, Stoneking, and Wilson, 1987). Human anthropology, in particular, would be revolutionized by the availability of a complete map of the human genome. It should then be possible to give much more precise estimates of the biological relationships between various subpopulations of the human species.

B. Benefits for diagnosing disease and disability

Established genetic disorders now account for almost 50 percent of all childhood deaths in the United States. They also account for as much as 25 percent of all hospital admissions for children. The ability to diagnose the genetic contribution to disease and disability will, according to many of those who concluded the genome project was worth funding, greatly enhance understanding of the role heredity plays overall in causing childhood death, disease, and impairment (Office of Technology Assessment, 1988). Acquiring new knowledge of the genome should also lead to earlier diagnoses of which couples and children are at risk of encountering various genetically mediated medical problems.

Having a complete, high-resolution map of the human genome will allow scientists to undertake careful studies of inheritance patterns for various diseases in order to obtain more precise estimates of the extent to which genetic anomalies and mutations are responsible for medical problems and impairments within specific family lineages and in the general population. Since many widely prevalent disorders have etiologies in which heredity plays a major role, the creation of a high-resolution map will, proponents claim, have a major impact on medicine's ability to warn persons of the risks they face of contracting various diseases relative to their lifestyle and the environment in which they work or live. Diseases for which greater diagnostic precision might be possible include some forms of Alzheimer's disease, some forms of coronary heart disease, various forms of cancer, allergies, hypertension, schizophrenia, obesity, metabolic disorders, asthma, alcoholism, dyslexia, some forms of diabetes, and some forms of Parkinsonism, to name but a few (Lappe, 1987; National Research Council, 1988).

C. Benefits for prevention and therapy

There are a number of ways in which the sequencing and mapping of the human genome could, according to those who want to see the genome project proceed quickly, produce benefits for the prevention and treatment of disease and disability. A map could be used directly in the creation of vectors for inserting other genes where the analysis of a person's genotype reveals dysfunctional genes. Early forms of gene therapy are already being tested for the treatment of cancer and immunological disorders. Within a few years, there will probably be experimentation with other methods of transplanting genetically engineered marrow cells for various diseases caused by inborn errors of metabolism, such as Hunter's, Hurler's, and Sly's syndromes.

In addition to the replacement of cells or the substitution of genetically altered cells, genetic maps may prove useful in allowing for the direct manipulation of the genome. Genetic microsurgery, while still a technically daunting feat, will become at least a theoretical possibility with a detailed map of the genome in hand.

Indirect benefits are also prominently mentioned as following from the decision to push ahead with the genome project. It should be possible to create drugs and hormones in large amounts so as to correct inadequacies in the natural production of these substances resulting from genetic anomalies. The ability to detect genetic anomalies from tissue samples derived in utero may allow for the early use of surgical, medical, or pharmacological interventions (perhaps also in utero) which may prevent some of the morbidity and mortality associated with certain genomes. And a high-resolution map of the genome should make it possible to create cells with desirable characteristics which can then be cultured and used for purposes such as vaccine development or toxicity testing (Office of Technology Assessment, 1988).

Recent breakthroughs in genome mapping have allowed scientists to detect markers for Huntington's disease, polycystic kidney disease, retinoblastoma, neurofibromatosis, Duchenne's muscular dystrophy, and cystic fibrosis (McKusick, 1989). An ability to screen for such diseases may influence a couple's reproductive choices as well as procedures such as artificial insemination by donor and in vitro fertilization.

There ought be no doubt that application, not knowledge for knowledge's sake, was the critical consideration in securing funding for the genome project. The promise of benefits has a long history in the funding of genetic research throughout this century (Kevles, 1985) Yet, despite the overwhelming potential for benefits resulting from the genome project, many of those who support the genome project say they are befuddled by the ethical worries that have been raised about it.

III. Are there ethically distinct issues raised by the human genome project?

An obvious question has dominated a lot of the ethical discussion surrounding the genome project (Office of Technology Assessment, 1988; National Research Council, 1988): Now that the policy decision has been made to sequence and map the genome, how can the project be completed in an expeditious but socially responsible manner (Lappe, 1987)? How many and which institutions and scientists should receive support to undertake various aspects of the project? Is the public or private sector or some combination of the two best suited to undertake the work involved so as to obtain the benefits desired from the project in the shortest period of time? To what degree should those involved in the project feel obligated to share their findings freely with other scientists and with commercial firms both in the United States and other nations (McKusick, 1989)? One of the most vexing questions of all, at least to judge by the amount of attention that has been devoted to it (Office of Technology Assessment, 1988; National Research Council, 1988; Smith, 1988), is the property and patent status that ought be assigned to knowledge about and techniques for manipulating the human genome.

Finding answers to these questions requires a careful examination of the evolution of commercial biotechnology in the United States and other nations. Those responsible for organizing and funding the genome project also need to know what lessons can be learned from analogous "big science" efforts in chemistry, agriculture, medicine, computer science, oceanography, physics, astronomy, and space exploration. These are all important issues, but they are not especially questions of ethics.

There is a long history of commercialization of scientific knowledge and of university/industry cooperation for profit in many fields of inquiry. While moral concerns and legal regulations are in evidence in computer science, chemistry, engineering, and agriculture, people working in these fields are not subject to special or unique moral codes, regulations, or legal oversight. Why, some of those involved in the genome project wonder, would the application of new genetic knowledge require special ethical or policy attention?

If the mores of the marketplace and the conscience of individual researchers are adequate to the task of guiding research in most areas of scientific inquiry, why should genetics be subject to a special, more exacting set of norms? In other words, if there is nothing ethically distinctive about the financing, organization, and administration of efforts to map the genome, is there any reason to believe that scientists working on this project ought to be subjected to—or impose on themselves—a set of moral norms that are "strongly differentiated" (Goldman, 1980) from the moral and legal norms which society and scientists ordinarily accept as adequate for guiding scientific conduct? Questions of patents, data sharing, and trade secrecy are important, but they are also important in many other areas of science and industry. Is there any reason for special ethical concern about the genome project or to believe, as many do (Rifkin, 1983; World Council of Churches, 1989), that special moral norms must be adopted by or imposed on those who conduct research in this area?

There are ethical considerations which do justify making human genetics the object of special moral concern and, perhaps, special moral norms. None of them have anything to do with the organization of the genome project, its funding, or the patent status of its techniques. They have everything to do with the application of new genetic knowledge.

The applicability of genetic knowledge to human reproduction through clinical application and public health programs of various sorts raises a number of important ethical issues. The case for special concern and sensitivity about the application of genetics to human reproduction is cemented by the history of abuse and murder conducted in the name of genetics by competent and sometimes illustrious scientists and physicians in Nazi Germany and, to a lesser extent, in the United States, the United Kingdom, the Soviet Union, and other nations (Graham, 1978; Kevles, 1985; Muller-Hill, 1988; Proctor, 1988; Wolper, 1989)—all in this century.

Another reason for special ethical attention is that expanding knowledge of human genetics is likely to cause a conceptual revolution in our understanding of human nature and in human self-perception. Concepts such as normality, unnaturalness, disability, personal responsibility, equal opportunity, paternity, parentage, race, ethnicity, instinct, and family are closely tied to beliefs and opinions about the biological constitution of human beings (Hardin, 1977; Midgley, 1978; Wilson, 1978). Our sense of who we are in relationship to other species and how we came to exist, both as members of a species and as individuals endowed with characteristic traits and behaviors, are all linked to beliefs about our ontogeny, phylogeny, history, and heredity. Other sciences can and have shaken common-sensical beliefs about the place of human beings in the natural world. New knowledge resulting from mapping the genome has the potential to force shifts in our metaphysical and ethical self-understanding.

Lastly, the notion of the perfectibility of humankind (Passmore, 1970; Ramsey, 1970; Harris, 1981) is one that has long prevailed in and shaped Western culture. Biology in general and genetics in particular are often seen as setting the limits of what can and cannot be done to perfect, or at least improve, the human condition. The consequences of learning more about our own genetic makeup are not confined to the prospect of being able to intervene to repair or compensate for defects and disorders.

The same door which leads to these opportunities also opens onto a path which can lead to systematic attempts to improve, enhance, and optimize human traits and functions (Kass, 1975; Caplan, 1980). New genetic knowledge of the sort inherent in mapping and sequencing the genome forces a confrontation with the question of what is ethically wrong with social policies or medical efforts which aim at achieving goals consistent with positive eugenics. Such knowledge and the ability to act on it to enhance or improve the genetic makeup of our species also raises questions about the rights of individuals visa-à-vis the state with respect to such fundamental matters as procreative choice, quality of life, personal autonomy, equality of opportunity, and liberty. The opportunity to design our descendents with a greater degree of accuracy raises the most morally distinctive issue arising from the genome project.

IV. Ethical issues arising from the application of new knowledge concerning the human genome in reproduction

Control over one's procreative decisions has been recognized as a basic human right by American and international courts. Information about the human genome could be used to restrict that freedom. Singapore, for example, has adopted a policy of providing financial incentives for couples who are seen as having desirable traits to have more children, while others are encouraged to limit family size (Chan, 1987). Genetic screening for sex selection is apparently a thriving industry in some cities in India.

Information about the human genome could also be used to enhance reproductive opportunities and choices. In utero fetal surgery has emerged as an alternative to abortion for hydrocephaly detected in the fetus in utero. The early detection of other congenital anomalies using a comprehensive genome map might allow for other antenatal prophylactic interventions. Screening for PKU and related metabolic disorders allows for the early utilization of dietary therapy for conditions that are life-threatening if not detected early after birth. Mapping the genome may permit a broad range of prophylactic regimens to be instituted soon after birth for disorders that are life-threatening or that severely compromise the quality of life.

But genetic information can also be misunderstood or misapplied, as was the case during the early 1970s in efforts to undertake mass screening for sickle cell disease and sickle cell trait (Bergsma, 1974). Some states enacted laws which required those with sickle cell trait to be immunized against the disease prior to admission to public school! Some of those diagnosed as having sickle cell trait were excluded from certain jobs in the armed services. Without massive efforts at public education, there is a very real danger that persons who have certain genetic propensities or carry certain genetic traits could be stigmatized or made the victims of restrictive laws concerning reproductive freedom.

Some scientists dismiss concerns about the misapplication of genetic knowledge as overblown. They reject as scientifically naive the scenarios spun by some critics of the decision to map the genome, dire visions of human-animal chimeras created to do the dirty work of society or the propagation of a subpopulation of human beings cloned for their leadership skills, appearance, or athletic abilities.

These scenarios are both implausible and by no means the necessary end products of mapping and sequencing the human genome (Boone, 1988). But this century has witnessed two sustained efforts by totalitarian regimes, one in Germany and the other in the Soviet Union, to bend the practice of clinical genetics to serve the eugenic goals of the state (Graham, 1978; Harris, 1981; Kevles, 1985; Muller-Hill, 1988; Proctor, 1988). The legacy of abuses perpetrated in the name of the science of genetics in Germany and the Soviet Union lends credibility to worries about the consequences of the decision to aggressively pursue knowledge about the human genome, regardless of how well such a project is organized and administered or how impeccable the scientific credentials of those who conduct and supervise the actual work. The fact that during the first few decades of this century public officials in democracies such as the United States, the United Kingdom, Australia, and Canada were quick to seize upon early findings concerning the genetic basis of human variability, disease, disability, and intelligence to create policies that were consciously intended to discriminate against (and in some cases sterilize) the members of certain ethnic, racial, and disabled groups (Hofstadter, 1955; Kamin, 1974; Chase, 1977; Chorover, 1979; Kevles, 1985; Muller-Hill, 1988; Proctor, 1988; Wolper, 1989) shows that the abuse of knowledge in the realm of genetics is not limited to authoritarian or totalitarian states or to those who espouse overtly racist or discriminatory views.

Medicine and public health have had to struggle with the legacy of abuse and murder that continues to haunt efforts by well-intentioned scientists and physicians to utilize genetic knowledge for the good of patients or society (Wolper, 1989). The problem of living with the tragic record of abuse on the part of medicine and science in Germany and other nations in creating and implementing lethal or discriminatory social policies inspired by beliefs based upon genetics has made concerns about the application of genetic information something more than a subject fit only for those with fervid imaginations or an anti-science bent. The Lebensborn program administered by the Office of Eugenics in the Third Reich and the sterilization of the "Rhineland bastards" during the 1930s for genetic reasons are not the products of the overheated imaginations of the contemporary critics of the human genome project. They were real social policies, instituted and overseen by scientists and physicians, and aimed at modifying the genetic makeup of future generations based on prevailing beliefs about genetics (Kevles, 1985; Muller-Hill, 1988; Proctor, 1988; Wolper, 1989).

Of course, the acquisition of genetic knowledge has already raised questions about its application in the domain of reproduction. Efforts in health care to evolve and follow moral norms that will limit abuses and misunderstanding may be instructive in thinking about how to grapple with the application of new knowledge arising from the mapping and sequencing of the human genome in the years to come. In clinical medicine, the most important moral norm which has evolved for coping with the ethical challenges of an individual's or a group's genetic constitution is to adopt a conscious stance of ethical or value neutrality.

V. Value neutrality as the moral foundation for clinical genetics

The view that those involved in clinical human genetics should adopt a posture of value neutrality—a kind of carefully inculcated agnosticism—concerning reproductive decisions commands broad assent within both the professions of clinical genetics and genetics counseling. The central ethical dogma espoused by those involved in screening, counseling, and therapy in the realm of human genetics is (and has been since the end of World War II) that the provider of services should not impose his or her values on those seeking or receiving genetic information (Bergsma, 1974; National Academy of Sciences, 1975; Reed, 1980; Steinbrook, 1986; World Medical Association, 1987; West, 1988).

Within the domain of human genetics, value neutrality is deemed appropriate where matters of screening, diagnosis, and therapy are concerned—whether the information available is rough, partial, and crude, as is true today, or precise and refined, as may be true a decade or two from now. Practitioners who do counseling are especially vocal in espousing the view that they must strive to remain neutral in the face of the moral choices raised by genetic knowledge. They teach their students and try themselves to take every reasonable precaution against allowing their personal values to influence opinions and decisions on the part of those in their care (Reed, 1980). Patient values are to be determinative whenever hard choices have to be made on the basis of genetic information (West, 1988)

The question of whether value neutrality is desirable on the part of those doing genetic screening and counseling is one that has received a negative answer in some quarters in recent years. Some members of advocacy groups for the disabled have become increasingly leery of the alleged value neutrality of those who provide genetic screening and counseling services (Saltus, 1989). Former Surgeon General C. Everett Koop on numerous occasions criticized genetic testing as nothing more than "search and destroy missions" aimed at aborting the disabled.

A number of studies have been published (Sorenson, Swazey, and Scotch, 1982; Fletcher and Wertz, 1988) which examine the practices of genetic counselors and clinical geneticists concerning such issues as whether information ought be provided to patients as to the sex of a fetus, the presence of XYY syndrome, and what sort of information should be presented in terms of the risks posed for the quality of life of those with spina bifida and other neural tube disorders (West, 1988). These studies reveal sufficient variations in both attitudes and practice from hospital to hospital and nation to nation to raise suspicion about the degree to which those who now offer genetic screening and testing services actually act in conformity with their self-imposed ideal of value neutrality. Variability in what patients are or are not told—sometimes as a matter of institutional policy, sometimes as a matter of individual practitioner conscience—raises doubt as to whether anything close to a consensus exists as to what activities are compatible with the norm of value neutrality.

The question of whether those now doing clinical genetics live up to (or are even in agreement about) their normative ideals in their professional practice does not address the more fundamental question of whether it is desirable to have a moral norm of value neutrality in place with respect to human clinical genetics. This question seems beyond dispute for many who provide genetic services and counseling using current knowledge about the constitution, components, and relative ordering of the human genome. Since even the partial completion of the sequencing and mapping of the human genome will greatly enhance current capacities to test, screen, and predict genetic disorders, it is critical that the norm of value neutrality receive a close look both for its desirability as well as for its practicality.

VI. Value neutrality, screening, counseling, and the disclosure of information about genotypes

The question of whether or not those who now offer clinical services in the area of genetics can or should strive to remain value neutral in their behavior and counseling is pivotal in understanding the ethical issues raised by the availability of new knowledge resulting from mapping and sequencing the human genome. Many commentators have noted the uncertainty which surrounds questions of responsibilities and duties in such areas as the protection of privacy and confidentiality, the duty to warn potential parents of risks to the health of any offspring they might choose to create, when testing or screening is appropriate and when it is mandatory, and the determination of what conditions or disorders are appropriately classified as defects, diseases, anomalies, and abnormalities (Steinbrook, 1986; Lappe, 1987; Boone, 1988; West, 1988). The answers given to all of these moral questions hinge on the desirability of adhering to an overarching norm of value neutrality for those providing clinical genetics services.

In order to understand whether it is desirable to adhere to and insist upon a norm of value neutrality with respect to clinical human genetics it is necessary to address a number of questions: How should the norm of value neutrality cash out in terms of actual practice and policy? Do those who provide genetic services strive to be value neutral in their practices and policies? Are those who provide genetic services value neutral in their practices and policies? Is it possible to provide genetic services and adhere to a norm of value neutrality? Is value neutrality appropriate as a norm at the bedside or as a matter of public policy or both?

Philosophers sometimes say that in trying to prescribe how it is that persons ought to act it is important not to call for norms which are impossible for fallible human beings to fulfill. If "ought" implies "can" and it is reasonable not to ask people to aspire to normative principles that they cannot, for practical reasons, come close to meeting, then is value neutrality a norm that is feasible and practical in the realm of clinical genetics, either in the doctor's office or as a part of public health programs?

A. Is value neutrality possible in clinical genetics?

There seems to be a great deal of evidence that those who provide testing, screening, and counseling strive very hard to remain value neutral. Those who do counseling are adamant in their view that value neutrality is a norm that ought to guide their behavior at all times with patients (West, 1988). They consciously see themselves as serving the role of only providing information to those who (usually voluntarily) seek to have it. The hallmarks of value neutrality as an ideal (if not always a reality) of human clinical genetics are (1) a willingness to provide testing and counseling to all who voluntarily seek it, (2) the presentation of information concerning findings in a manner that is balanced and comprehensible to patients or clients, (3) the fair and balanced presentation of all options for action if a problem is discovered, (4) a willingness to answer all questions asked by those seeking services, and (5) an obligation to protect privacy and confidentiality at all times regardless of societal needs or benefits (Bergsma, 1974; West, 1988). What value neutrality means, at least in the context of clinical human genetics, is that those who seek services do so freely and without pressure or coercion, that there is no judgment offered as to the appropriateness of seeking services, that the counselor must protect the rights of those seeking services—especially the right to privacy and confidentiality—and, most importantly, that the sole aim of clinical genetics screening, testing, and counseling is to provide comprehensible information.

Numerous studies of the practice of clinical human genetics cast doubt on the claim that those who provide testing and counseling do so in a manner that is in conformity with this view of value neutrality (Fletcher and Wertz, 1988). For example, those who have access to genetic services tend to be middle and upper class. The poor and minorities rarely receive genetic counseling and testing. The same is true of those who are dependent on Medicaid or who lack health insurance. So there are financial pressures at work in determining who can "voluntarily" seek to obtain information about genotypes and in evaluating who needs testing and counseling.

Further evidence against the practicality of value neutrality in clinical and public health practices are findings which show that many institutions have adopted policies which prohibit the release of information about the sex of a fetus following a prenatal test while others routinely release such information to parents who request it (Fletcher and Wertz, 1988). Some states believe that it is either not cost-effective or constitutes too great an infringement of parental authority to require all infants to undergo postnatal tests for detectable metabolic disorders, while others require such testing, with no exceptions permitted for any reason. Some genetics counselors will present information about the association between XYY syndrome and criminality, while others think the reported association so weak and ill-supported as not to be worthy of comment (personal communications, genetics counselors at Columbia, Minnesota, and Yale). Similar diversity of opinion seems to exist about whether and how to present information concerning mild forms of genetic mosaicism. The views in England and the United States about the significance of the detection of chromosomal abnormalities such as Down's Syndrome or neural tube defects such as spina bifida in terms of counseling parents and the need for testing those at risk, and in identifying who is at risk, vary a great deal (Steinbrook, 1986; West, 1988). Strong differences of opinion exist among clinical genetics professionals about the impact of low IQ on the quality of life that people can enjoy. These variations in practice, belief, and attitude call into question the claim that the actual practice of human clinical genetics is value neutral, even if one defines the norm for value neutrality according to the terms advanced by its advocates.

Genetics counseling programs face a greater demand for their services than their resources can support, forcing choices as to who ought to receive priority of access for services. Since there are important variations in actual counseling practices from center to center in different parts of the United States as well as internationally, it is hard to defend the claim that genetics screening and counseling are or can be value neutral. Nonetheless it also seems true that those in the field strive to achieve value neutrality within the boundaries set by resource constraints and institutional and public policies. Is this a reasonable norm or ideal to aim for where matters of reproduction and health are concerned?

B. Is value neutrality desirable?

It would be odd to hear physicians who practice internal medicine or family medicine say that they are striving to be value neutral with respect to the care of their patients. Physicians are taught—and their patients to some degree expect—that they will not only inform those in their care about the risks and dangers of alcohol, smoking, unprotected promiscuous sexual practices, and the recreational use of narcotics, and about the benefits of exercise, wearing seatbelts, and sound dietary practices, but that they will actively discourage other risky behaviors and aggressively promote and encourage other healthful behaviors. Physicians, nurses, and psychologists in many areas of clinical practice and public health adhere to professional norms that go beyond value neutrality—they are zealous advocates of the value of health and prevention of disease and disability. Is there any reason to think that this sort of normative stance is inappropriate or unethical in the realm of human genetics?

Three problems facing those in the field of genetics are likely to become more vexing as knowledge of the human genome grows. First, there has been no sustained effort to obtain consensus as to what constitutes genetic health or genetic disease. Second, to date, the range of therapeutic options available for many congenital anomalies—abortion, forgoing reproduction, artificial insemination, chronic dependency on supportive technologies such as respirators—are fraught with negative evaluations and moral connotations. It is difficult to explicitly avow a commitment to genetic health or to combat genetic disease knowing the nature of the therapeutic options currently available. And third, at present too little is known about the function of the genome to permit any confident prediction of what will result from attempts to alter the genome of either somatic or germline cells.

Mapping and sequencing the genome is likely to change the range of therapeutic options and interventions that are available for repairing, modifying, or ameliorating a wide range of conditions and behaviors. In the not-too-distant future, it is likely that those who might wish to promote genetic "health" will not be so constrained by uncertainty as to what will happen if efforts are made to engineer changes in the human genome.

As therapeutic, palliative, and adaptational options for responding to genetic anomalies, disorders, and defects expand, consensus will begin to emerge among the medical and scientific community as to what constitutes normality, disease, and health with respect to the human genome. This in turn may lead to a shift in normative attitudes on the part of clinicians and public health officials from a stance of value neutrality to the espousal of norms that are more prescriptive in terms of health promotion and disease prevention.

If mapping and sequencing the genome does make it possible to detect the genetic components of cancer, depression, or heart disease, then consensus will begin to emerge that those with genetic endowments less prone to the manifestation of these diseases are "healthier," just as those who now possess acute vision and hearing or ample strength and stamina are seen as healthier than those who must rely on glasses or who cannot walk up three flights of stairs without resting. If we know that a particular genome disposes a person to cystic fibrosis, breast cancer, schizophrenia, or any other dysfunctional or disadvantageous condition, then there will be a tendency to see these diseases as manifestations of underlying diseases or disorders which have their basis in a physical lesion or programming error in the human genome. Medicine and public health will rapidly orient themselves toward the detection and correction of these lesions.

Value neutrality in clinical genetics and in public health programs that focus on the genetic contribution to disease, disability, and disorder is likely to shift from a normative stance of value neutrality toward an ethic in which the promotion of genetic health and the amelioration, prevention, and correction of genetic disease are the foundations of clinical and public health practice. The question facing society will be whether a normative shift of this type is ethically defensible.

If it is possible to obtain reasoned consensus among the members of society that certain physical or behavioral traits restrict the abilities, capacities, and opportunities open to those who possess them—and if it is possible to discover interventions consistent with the values that society places on the worth of human life and autonomy—then it is not clear that society will be troubled if those in the realms of clinical genetics or public health espouse norms that favor genetic health and discourage genetic disease. Neither is it at all obvious that there is anything inherently unethical about a moral commitment to health and disease at the level of genetics. If serious and debilitating diseases and disorders can be corrected or palliated with a high degree of safety and certainty by direct intervention in the human genome, be it in somatic cells or reproductive cells, there would not appear to be any reason to discourage such interventions. Interventions at the level of the genome in and of themselves have no particular ethical uniqueness. The only relevant questions are those of safety, efficacy, reliability, and risk. If these questions can be answered in ways that those seeking medical care find appropriate, then there would not appear to be any special ethical reason to insist upon moral neutrality on the part of clinicians and public health officials where matters of human genetics are concerned.

A shift from value neutrality to an explicit prescriptive moral stance promoting health and disvaluing disease in human genetics must, however, retain some aspects of the component elements which constitute the current ethic of value neutrality. While mapping and sequencing the genome may lead to greater consensus as to exactly which genomes represent health and which represent disease, it seems reasonable to retain the norm that information about health and disease and decisions as to what to do in response to such information ought remain in the hands of patients or, if the patients are children, their parents.

Similarly, while the promotion of health and the prevention of disease may be valid norms to guide the practice of medicine and public health, it is essential that participation in either realm remain voluntary. No competent adult ought feel any obligation to be a patient. The circumstances under which either clinicians or public health officials can compel compliance with their prescriptions are restricted to emergencies or situations in which a condition poses a clear and direct threat to the life of others or a remediable threat to the life of a dependent and incompetent person. Genetic conditions are not emergencies, nor do they often pose imminent, direct threats to the lives of others. In those cases where they do pose a remediable threat to the life of an incompetent person, interventions may be required or compelled by legal or legislative authority. Even in such cases, the evidence is persuasive that voluntary participation by parents or guardians will lead to greater compliance and thus greater benefits for those at grave risk than will compulsory policies (Bergsma, 1974). The State of California's experience with mass screening for neural tube defects for pregnant women represents an exemplary effort to assure the availability of genetic screening and counseling while keeping actual participation in screening and counseling voluntary rather than mandatory (Steinbrook, 1986).

Some elements of the ethic of value neutrality also make sense with respect to clinical genetics insofar as the presentation of information ought be comprehensible and complete. Every person involved in testing and counseling must realize that the dependency of those seeking testing, counseling, or therapy requires the presentation of clear, accurate, and complete information. Providers of genetic services must subordinate their values to the norm of value neutrality in the sense that they must give patients information about all reasonable options and courses of action and answer all questions to the best of their ability. Patients expect value neutrality with respect to the presentation of information, not because they believe health care providers ought to remain indifferent to health and disease but because they want to be assured that every provider can be trusted to present all facts and options concerning care, even if the provider's personal values favor some options over others.

Some elements of value neutrality are appropriate in the provision of information about a person's genome or about the hereditary contribution to various traits and behaviors. But public health officials and those involved in making public policy with respect to genetics must be wary of allowing the prevailing norm of value neutrality, which is rooted both in the history of abuses conducted in the name of genetics and in moral ambivalence about current options for intervening with respect to genetic problems, to distort the stance they adopt toward genetic screening and testing as knowledge of the human genome increases. From the point of view of social policy, it is surely wise to make information about the genetic contribution to disease and disability widely available. Social resources ought to be committed to those activities which can help maximize the potential for health and minimize the risk of disability and disease. And there should be no reluctance to commit social resources to the alleviation and treatment of genetic diseases and disorders.

Moreover, public health and social policy should not be seduced by the rhetorical pull of the ethos of value neutrality which pervades discussions of the ethics of genetic screening and testing into believing that prescriptive advocacy concerning the manner and methods of screening and testing is somehow inappropriate in the area of genetics. Testing and screening which are not linked to sound programs of counseling are likely to cause more harm than good. As those involved in public health efforts with respect to AIDS have learned, public participation and compliance are greater when those receiving information are given assistance in interpreting and understanding it. Not only must genetic screening and testing be voluntary when the condition being tested poses no direct, imminent threat to the lives and health of others, but testing must always be linked to counseling. It is not reasonable or consistent with current general understanding of human genetics or with existing analyses of informed consent to allow or encourage public health programs which merely disclose complex and potentially disturbing information. Fact dumping is not informing. Counseling which helps to interpret information and to address misunderstanding, fear, and stigma is an essential (although, of necessity, not purely value neutral) element of public health programs. It is certainly not value neutral for those making public policy to insist that the clinical application of new knowledge of the human genome be carried out in a manner consistent with respect for the values of personal autonomy, dignity, and comprehension.

VII. Normalcy, deviance, and perfection

In some respects the prospect of new knowledge of the human genome is disturbing precisely because of the benefits in terms of diagnosis, prevention, and therapy that make the mapping and sequencing project so attractive. The greater our knowledge of the genetic contribution to various diseases, disorders, and disabilities, the greater the stigma may be for those who have such traits, are at risk of exhibiting them during the course of their lives, or are likely to pass these traits on to their offspring. Those with disabilities already face significant obstacles to securing equal opportunities and being treated with basic consideration in our society and in many others. Greater knowledge with the potential for application carries with it the danger of expanding the discrimination that already exists between those who are relatively healthy and able-bodied and those who are not.

Moreover, the possibility of intervening to prevent disease, disorders, and disabilities based upon greater knowledge of the human genome holds out obvious possibilities for application in such arenas as employment, insurance, and even marriage and reproduction. It would be ironic if an increased understanding of the role of genetics led to further restrictions for those who are at greatest risk of facing problems of at least partially genetic origin. If the cost of mapping and sequencing of the human genome is in part justified on the basis of the applications such information will have for benefitting human-kind, then there would seen to be a strong obligation to insure that the distribution of these benefits is equitable.

Not only will greater knowledge of the human genome challenge our understanding of normality and deviance and our societal ability to respond to human differences in a just and humane manner but increased knowledge will also challenge the commitment of American society and that of many other nations to the norm of perfectibility both of the individual and of the society. As the British journal *The Lancet* noted in an editorial on worries that gene therapy might be used for the improvement of the human species, "Self improvement is a highly valued social attribute" (1989). The desire for self-improvement is valued by many, not only as a social attribute but also as a norm toward which societies ought to strive.

Despite the allure of the goal of self-improvement and the com-mitment (especially powerful in the tradition of Western society) to human perfectibility (Passmore, 1970), it is not self-evident that im-provement is a concept that ought to command respect or social re-sources. The positive value associated with the concept of improvement very much depends on the explication that is given of the concept.

When the *Lancet* editorialist extols the virtue of self-improvement, what is being praised is not a specific goal or end-product but a character trait. It is virtuous, many would hold, to be the kind of person who wants to better himself or herself. But it is not obvious that the desire for self-improvement is a good if it is the only desire that is present. Those who wish to improve their lot with little regard for the welfare of others might be thought of as self-centered or even cruel rather than virtuous. And those who seek self-improvement only in terms of physical beauty or monetary gain are appropriately viewed as egotistical, vain, or greedy. The desire to improve oneself is a valued trait but its value is a function not only of the good associated with improvement but of the degree to which the goal or end-state sought is viewed as good. The value of self-improvement is also contin-gent upon the degree to which the pursuit of personal improvement is respectful of the needs and interests of others.

Similarly, it might be said that there is nothing intrinsically wrong and much that is morally right with social policies in the realm of genetics that aim at improvement of the genetic health of the society or at the positive enhancement of the genomes present in the population. After all, improvement is clearly a good and many of the political and social activities society expects of government are aimed at improvement. But again, conceptual caution is in order where matters of improvement or enhancement or perfectibility are concerned. Improvement is generally a desirable goal for social policy. But, in and of itself, improvement is not admirable or even practical. The question which can no longer be avoided as the understanding of the human genome increases is this: "Improvement with respect to what goals or end-states?".

In thinking about improving the genetic health of the population, we must also ask what this improvement or perfection will cost if some are likely to enjoy the benefits of social policies which aim at improvement while others do not or cannot. The complicated nature of the value associated with improvement or perfection as a matter of social policy is illustrated by an emerging controversy over the use of human growth hormone.

Recently, genetic engineering has made it possible to synthesize relatively large amounts of human growth hormone. Until this synthesis became possible, those who suffered from a deficiency of this substance had to scramble to obtain a share of the small amount of hormone that could be reclaimed from cadaver sources. The supply of hormone was so tight that only those suffering from the greatest deficiency, who were at the greatest risk of not growing, could obtain access.

All that is beginning to change. The supply of hormone is increasing, and those who can pay for it can have access. This has been a great benefit to those children who are at risk of not growing because of a lack of the hormone. But some parents of children who do not suffer from any deficiency in the amount of growth hormone they secrete have begun to seek access to the synthetically produced substance. They wish to provide this hormone to their young children in the hope that they will grow taller. Some parents hope that the hormone will bestow a height advantage on their child, such that they will fare better in the worlds of business or athletics than people who are less tall.

Should society tolerate or encourage the "cosmetic" use of synthetic growth hormone? If it is true that improvement or perfection is a laudable social aim for public policy, then should society merely tolerate the use of growth hormone in children who have no discernable deficiency or disorder in hormone production? Should social policies be instituted to require or at least encourage parents to consider administering growth hormone to each of their children at appropriate times in their development?

But why should society tolerate or encourage practices aimed at increasing the height of children who are not known to suffer from any specific biological or genetic anomaly? What is it about the pursuit of improvement, enhancement, or perfection that makes height of value? In part it is that society has chosen to reward those who are tall with various benefits, the vast majority of which are tacit and rooted deeply in cultural traditions. But of course it would be just as easy to urge educational programs and social reforms that aim at minimizing the role of height in daily life as it would be to encourage social policies which try to maximize the height potential of every child. Being tall is, at least according to most social psychology studies, a good thing in this and many other societies. But the good is a function not of height but of what society chooses to make of height. Even putting aside the issues raised by inequities in access to synthetic growth hormone due to high cost and even knowledge of its existence, improving or enhancing height may not be good or commendable since height is really of instrumental rather than intrinsic value.

It is quite likely that, as knowledge of the structure and function of the human genome expands, social pressures will arise not only to repair defects and disorders that are detected in both structure and function but to undertake interventions aimed at improving or perfecting the structure and function of the genome. There is a grave danger that our society or others will be seduced by the language of improvement, enhancement, and perfection into thinking that any change conducted in the name of these goals must be good and desirable. But this is by no means the case. Improvement or perfection as social policies are good only to the extent that society is in general agreement that the ends which they serve are good. Moreover, improvement is a good as a matter of social policy only to the extent to which efforts conducted in the name of improvement or perfection are sensitive to the impact they have on all members of society. Social policies which create a society in which there co-exist two castes, the very tall and the short—or, for that matter, policies which create divisions with respect to intelligence, susceptibility to disease, or overall appearance—may or may not be good or desirable, depending on whether the means taken to achieve them are fair and equitable.

The language of improvement and perfection is seductive. In part, it is the language that proved persuasive in securing funding for a "big science" project at a time when money is tight and the competition for it fierce. The prospect of intentionally changing and even trying to perfect the human genome (a notion enunciated while securing funds for the project) also assures ethical insecurity about the project. The greater the prospect for application, the more reasonable worries about the morality of what is being done will appear.

References

American Association for the Advancement of Science. 1988. *Biotechnology.* Washington: AAAS.

Bergsma, D. (ed). 1974. *Ethical, Social and Legal Dimensions of Screening for Genetic Disease.* New York: Stratton.

Boone, C.K. 1988. "Bad axioms in genetic engineering," *Hastings Center Report,* 18,4:9–13.

Cann, R.L., Stoneking, M., and Wilson, A.C. 1987. "Mitochondrial DNA and human evolution," *Nature,* 325: 31–36.

Caplan, A.L. 1980. "The unnaturalness of aging—a sickness unto death?" in A. Caplan and H. Engelhardt, eds., *Concepts of Health and Disease.* Reading, Mass.: Addison-Wesley.

Chan, C.K. 1987. "Eugenics on the rise: a report from Singapore," in R. Chadwick, ed., *Ethics, Reproduction and Genetic Control,* London: Routledge: 164–172.

Chase, A. 1977. *The Legacy of Malthus.* New York: Knopf.

Chorover, S. L. 1979. *From Genesis to Genocide.* Cambridge: MIT Press.

Fletcher, J., and Wertz, D. 1988. *Ethics and Applied Human Genetics: A Cross Cultural Perspective.* Heidelberg: Springer-Verlag.

Goldman, A.H. 1980. *The Moral Foundations of Professional Ethics.* Totowa, NJ: Rowman and Littlefield.

Graham, L. 1978. "Attitudes toward eugenics and human heredity in Germany and the Soviet Union in the nineteen twenties" In H. Engelhardt and D. Callahan, eds., *Morals, Science and Sociality.* Hastings-on-Hudson, NY: Hastings Center: 119–49.

Hardin, G. 1977. *The Limits of Altruism.* Bloomington, Ind: Indiana University Press.

Harris, C.L. 1981. *Evolution: Genesis and Revelations.* Albany, NY: SUNY Press.

Hofstadter, R. 1955. *Social Darwinism in American Thought* (rev. ed.). Boston: Beacon.

Kamin, L.J. 1974, *The Science and Politics of IQ.* New York: Halstead.

Kass, L. 1975. "Regarding the end of medicine and the pursuit of health." *The Public Interest,* 40 (Summer).

Kevles, D.J. 1985. *In the Name of Eugenics.* Berkeley: University of California Press, 1985.

Lancet. 1989, i: 193–94.

Lappe, M. 1987. "The limits of genetic inquiry." *Hastings Center Report,* 17, 4:5–10.

McKusick, V. 1989. "Mapping and sequencing the human genome," *New England Journal of Medicine,* 320, 14: 910–915.

Midgely, M. 1978. *Beast and Man.* Ithaca: Cornell University Press.

Muller-Hill, B. 1988. *Murderous Science.* Oxford: Oxford University Press.

National Academy of Sciences. 1975. *Genetic Screening.* Washington: National Academy of Sciences Press.

National Academy of Sciences. 1986. *Biotechnology: An Industry Comes of Age.* Washington: National Academy Press.

National Research Council. 1988. *Mapping and Sequencing the Human Genome.* Washington: National Academy Press.

Office of Technology Assessment. 1988. *Mapping Our Genes.* Washington: USGPO.

Passmore, J. 1970. *The Perfectibility of Man.* New York: Scribners.

Proctor, R.N. 1988. *Racial Hygiene.* Cambridge: Harvard University Press.

Ramsey, P. 1970. *Fabricated Man.* New Haven: Yale University Press.

Reed, S. 1980. *Counseling in Medical Genetics.* New York: Alan R. Liss.

Rifkin, J. 1983. "Resolution," June 8, Foundation on Economic Trends.

Saltus, R. 1989. "Paradox in gene therapy debate," *Boston Globe.* February 6:31, 34.

Smith, G.P. 1988. "Biotechnology and the law: social responsibility or freedom of scientific inquiry?" *Mercer Law Review,* 39,2:437–60.

Sorenson, J.R., Swazey, J.P., and Scotch, N.A. 1982. *Reproductive Pasts, Reproductive Futures,* New York: Alan R. Liss.

Steinbrook, R. 1986. "In California, voluntary mass prenatal screening." *Hastings Center Report,* 16,5:5–7.

West, R. 1988. "Ethical aspects of genetic disease and genetic counseling" *Journal of Medical Ethics,* 14: 194–97.

Wilson, E.O. 1978 *On Human Nature.* Cambridge: Harvard University Press.

Wolper, L. 1989. "The social responsibility of scientists," *British Medical Journal:* 298, 941–43.

World Council of Churches. 1989. *Biotechnology: Its Challenges to Churches and the World,* Geneva, Switzerland.

World Medical Association. 1987. "Statement on genetic counseling and genetic engineering." *IME Bulletin,* 31: 8–9.

Part IV

Transplants and other
unnatural acts

9.

Requests, gifts, and obligations
The ethics of organ procurement

The inadequacy of present methods
of procuring organs

The field of organ transplantation has enjoyed remarkable progress since the 1960s. Early in the decade, the first attempt was made to transplant a kidney between identical twins. Since that initial attempt surgeons have perfected their techniques, immunologists have developed powerful new immunosuppressive drugs and tissue-matching capabilities, and health care professionals have learned how to manage the complications that often ensue once a transplant has been performed. Today it is possible to transplant many different organs and tissues using both cadaver and living sources to both related and nonrelated recipients. More than 400,000 transplants were performed in the United States in the 1980s, including kidneys, hearts, livers, corneas, skin, bone, and lungs.

As the ability to transplant organs and tissues has grown, the demand for these procedures has increased as well. In the early days of kidney transplant surgery the technique was seen as so experimental that many physicians would not even consider a transplant from a nonrelated or cadaver source.

While renal dialysis was developed primarily as an adjunct to kidney transplantation, the poor rates of success associated with transplant surgery in the early and mid-1960s led many physicians to recommend dialysis as the treatment of choice for those afflicted with renal failure who lacked a willing living donor. This was true despite the fact that dialysis itself was known to have many serious and even potentially lethal side-effects.[1]

As better surgical techniques and more powerful immunosuppressants were perfected and as success rates utilizing cadaver organs in nonrelated recipients improved, more and more individuals were viewed by their physicians as potential candidates for transplants. In the early days of the Stanford Heart Transplantation program it was unusual for someone over the age of 45 to receive a transplant. Today that age range has been extended to 55. Some centers believe that even this age restriction is merely arbitrary and have extended the pool of heart recipients to include those 60 and older.

The demand for organs and tissues from cadaver sources has grown to the point where it far exceeds the available supply. While approximately 5,500 kidneys were transplanted in the United States in 1984, the waiting lists at dialysis centers around the country included the names of more than 10,000 persons who were actively seeking a transplant. Similar shortfalls exist for those seeking corneas, livers, hearts, bone, and pancreases.

The gap between the supply of cadaver organs and the demand for them is not adequately reflected by figures citing those actually on waiting lists to receive an organ or tissue. Many potential recipients are not even placed on waiting lists.

Physicians are well aware of the fact that there is an insufficient supply of organs to meet the demand for them. They cope with the shortage by denying access even to waiting lists on the grounds that some possible recipients are medically unsuitable candidates. This "scientific" judgment is often based upon a hodgepodge of physical, economic, and psychosocial factors.[2]

The reality is that the waiting lists for cadaver organs have grown so long that a quiet form of triage is currently undertaken in order not to raise false hopes among those dying of organ failure. For infants and children the lack of cadaver donors is so severe that for many organs the only viable source of a transplant appears to be other species. There is little doubt that if more organs were available the lists of those deemed "medically suitable" for various types of transplants would expand dramatically.[3]

Many difficult ethical questions arise whenever scarce resources cannot be given to all who might benefit. It is not clear what standards or criteria should be followed when not all who might be helped can be helped.

Uncertainty about the principles to utilize in allocating the inadequate supply of organs from cadaver sources is further complicated by the growing suspicion that there are gross inequities in the way organs are currently being allocated by various transplant centers both in the United States and in other countries. Heated controversies have emerged about the moral acceptability of using what might be termed a "green screen" to select who will and will not be transplanted. Other debates have swirled around the revelations that some centers have given priority on their waiting lists to wealthy foreign nationals.

Issues of what constitutes just and equitable standards of allocation and a fair distribution of the enormous costs involved in transplantation are obviously complex and important. Furthermore, since there is likely to be a scarcity in the supply of cadaver organs for the foreseeable future, there is a real need for both professional and public discussion of the kinds of policies that should prevail in allocating organs to those in need.

Nonetheless, it is difficult to know how to address the matter of social and professional responsibility with respect to the allocation of organs unless one is certain about the degree to which something might be done to diminish the gap between supply and demand as well as about the moral presuppositions that govern organ donation. In order to know whether anyone or any group has a special claim upon organs and tissues, it is necessary to know the moral circumstances under which they were originally obtained. Before any serious argument can be entertained concerning the best policy to use to distribute scarce resources such as hearts and livers, it seems reasonable to make sure that our social policies are such as to maximize the supply of organs and tissues available for transplantation. Unfortunately, there are many reasons for believing that our system of organ procurement is not as efficient as it could be in obtaining organs from cadaver sources. Moreover, part of the reason for a lack of efficiency under the prevailing system is an inadequate examination of the moral status of organ donation.

It is generally estimated that about 100,000 persons die each year of accidents and strokes. Of this number about 20,000 are medically suitable candidates for organ or tissue donation.[4] While age and other medical criteria for acceptability severely limit the number who might serve as a donor of a heart, lung, or liver, most of this group could serve as a donor of bone, corneas, and other tissues.

Yet no more than 3,000 of this number actually served as a donor of any tissue or organ in 1984. Our present system of relying on voluntary donations as indicated on a "donor card" or living will on a driver's license, or the permission of a family member if the deceased's wishes are not known, yields no more than 15 percent to 20 percent of the available pool of donors of corneas, kidneys, and other life-saving and life-enhancing organs and tissues.[5]

The poor performance of the system is particularly disturbing in light of the enormous amount of time, money, and effort devoted to educating the American public about the importance of donation. Since recent advances and experiments in the field of transplantation have hardly been lacking in media coverage in recent years, there is little reason to assume that more time, money, and effort will significantly increase public awareness about organ donation. The fact is that the prevailing public policy established by the recommendations contained in the Uniform Anatomical Gift Act of 1968 has not worked. What I have termed elsewhere "encouraged voluntarism"— using public education to urge people to consider organ donation and to use donor cards to make their wishes known—has not been effective as a means of procuring organs from cadaver sources.[6,7]

Why has encouraged voluntarism failed?

The reasons for the failure of the policy of encouraged voluntarism are many. Most people still do not carry a donor card or other written directive governing the disposition of their bodies when they die. Only 20 percent of Americans have a signed donor card. In only a few states does the percent of persons completing a checkoff box on the driver's license exceed this figure. Some experts estimate that as few as 3 percent of all those who serve as organ donors are actually carrying a donor card at the time they are pronounced dead.

In one sense this is not surprising since most people are loath to contemplate their own deaths, much less make plans for the disposition of their property and bodies once they are gone. While it is all well and good to promote public education and awareness where organ donation is concerned, the fact remains that it is a subject that lacks intrinsic attraction for a large number of people.

Reservations and fears about death are not the only reasons for the low number of persons carrying written directives of some sort concerning organ donation. There are still some states where "brain death" has not been recognized by legislative statute as the definition of death. This leads to confusion on the part of both physicians and the public as to when and whether organ donation is appropriate.

The fact that health care has in recent years become increasingly centralized in large, impersonal, institutional facilities undercuts the trust that exists between patients and health care providers.[8] It is very difficult to trust in the good intentions of strangers, and many people are still afraid that if they carry a donor card they may not receive aggressive medical care if they need it.

The failure to secure high rates of compliance with respect to written directives and the mistrust of hospitals and health care providers are, however, only part of the explanation for low procurement rates. The reality of organ procurement in the United States today is that many hospitals fail to raise donation as a possibility when a death occurs. If hospital personnel do not wish to become involved in organ procurement for any reason—legal, economic, or simply out of laziness—they are under no obligation to do so. This means that even if a person has a donor card there is a good chance it will not be discovered since the possibility of donation is often not raised by those caring for the critically injured and the dying.[9]

The fact that many hospitals and physicians do not ask family members or legal guardians about organ donation means that the present system of encouraged voluntarism through written directives is not only ineffective in terms of obtaining organs and tissues, but it is ethically suspect as well. Those who carry donor cards may not have their desire to donate respected because no one bothers to locate their donor card or to ask family members about the existence of a card or written directive. Those who have not signed a written directive but who have no objection to donation will not be utilized because their family, friends, or guardians are not given the opportunity to consent to donation.

Even those who have objections to donation for religious or personal reasons cannot be assured that their wishes will be respected after their deaths under the present system. In Florida, tissues were taken from prisoners executed at the state prison without prior consent of the prisoners or the consent of their family members or legal representatives, highlighting the fact that prevailing public policy is not always adequate either with respect to honoring desires to donate or in not harvesting organs when possible objections exist.

Possible reforms of the existing policy for organ procurement

Present public policy based upon voluntary participation in organ procurement on the part of both the medical profession and potential donors and their families does not appear adequate in light of the current state of the art with respect to the successful transplantation of such organs as corneas, bones, kidneys, and hearts. These types of transplants work well, there are many persons currently in need of the procedures, and there are potentially thousands more who might benefits if the supply of organs could be increased.

It is important to realize that the prevailing policy of encouraged voluntarism utilizing written consent evolved at a time in the late 1960s when success rates for transplants utilizing cadaver donors were low, when the number of candidates awaiting such surgery was small, and when many of the potential donors of organs and tissues were alive rather than dead. Courts and legislatures were, during this period, rightly concerned with protecting the autonomy and free choice of living donors, especially children and mentally incompetent persons. The danger of coercing living donors against their will to undergo risky surgery of uncertain benefit as well as the need to guard against surreptitious removal of organs and tissue loomed large in the minds of those responsible for developing public policy with respect to organ procurement.

The Uniform Anatomical Gift Act, which was adopted in all fifty states and the District of Columbia during the early 1970s, made every effort to ensure that coercion and surreptitious harvesting of organs would be kept to a minimum. It insisted upon individual free and autonomous choice as the basis for donation from both living and cadaver sources.[10]

The question obviously arises as to whether a public policy that was formulated to cope with transplantation as it existed in the late 1960s is adequate for coping with transplantation today. Fifteen years ago most organs were obtained from living, related donors, but that is hardly true today. Fifteen years ago no form of transplantation was particularly successful. Today survival rates of cadaver grafts of hearts and kidneys have reached 50 percent at five years, a rate comparable to or better than that achieved with many other surgical and medical treatments. Fifteen years ago few persons were deemed medically able to withstand the rigors of a highly experimental surgical procedure. Today medical skills have evolved to the point where the very young, the old, the mentally ill, and those with various medical complications can be considered possible recipients of various types of transplants.

There are a number of social policy options that might be considered in seeking an alternative to the present policy of encouraged voluntarism. One is to allow a market in organs in order to encourage donations through financial incentives either to the living or to the next of kin of the dead. Another policy option is to modify public policy so that the burden of consent is shifted to those who do not wish to serve as donors. Rather than asking people to "opt in" to organ donation by carrying a written directive, we could simply require those who wish to "opt out" of donation to carry a written directive or so notify their next of kin.[6,11]

The problem with these alternatives is that they appear to subjugate individual autonomy and free choice to the socially useful purpose of obtaining more organs. Creating a market in organs would give incentives to the poor and disadvantaged to sell their body parts in ways that might adversely effect their health and well being. And even if markets were restricted to sales from the dead, the potential for conflict of interest among physician and patient, family members and the dying would appear to threaten the ability of individuals to do with their bodies as they wish.

Nor is there any guarantee that creating a market in organs would lead to an increase in the supply. Since some persons seeking organs are likely to be willing to pay any price in order to obtain them, the poor and the middle class might not be able to afford the huge amounts demanded by those with organs to sell. There are likely to be far fewer persons willing to give away what can in theory be sold for astronomical prices, so the overall effect of a market might actually be a decrease in the number of organs and tissues available for transplantation.

Putting the burden of proof on those with objections to organ procurement under a system of what is often termed presumed consent might yield more organs, but such a policy would be costly and difficult to administer. In order to assure the rights of every person to control his or her own body, it would be necessary to create a large and centralized registry that could be rapidly searched when a death occurred. The system would also have to be continuously updated to allow for modifications in the desires of each individual.

Most worrisome from an ethical point of view is that a policy of presumed consent can protect the rights of those opposed to transplant only by forcing them to indicate in some public manner their objections to the harvesting of organs. In order to assure that procurement is limited to only those without objections, it would be necessary to require each person with objections to record publicly their unwillingness to serve as a donor since this is the only way to assure compliance with their wishes. Ironically an approach intended to protect free choice might well hinder autonomous behavior rather than encourage it, since those with objections would have to state them and state them publicly rather than having the right to make no decision or to leave the decision to others if a tragedy were to occur.

A viable policy alternative: required request

There are many reasons, both ethical and practical, for skepticism about either a market or presumed consent as policy alternatives to the current policy of encouraged voluntarism. Perhaps the most serious of all is that neither of these policies takes seriously the fact that the low yield of organs obtained in the United States from cadaver sources is not attributable to the unwillingness of Americans to help those in need of transplants. If public opinion surveys can be trusted, most Americans still believe that transplantation is important, and they indicate a willingness to serve as a donor or to have a loved one donate. More impressive still are the figures associated with actual consent rates when family members are asked their permission for donation. In some hospitals, well over 60 percent of those families asked consent to donation. While one might raise questions about the competency of those asked to give a truly valid consent to donation in light of the terrible circumstances they face when an unexpected death occurs, the fact remains that the level of altruism on the part of the public in both theory and deed is high. The problem is that encouraged voluntarism using donor cards does not seem to be able to tap this powerful sentiment. A policy of a free market in buying and selling organs simply overlooks this valuable moral source of organs. A policy of presumed consent recognizes the prevailing desire of most people to help others upon their deaths but removes the moral dignity of donation by making it mandatory.

There is another way of modifying existing policy that would respect the dignity and value of individual choice while at the same time holding out the prospect of greatly increasing the number of organs and tissues obtained from cadaver sources for transplantation. It is a policy option that seems far more consistent with the contemporary realities of transplantation both in terms of need and efficacy.

If each state were to modify its existing law with respect to organ donation to require that family members or guardians be given the opportunity to make a donation when a death has occurred, this might go a long way toward both increasing the supply of available organs and tissues from cadaver sources as well as maximizing the opportunity for free choice where the harvesting of organs for transplantation or other purposes is concerned.

This policy option, which I have dubbed "required request,"[7,12] would restrict voluntarism but only on the part of hospitals and health care providers, not individual prospective donors and their families. A policy of required request would mandate that hospitals be responsible for designating an appropriately trained person to inquire about organ donation at the time death is pronounced. Such a request would be noted in writing on every death certificate in order to assure full and zealous compliance with the policy. A required request approach can permit exceptions to requests when there is reason to believe that a request would not be in the best interest of the next of kin of the deceased, but these exceptions would also have to be noted in writing on the death certificate.

A policy of legally mandating requests at the time of death addresses many of the failings of the current approach to cadaver organ procurement. It maximizes the opportunity to make a donation by way of a donor card or written directive since it ensures that some effort will be made by health professionals and family members to find a donor card if one exists. When no card exists, a required request approach allows families and guardians to make donations that now are simply lost due to a failure to ask.

Most importantly, routinizing a policy of requests for organ donation when death is pronounced will help ensure that better decisions are made about organ donation. If requests are customary and therefore routine, the public will soon come to expect such requests as a normal part of the process of death in hospital settings. By creating such an expectation, members of the public can be encouraged to discuss their wishes with family members, friends, or legal guardians in order to assure compliance with their wishes. Rather than coming as a surprise, as is now all too often the case, requests for donation would be routine. The decisions that are made would therefore be more likely to reflect the values and choices of all parties involved rather than the desperate, pressured reactions of unprepared and grief-stricken family members.

A policy of requiring requests about donation does give family members greater say in the process of organ donation if for no other reason than their greater involvement in terms of gross numbers in considering requests. However, there is no reason to assume that a required request policy will threaten or infringe upon the rights of individuals to control the disposition of their tissues and organs.

Family members would still be bound to honor the known objections of their loved ones to organ donation if such objections exist. They would also be responsible for helping to locate donor cards or call to the attention of health care providers the oral statements of the deceased about donation. Since most persons do not carry cards or complete written directives, a policy of required request places the burden of considering donation squarely on family members. Since these persons are generally responsible for the disposition of the body, there is little reason to assume that adding an additional inquiry about organ donation will constitute an undue burden when death occurs.

A final benefit of a required request policy is that it adds an additional level of protection for those with objections to organ donation. By requiring requests of family or guardians, individuals who are opposed to donation are afforded greater protection that nothing will be done to their bodies that they would not want done were they in a position to make their views known. This protection can be optimized by simply restricting donations to those cases in which family or guardians (or donor cards) can be located.

A policy of required request aims directly at the altruism that plausibly exists on the part of the public with respect to organ donation. It attempts to realize the effects of this altruism by ensuring that someone will ask about donation when a death occurs. The policy respects individual choice but also acknowledges the fact that giving will not occur unless someone remembers to ask.

Organ donation—charity or obligation?

Requiring requests about organ donation when death occurs is a policy that will help increase the supply of organs available from cadaver sources. However there is another aspect of the present system for procuring organs that merits examination if the number of organs available is to increase drastically.

For many years the rhetoric of public education in the organ procurement field has been that of charity. The public is constantly being urged through public service advertisements in magazines, in newspapers, and on radio and television to "make the gift of life."

What is interesting about the language of gifts in the area of organ donation is that the moral force of such language is not particularly strong. Gifts are a form of charity. Most moral theories recognize a strong moral obligation or duty not to harm others. But few theories posit the existence of an obligation or duty to give gifts to other people. Gift-giving behavior is viewed as morally laudable, even heroic, but it is not often seen as mandatory.[13]

The question raised by the use of the language of gifts in the context of organ donation is whether our society really wants to view donation exactly as that. Is organ donation a matter of preference and whim like some forms of gift giving? Or is it a morally superrogatory act—praiseworthy and admirable but not something we can reasonably expect people to do?

One way of answering these questions is to examine the ways in which positive obligations or duties to aid other people are usually generated. Some duties to help others arise as a result of particular roles or jobs in society. Fire fighters, parents, and nurses all have special duties to render positive aid to others even when helping requires sacrifice and even risk.

Another way in which duties to help others can arise is through the act of contracting or promising. I can voluntarily promise to help someone else if the need should arise, and I can be blamed for my failure to do so under the appropriate circumstances.

Unfortunately, neither of these positive obligations seems applicable to the situation that prevails with respect to organ donation. Unless I have promised to donate an organ to another and have reneged on my promise, there would seem to be no ground for saying that I ought to be an organ donor in any sense stronger than charity.

There is, however, another way in which duties to help others can go beyond exceptional cases of charity or gift giving. If it is possible for someone to do a great deal of good for another person without facing the prospect of a great deal of risk or even inconvenience, and if there is a strong likelihood of benefit for the recipient, most philosophers and theologians would argue that a duty to help arises that is stronger than the relatively weak obligations associated with charity and other generous acts.[13,14] If, for example, a strong swimmer can save the life of a drowning child merely by swimming twenty feet out into a calm lake, it would seem morally reprehensible and blameworthy for the swimmer not to do so. Indeed, it would seem odd to describe such a rescue as a charitable act or even a gift from the swimmer to the drowning child!

Much more discussion and debate are in order with respect to organ donation. Is donation closer to an obligation of the sort described above than it is to an extraordinary act of moral beneficence or charity? If it is true that many people can be helped by an increase in the supply of organs, and if it is also true that the dead can suffer no harm through the utilization of their tissues and organs for transplantation or other educational or research purposes, then is it correct to describe a decision to donate as a gift that is praiseworthy if offered but not blameworthy if withheld or as an obligation that is both?

It is possible that different people may answer the question about the moral status of organ donation differently; however, the time has surely come for encouraging debate about whether a reevaluation of the prevailing moral rhetoric of gift giving is in order. In order for this discussion to come about, both health care providers and other citizens will have to make every effort to reassure the general public that organs that are obtained are distributed fairly and efficiently. While it is true that allocation criteria are closely tied both to the availability of organs and to the system used to obtain them, it is also true that the connection between the ethics of procurement and allocation is reciprocal. Few people will feel obligated to help those in need if they perceive inequities in the system used to designate exactly who is most in need and most deserving.

References

1. Caplan, A. *J Health Politics, Policy, Law* 6:488, 1981.

2. Caplan, A. *Br Med J* 283:727, 1982.

3. Evans, R. et. al. National Heart Transplantation Study. Final Report. Seattle. Battelle Human Affairs Research Centers, 1985.

4. Bart, K. et al. *Transplantation* 31:383, 1981.

5. Caplan, A., Bayer, R. Ethical, Legal and Policy Issues Pertaining to Solid Organ Procurement. New York, Empire Blue Cross/Blue Shield, 1985.

6. Caplan, A. *Hastings Center Rep* 13:23, 1983.

7. Caplan, A. *Hastings Center Rep* 14:6, 1984.

8. Starr, P. *The Social Transformation of American Medicine.* New York, Basic. 1984.

9. Prottas, J. Obtaining Replacements. Hearings on Organ Transplants before the Subcommittee on Investigations and Oversight of the Committee on Science and Technology. U.S. House of Representatives, April 1983, pp. 714–751.

10. Sadler, A., Sadler, B. *Hastings Center Rep* 14:6, 1984.

11. Dukeminier, J., Sanders, D. *New Engl J Med* 280:862, 1969.

12. Caplan, A. *Midwest Med Ethics* 1:2, 1985.

13. Beauchamp, T., Childress, J. *Principles of Biomedical Ethics.* New York, Oxford, 1979.

14. Goodin, R. *Protecting the Vulnerable.* Chicago, University of Chicago Press, 1985.

10.

If I were a rich man could I buy a pancreas? Problems in the policies and criteria used to allocate organs for transplantation in the United States

I. The fragility of societal support for transplantation

Those in the field of transplantation have many reasons for taking pride in their field. In 1950 solid organ transplantation was a fantasy. In 1960 the kidney was the only vital organ that could be transplanted, since transplants could be performed only between living, genetically identical siblings. In 1970 liver and heart transplantation from cadaver sources were in their infancy, and it was far from certain that they would ever make it to maturity.

Only since 1980 has Cyclosporine emerged as a major weapon

in controlling rejection, initial attempts have been made to transplant lungs and multiple organs, the first attempt was made to perform a heart xenograft in an infant, the first successful infant heart transplants were performed, the first partial liver transplants in children were performed, and the first successful heart transplant using an infant with anencephaly as a donor was accomplished. Heart-lung, kidney, pancreas, and non-related transplants were introduced and are becoming established, if still innovative, therapeutic options. Better drugs and technologies for storing organs, reversing acute rejection, transporting organs, and performing antigen screening and typing have been found.

The field has also seen numerous advances in public policy and legislation since 1980. Forty-eight states have either laws or appellate court decisions recognizing brain death. Numerous state and federal laws aimed at increasing the supply of organs available for transplantation have been enacted (Caplan, 1986). Medicare has expanded its coverage to include heart and liver transplants. A national network for obtaining and allocating organs has come into being.

These are wondrous achievements. They have taken place in what is, from the point of view of both the history of medicine and public policy, the blink of an eye.

But no one in or outside the field of transplantation should be lulled into complacency by these accomplishments. The entire practice of organ transplantation rests upon a very fragile base—the willingness of the public to support the procurement of organs for transplantation to others (Caplan, 1983; Caplan and Bayer, 1985; Caplan, 1986). Transplantation also relies upon the willingness of the public to pay—either directly through tax-supported public programs or, indirectly, through private insurance plans—the tremendous costs associated with organ transplants. There are, sadly, important reasons to worry that the public trust requisite for both the provision of organs and the money to pay for them is eroding.

There has been no public enthusiasm for proposals to grant physicians the authority to remove organs from cadavers whenever others might benefit prior to returning control of the body to next of kin. Even so-called "presumed consent" policies, which merely shift the burden of organ procurement from an "opt in" system to an "opt out" approach, have generated no groundswell of public support (Caplan, 1983).

The public has accepted the concept of brain death but still remains wary of the process by which it is diagnosed. How many Americans still hesitate to check the box on their driver's license indicating they will be donors, how many refuse to carry a donor card for fear that they will not receive aggressive care should they wind up in an emergency room? Fears and doubts are expressed about proposals to routinely utilize infants born with anencephaly as organ donors. Are doctors killing infants to take their parts? What infants with congenital defects will surgeons target next as prospective organ donors? These fears show how much the public distrusts the transplant community (Caplan, 1989a).

Most disturbing of all is the failure of the public, including the medical community outside the realm of transplantation, to support organ donation (Caplan, 1988b; Caplan and Welvang, 1989b). Positive responses to requests to donate average about 25 percent. In many states physicians and nurses are simply refusing to comply with newly created state and federal laws requiring that the option of donation be offered when a death occurs in a hospital setting (Caplan and Welvang, 1989b).

The trust that is essential for public support is a product of a key ethical value—equity. The values of altruism and autonomy—the foundations of organ procurement—rest on the presumption that organs which are given freely, voluntarily, and altruistically will be distributed in a fair and impartial manner to those in need. Any policies, practices, or activities that suggest otherwise imperil the entire enterprise of organ donation and, thus, transplantation. There is sufficient evidence of inequity in the allocation of organs to raise doubts about the fairness of the existing system.

The ever-present news stories (Caplan, 1987; Aleshire, 1989) of families desperately seeking funds, begging for money to pay for transplants, leave an especially bitter taste in the mouths of a public that expects altruism. What must the impact on the public be of spectacles such as that of Coby Howard of Oregon and Danny Bradley of Texas dying while trying to raise money to qualify for admission to a transplant center? If organs are taken from the rich and poor alike but given only to the rich, how long can we expect the public to support transplantation with either organs or money?

Stories about families who have used publicity to manipulate their access to transplants—sometimes intentionally, sometimes inadvertently—do nothing to convince the public that equity prevails in the distribution of organs for transplantation. When the public sees that a family can go on a national television program and secure a heart for their dying child ahead of other children with equal or more critical needs (Caplan, 1985), or when they read stories about Soviet citizens coming to the United States to seek heart-lung transplants when Americans in need of the very same operation are not deemed worthy of publicity either by transplant centers or by the media (Aleshire, 1989), questions naturally arise about the fairness of the procedures and criteria used by surgeons, hospitals, and medical centers to select transplant recipients.

The question of whether the allocation of organs for transplantation is equitable is not based only on anecdotes. An impressive number of papers have appeared in the past few years in professional journals, some of which have received prominent attention in the media, maintaining that women, the elderly, the disabled, the retarded, and minorities are not represented in the ranks of those receiving transplants to the extent that they could and should be (Blakeslee, 1989; Kifner, 1988b; Kjellstrand, 1988; Van Thiel et al., 1988; Arenson and Forde, 1989; Held et al., 1988; Coburn, 1988; Jonasson, 1989; Monaco, 1989).

Policies which give priority of access to patients on artificial hearts or requiring multiple organ transplants or retransplantation leave plenty of room for doubt about what values are being used to allocate scarce organs. Explicit policies at some centers which exclude those who are alcoholic, mentally ill, severely retarded, poor or elderly from the prospective recipient pool (Coburn, 1988; Kifner, 1988b; Van Thiel et al., 1988) give further reason for doubt about equity in the allocation of organs.

Even seemingly objective medical criteria such as antigen matching can produce inequities in who can and cannot obtain a transplant. The emphasis on tissue matching in evolving United Network for Organ Sharing (UNOS) policies means that, de facto, minority groups are at a disadvantage in receiving transplants due to the underrepresentation of minorities in the donor pool and the difficulty of doing accurate tissue typing for rare antigens (Van Buren et al., 1988; Salvatierra, 1988; UNOS, 1989; Starzl, 1989).

Even the fact that so many hospitals and medical centers have rushed into the transplant field raises legitimate doubts about the fairness of the system for distributing organs. The United States now has more than 125 centers doing heart transplants. The competition in some states and cities between these centers is certainly not in the public interest. Few persons can be found who think that the United States needs more than 125 centers doing heart transplants or that this number of centers will assure the most efficient and equitable use of the scarce supply of donor hearts.

No other country has anything close to our ratio of heart transplant centers to inhabitants. Yet the proportionate volume of transplants done and the success rates in the Netherlands (3 centers), Germany (12 centers), Canada (8 centers), Sweden (3 centers), Switzerland (2 centers), and France (14 centers) are not significantly different from those which prevail in this country (Transplant Lifelines, 1989).

The demonstration or even the suggestion that the allocation of organs is based on bias, prejudice, favoritism, greed, or publicity is enough to destroy public confidence that the system is equitable. Flat or falling rates of organ donation (Callender, 1987; Caplan and Welvang, 1989b) may indicate that the public's confidence is weakening.

II. Is it really fair to give everyone in need an equal chance to get a transplant?

In order to know whether the distribution of organs for transplants in the United States is fair and equitable, it is not sufficient to look at data on who did and did not get transplanted in any given year. This information is necessary but not sufficient for evaluating the fairness of the distribution.

All that any pattern of distribution proves is that there may be reason for concern about inequity. The underrepresentation of minorities, women, the poor, the disabled, or the elderly in the ranks of transplant recipients might be unfortunate but it might not be unfair (Engelhardt, 1986).

In order to know whether the distribution of organs is fair, it is necessary to know the pattern of need for transplants. If every person is at equal risk of end-stage organ failure, or if those who actually suffer organ failure of various kinds represent a microcosm of the overall American population, then any deviation from this average in the distribution of organs gives reason for concern about fairness.

A final assessment of the equity of the distribution of organs will depend upon an examination of the criteria and rules (or lack of them) being followed by transplant centers. It might be fair to give men more organs than women or whites fewer organs than blacks if the allocation were based on a set of criteria and rules that men and women and blacks and whites could all agree are fair, even if the rules work to the disadvantage of some persons or groups.

It may be fair to give every American who has organ failure an equal chance at a transplant. Or it may not. The answer to what is fair will depend upon the reasons that are given for following policies that produce anything other than a purely egalitarian distribution of organs, a distribution in which everyone, or perhaps everyone in need, has exactly the same chance of getting a transplant (Priester and Caplan, 1989). Fairness will also depend upon the degree to which the public has been given a chance to review existing policies and to hold those who use them accountable.

Most theories of justice accept distributions in which not everyone gets an equal share of a resource as fair. Some argue that, as long as everyone has an equal chance at getting a minimal share of goods and services, then outcomes which vary from pure egalitarian distributions are fair. Other theories of justice hold that those with the greatest need are entitled to the greatest share or to priority in access to scarce resources. Still other theories of justice accept some inequality in distribution if the inequity is aimed at rewarding merit, benefiting the least well off or maximizing the common good. The real issues in thinking about fairness with respect to organ transplants are what reasons govern the policies that exist, whose values they reflect, and what means exist for challenging the policies and for holding those who enforce them to account.

III. Who gets a transplant?

In asking what criteria, policies, and procedures are used to allocate organs, it is tempting to seek the answer by examining what happens to a particular organ that is donated or what decisions are made on any given day in the case of a particular transplant program. But looking only at such situations conveys a very misleading impression of how allocation decisions are actually made.

The question of who gets organs is a function of numerous factors. How many transplant programs there are, how many organ donors there are, what standards exist for evaluating the suitability of organs for transplant, and a host of other variables. It is simply wrong to suppose that any one person or organization determines who will receive a transplant and who will not.

But more important is the fact that we cannot evaluate the fairness of organ allocation—or even come to understand the criteria used to allocate organs—simply by watching what various surgeons or transplant centers actually do when they have the opportunity to transplant a donated organ. Transplant centers, and the surgeons who administer particular organ transplant programs within them, need to deal only with those patients who have actually made it through their doors. But many potential recipients never appear on any center's waiting list. The most important ethical decisions about allocation take place long before an organ actually arrives to be used at a particular transplant center.

IV. How big is the top end of the funnel?— eligibility for transplants

Perhaps the best metaphor for describing the process by which people are deemed potential recipients for organ transplantation is a funnel (see figure). At the top end of the funnel are all those who are seen as possible candidates for transplantation.

At first it might seem obvious that only those persons whom surgeons view as being in need of a transplant will be present at the top of the funnel. But this is not so. The number of persons at the top end of the funnel is determined by public opinion, the availability of doctors capable of diagnosing end-stage organ failure, political considerations, individual self-perceptions of health, and general beliefs within the medical community about the utility of various kinds of transplants.

We often assume that the pool of persons who might receive transplants is limited only to American citizens. But of course this need not be true.

The pool of potential recipients of transplants in the United

The funnel of organ allocation

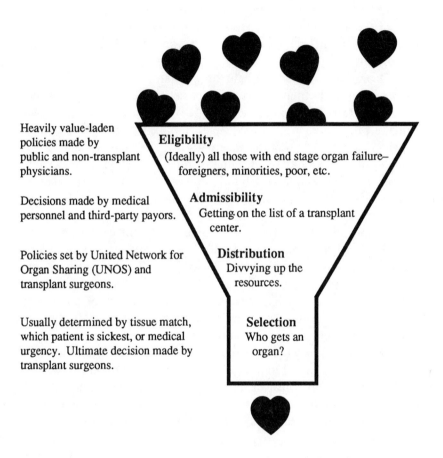

Heavily value-laden policies made by public and non-transplant physicians.

Eligibility
(Ideally) all those with end stage organ failure– foreigners, minorities, poor, etc.

Decisions made by medical personnel and third-party payors.

Admissibility
Getting on the list of a transplant center.

Policies set by United Network for Organ Sharing (UNOS) and transplant surgeons.

Distribution
Divvying up the resources.

Usually determined by tissue match, which patient is sickest, or medical urgency. Ultimate decision made by transplant surgeons.

Selection
Who gets an organ?

States often includes resident aliens and even illegal aliens. Some people living elsewhere do manage to obtain transplants in the United States as well.

In fact the potential pool of prospective recipients who could be put into the top end of the transplant funnel includes anyone in the world with end-stage organ failure, whether diagnosed by a doctor or not. Of course we rarely consider those dying of kidney, heart, or liver failure in Bangladesh, the Sudan, Paraguay, or Chad as eligible for consideration as a transplant candidate at a transplant center in the U.S. Our focus at the top end of the funnel is on Americans.

But the decision to think about Americans as exhausting the pool of those eligible for transplantation is entirely a political decision. When it suits our purposes, we can and do modify the boundaries of eligibility.

Occasionally, the president or a senator will go to some faraway (and usually medically impoverished) land and return with a child who desperately needs a transplant. When there is a disaster and the provision of advanced medical care ties in with our own political agenda—as was the case with the 1989 earthquake in Armenia—then Soviet citizens dying of renal failure may be deemed eligible for treatments they could not have hoped to receive in their own country or here under any circumstances only a few years earlier.

A hospital administrator at a large transplant center once permitted me to listen in on one end of a phone call between him and a high-ranking official in the State Department. The government official wanted a resident of an important Middle Eastern nation admitted for a kidney transplant because he was a relative of one of the leaders of that nation. The State Department official said it was in our national interest to give this man priority for a transplant. And he was given top priority for an operation that otherwise would not have been available to him. Eligibility is very much a function of what are indisputably non-medical criteria such as beliefs about the obligations we do or do not have to try to help those from other countries or what uses of our medical capacities we think serve our national interests.

Medical assessment and opinion also play key roles in determining eligibility. It is just that they do so in ways very different from what surgeons do in trying to decide whom to transplant on a given day at their hospitals and medical centers.

Few people, even very sick people, go directly to a transplant center. In many cases those who need transplants are not even aware that they have a serious medical problem that might be amenable to treatment by transplantation. Those who get transplants almost always arrive in a transplant program as a result of a diagnosis by and a referral from a physician outside the program. Eligibility for transplantation is controlled and determined in large measure by doctors who normally have no direct connection with or special expertise in transplantation.

If one has no doctor—and since more than 30 million Americans have no health insurance, it seems fair to assume that there are many who do not—eligibility for transplantation may never become an option since no referral may be made. Or if one's doctor is not up on the latest breakthroughs in transplantation (say, in fields such as pancreas, heart-lung or single lung transplants) or if he or she holds values which lead to the belief that the chance of a high quality of life associated with a particular type of transplant is too uncertain (say, in an area such as infant heart transplantation), then no referral may occur. Referrals play a critical role in determining who does and does not get a chance at a transplant.

Money can play a role too. Doctors who have a vested interest in providing one form of therapy (say, renal dialysis) may not have as great an interest as they should in suggesting alternative forms of therapy (say, kidney transplants) to those in their care. Some doctors, knowing their patient lacks insurance or cannot hope to pay the costs of a lifetime on immunosuppressive drugs, simply do not raise a transplant as an option.

Personality can influence referral patterns as well. Patients who do not raise questions and seek out options or who are shy, fearful, non-compliant, or even abusive may not be referred with the same zeal and enthusiasm as are other prospective candidates.

Little is known about the criteria which determine referral patterns for consideration for a transplant in the United States. However, one recent survey of medical directors of dialysis facilities and kidney transplant programs (Kifner, 1988b) indicates that the majority weigh factors such as the psychological stability of prospective patients, age, quality of life, the availability of a supportive family, the cost of treatment, the need to advance knowledge through research, patient motivation, and even the social value of the patient to society in making decisions about access. If these values appear in the selection criteria for admission to dialysis facilities and if transplant directors say they weigh them as well, then it must be presumed that a large number of those making referrals take manifestly non-medical factors into account (also see Kjellstrand, 1987, and Bermel, 1983).

V. Getting into a transplant center—
Admissibility

The next stage in the process of narrowing the funnel, is that of admission to a particular transplant center's waiting list. There are many factors that influence admissibility, although again they have not been extensively or systematically studied (Caplan, 1987).

Age, geography, ability to pay, patient and referring doctor perseverance, whether someone is an interesting or unusual case, whether someone has the disease qualifications to enter into an ongoing research study, the presence of disability or mental illness, the availability of a supportive family, and having a "good" psychosocial profile—including the right (positive and, once in a while, grateful!) attitude—all play important roles (Kifner, 1988b).

There is no consistent set of standards for admission to organ (or tissue) transplant programs. Those who are referred but turned down may continue to "shop" for a center which will accept them. While there are sound reasons for some of the variations in admissions standards, their existence gives the public the impression that the pettiness or arrogance of providers can be decisive in determining who gains admission to a program.

Personal resources play a role too, since it is still possible for those in need to try and seek admission to more than one transplant center. It is not clear how many potential recipients pursue what can be a very expensive strategy, but some do. Pursuing multiple listings at different transplant centers is advantageous since different centers follow different allocation standards and many centers attempt to place organs they procure with patients on their own waiting lists before offering them to other centers. The ability to pursue multiple listing is not only expensive, but it is inherently unfair since only those with the resources to visit more than one center can gain the advantages conferred by being placed on lists at more than one center.

The gatekeepers who make admissions decisions at this stage of the allocation process have many identities. Many centers and hospitals operate with teams who regularly assess potential patients referred to them for suitability. More than purely surgical expertise is invoked since such teams often include social workers, transplant coordinators, psychologists, and psychiatrists. These teams each have their own medical criteria for admission. But there is more involved in the decision to admit than a medical diagnosis and evaluation.

Representatives of the business office, boards of trustees, institutional review boards (IRBs), ethics committees, local legislators, and third-party payors all have some say about who should or should not be taken into a particular program (Laudicina, 1988). All too often medical evaluations are recast for the purpose of persuading payors or the business office that a prospective patient really will benefit from access to a transplant. An operation that is described as experimental for the IRB is often termed "therapeutic" for the purposes of securing third-party payment for the person in need.

Admission decisions are closely tied to the experience of the transplant center and transplant team. The established centers pride themselves on taking on the hard cases, and often they do. However, the hardest cases sometimes wind up at the newest programs because these programs are competing against established programs and cannot attract referrals from physicians who want to send their patients to more established programs.

VI. Distribution: divvying up organs among centers and patients

Once someone has been entered on at least one waiting list, the process of allocation is then governed by two sets of distribution rules; those that exist in the particular hospital and those set by the United Network for Organ Sharing (UNOS).

UNOS, contrary to the hopes of some Federal legislators, and despite the claims of certain journalists, plays an important but still subordinate role in setting the rules governing the distribution of organs in the United States. UNOS has not claimed—and probably cannot yet get—total authority with respect to the distribution of organs among those on waiting lists at various transplant centers.

Individual transplant centers, despite the existence of UNOS, frequently claim first rights over organs they procure. Too many transplant programs in many parts of the country still view organs which they procure as "theirs" even if other centers might be able to make better use of them (Cicciarelli, Terasaki, and Mickey, 1987; Opelz, 1988).

This distribution policy has the advantage of giving individual centers an incentive to aggressively pursue organ donations. But it is a policy that also fails to assure that those who might be best suited to receive a particular organ actually receive it.

It is only when eligibility, admissibility, and distribution have been settled that a person actually becomes a candidate for selection for a transplant. The criteria and policies used in selection (the final stage in the process) are determined by individual transplant surgeons. The criterion that most surgeons and transplant teams have followed for decades is that of treating the sickest patients first when allowed to do so by the biology of the available donor organ. But exceptions to this criterion abound.

Consider a simple but relatively common example. The sickest patient in the pancreas transplant program may be so sick that only the best surgeon could hope to succeed with the case. But if that surgeon is sick, on vacation, or is too tired from a previous operation, then, even if a well-matched organ of the right size is available, the sickest patient may not get the transplant, a situation which is unfortunate but not unfair.

The allocation of organs moves through a process that involves four stages—eligibility, admissibility, distribution, and selection. Any assessment of the fairness of the current system for distributing organs must not simply look at the pattern of organ distribution among those getting transplants but also examine the values and principles that prevail at each of these stages in the allocation process.

VII. What are some of the policies, principles, and values at work at different stages in the process of allocating organs?

The overriding value that seems to govern eligibility is nationality. We simply do not make our scarce medical resources available to most of those who might benefit. Some argue that this is reasonable since what we should do is export the means to do transplants to nations that cannot do them (Evans, 1986). But this is not self-evidently the best policy to pursue. It might be more cost efficient to bring potential transplant patients here while at the same time exporting much cheaper public health programs to medically underdeveloped nations.

The moral norm which dominates the American view of eligibility is that we are obliged to take care of our own citizens first. In part, this view is linked to the values which govern the system we have for obtaining organs. Americans should be first in line for consideration as eligible recipients because we think that, ideally, altruism ought to be reciprocal—we feel a duty to share organs with those who are willing to share them with us.

For the most part, this means involving only North American donors and recipients. But our view of eligibility, insofar as it is tied to a tacit belief about the importance of reciprocity with respect to altruism, might well change in the near future. Emerging technologies will soon make it possible to procure, ship, and store organs anywhere in the world. But, whether our view of the importance of nationality does or does not change regarding eligibility for transplants, it is important to realize that it is a policy that has nothing to do with medical criteria. It is a moral view that, despite much rhetoric to the contrary, does not place an equal value on the worth of each human life.

The other major variable determining eligibility is the set of norms that governs referrals. One critically important variable is whether or not those in need of a transplant have a doctor who is both competent enough to know they might be benefitted and honest enough to fairly present transplantation as an option regardless of his or her own financial interests and personal views of the risk–benefit ratio facing the prospective patient (Bermel, 1983; Kjellstrand, 1988).

Since the poor, the uninsured, and the under-insured do not have the same access to high-quality primary medical care as do other members of our society, they are less likely to be referred for consideration at transplant centers or will be referred at a later stage of their disease than other patients are. The disabled and the elderly are not referred for consideration at the rates one would expect from the incidence of end-stage organ failure in these groups. The under-representation of the elderly, the disabled, and minorities on waiting lists is probably a result either of a lack of access to competent primary care or of substantive value disagreements between doctors and their patients about the value of a transplant for some members of these groups.

Money plays a major role in determining admissibility to waiting lists at hospitals and transplant centers in the United States. The rich and those who have comprehensive medical insurance have a better chance of being referred and admitted to transplant programs than do those who cannot demonstrate the ability to pay. Since health insurance is often provided in our society as a benefit of employment, those who are unemployed, who do not qualify for Medicaid but have an income below the legal definition of poverty, who work part-time or who are self-employed—in other words, the poor, minorities, the chronically ill, the disabled, and women—are at a significant disadvantage in gaining access to transplant centers. Unless our society wants to argue that the rich are entitled to easier access to the pool of altruistically donated organs and to explain this moral point of view to all potential organ donors and their families, the current underrepresentation of minorities, women, the elderly, and the handicapped in the recipient pool for transplants relative to their rates of end-stage organ failure is not an unfortunate or unlucky circumstance, it is simply unfair.

The criteria that dominate decisions about allocation at the levels of eligibility and admissibility are heavily weighted toward non-medical factors. Indeed, once the critical role of decision-making in determining the pool of candidates for transplants is understood, it is easy to see why non-medical factors predominate. The criteria that prevail at the levels of distribution and actual patient selection are also heavily value-laden.

The policies that have evolved to govern both distribution and patient selection are strongly weighted toward factors such as the following: size of donor organ and of recipient, blood and tissue matching, medical urgency, time on the waiting list, and logistics (UNOS, 1989; Salvatierra, 1988). Similar policies prevail at most centers for assigning priority to patients on waiting lists from week to week and from day to day.

There is no firm consensus within the transplant field about the importance of tissue matching for the success or failure of various forms of transplantation. Many transplant teams believe that tissue type plays a crucial role in determining the chances for a successful transplant, especially with respect to kidneys. Others believe that minor tissue mismatches can easily be overcome through prudent immunosuppression.

It is interesting to note that tissue typing has emerged as a critical variable for distributing kidneys that are offered to the national network (many are not, since they are used locally or regionally). Arguments in favor of tissue typing focus on the implication of close matches for efficacy. However, existing UNOS policies do not give equal emphasis to other factors that are associated with unfavorable outcomes such as being overweight, having lupus or diabetes or psychosocial facts concerning particular patients (e.g., Is this patient on the list because he or she elected to stop taking immunosuppressive medications? Is the candidate a drug addict?).

Emphasizing tissue type has the advantage of allowing an objective standard to be invoked in allocating organs. It is a standard which is relatively easy to assess and monitor. Other factors such as the existence of comorbid states or psychosocial complications are more difficult to assess and monitor.

However, the high priority given to tissue matching in current distribution policies may be more a function of the need to find a clear, objective, and nearly indisputable standard than it is the result of a well-established association with successful outcome. Furthermore, the cost of emphasizing tissue type in distributing kidneys in the national pool is to penalize those waiting for organs who have either rare (and sometimes hard to analyze) tissue types or who are members of racial groups for whom there are few closely matched donors. If there is no empirical basis or only a very weak one for the importance of tissue matching in determining successful outcomes (Starzl, 1989), then a distribution policy which emphasizes tissue type unfairly penalizes those with rare tissue types—minorities.

The other factor which seems to drive patient selection is medical urgency (Stevenson et al., 1987; UNOS, 1989). Both UNOS policies and individual transplant center policies tend to give priority to those who are in the greatest need of a transplant, "need" being defined as the likelihood of the patient dying unless a transplant is performed.

Such a policy can be defended as fair since medical urgency is not known to correlate with any particular characteristic of those patients waiting for transplant. People with a failing vital organ can suddenly take a turn for the worse and find themselves at death's door.

But is a policy which gives priority to the sickest fair? Does it represent the most prudent use of scarce, life-saving resources?

If one thinks of similar situations in which life-saving resources are in scarce supply, deciding whom to care for on the battlefield or who will receive food and water on a lifeboat, a strong case can be made for considering principles of distribution other than who is most likely to die. Indeed, following policies which favor those most likely to die in these situations would probably be seen as both unfair and illogical.

In facing rationing decisions (Priester and Caplan, 1989), there are many possible principles that can be used to allocate scarce, life-saving resources. There are theories of justice which would direct resources to those most likely to benefit from them, to those who are seen as most deserving, to those who are seen as likely to make the greatest social contribution in the future, to those willing to pay the highest price for them, to those who have the greatest responsibility for the lives of others, to those likely to enjoy the highest quality of life, or to persons selected through a random system of allocation that has the assent of those directly affected by the choices made (Childress, 1970; Rescher, 1969; Evans, 1983; Siegler, 1984; Churchill, 1987; Blank, 1988; Kifner, 1988a; Priester and Caplan, 1989).

There has not been a careful, systematic, and public debate about what theoretical premises ought to govern decisions on distribution of organs among patients who are on waiting lists at particular centers. Nor has there been a discussion of whether it would be desirable to set an explicit public policy with respect to such decisions. Nor has there been much effort to solicit the views of those waiting for transplants as to the policies they would consider fair or just.

I believe a strong case can be made for following a policy which will maximize the number of lives saved when distributing a scarce life-saving resource such as organ transplants when the effectiveness of the resource has been established. The criteria used to determine rationing schemes must be linked to the effectiveness of the resource, since the same standards may not be appropriate when one is trying to decide who gets access to a resource known to saves lives, e.g., heart transplants, as against granting access to resources whose effectiveness is uncertain, e.g., pancreas transplants or lung transplants (Caplan, 1983; Priester and Caplan, 1989).

Whatever criteria and norms are used, it seems clear that medical factors and judgments will have to play an important role. However, the role they play and the importance assigned to any particular factor will be a reflection of the particular conception of fairness that supports their use. Patient selection is no less a function of value judgments than is the determination of eligibility, admissibility, or optimal distribution.

Whether we like it or not, values determine who gets a transplant. The only question is which values will govern decisions at each stage in the allocation process and who will have input into determining the nature of those values.

Those who play a role in the process of allocation—legislators, third-party payors, referring physicians, transplant teams, UNOS, IRBs, boards of trustees, ethics committees, and patients—must make the assurance of equity in the allocation of organs their top priority. If the public does not believe the process by which organs are allocated to be fair, they will support neither the procurement of organs on a voluntary, altruistic basis nor the continuing commitment of public or private funds to pay for transplants.

References

Aleshire, P. "Organ transplant politics, luck may determine who lives, dies," *Arizona Republic*, February 6, 1989: 1–2.

Arenson, E. and Forde, M. 1989. "Bone marrow transplantation for acute leukemia and Down syndrome: report of a successful case and results of a national survey," *Journal of Pediatrics*, 114, 1: 69–72.

Bermel, J. 1983. "The Phoenix memo: rationing dialysis for Indian patients," *Hastings Center Report*, 13: 2.

Blakeslee, S. "Studies find unequal access to kidney transplants," *New York Times*, January 24, 1989, p.C1, 9.

Blank, R. 1988. *Rationing Medicine*. New York: Columbia University Press.

Callender, C. 1987. "Organ donation in blacks," *Transplantation Proceedings*, 19: 1551–54.

Caplan, A. 1983. "Organ transplants: the costs of success," *Hastings Center Report*, 13, 6: 23–32.

———. 1984. "Ethical and policy issues in the procurement of cadaver organs for transplantation," *New England Journal of Medicine*, 311, 15: 981–83.

———. 1985. Ethical issues raised by xenografts," *JAMA*, 254, 23: 3339–43.

——— and Bayer, R. 1985. *Ethical, Legal and Policy Issues Pertaining to Solid Organ Procurement*. Hastings-on-Hudson, NY: The Hastings Center.

———. 1986. "Requests, gifts and obligations," *Transplantation Proceedings*, 18, 3: 49–56. Reprinted in the present volume.

———. 1987. "Equity in the selection of recipients for cardiac transplants." *Circulation*, 75: 10–19.

———. 1988a. "Professional Arrogance and Public Misunderstanding," *Hastings Center Report*, 18, 2:34–37.

_____. 1988b. "Ethical issues in the use of anencephalic infants as a source of organs and tissues for transplantation," *Transplantation Proceedings*, 20, 4: 42–50.

_____. 1989a. "Fragile Trust" in H. Kaufman, ed., *Pediatric Brain Death and Organ Procurement*, New York: Plenum, 299–307.

_____ and Welvang, P. 1989b. "Are Required Request Laws Working?" *Clinical Transplantation*.

Childress, J. 1970. "Who shall live when not all can live?" *Soundings*, 53: 339–55.

Churchill, L. 1987. *Rationing Health Care in America*. Notre Dame, IN: University of Notre Dame Press.

Cicciarelli, J., Terasaki, P., and Mickey, M.R. 1987. "The effect of zero HLA Class I and II mismatching in cyclosporine-treated kidney transplant patients," *Transplantation*, 43, 5: 636–40.

Coburn, D. 1988. "Liver transplants for alcoholics," *Washington Post Health Magazine*, 4, 48, November 29: 12–15.

Engelhardt, H. 1986. *The Foundations of Bioethics*. New York: Oxford, 1986.

Evans, R. 1983. "Health care technology and the inevitability of resource allocation and rationing decisions," *JAMA*, 249: 2047–53, 2208–19.

_____. 1986. "The heart transplant dilemma," *Issues in Science and Technology*, 2, 3: 91–101.

Held, P., M. Pauly, R. Bovbjerg, J. Newmann, O. Salvatierra. 1988. "Access to Kidney Transplants," *Archives of Internal Medicine*, 148: 2594–2600.

Jonasson, O. 1989. "Waiting in line: should selected patients ever be moved up?" *Transplantation Proceedings*, 21, 3: 3390-94.

Kifner, J. 1988a. "Age as a basis for allocating lifesaving medical resources: an ethical analysis," *Journal of Health Politics, Policy and Law*, 13, 3: 405–19.

_____. 1988b. "Selecting patients when resources are limited: A study of US medical directors of kidney dialysis and transplantation facilities," *American Journal of Public Health*, 78, 2: 144–47.

Kjellstrand, C., and Logan G. 1987. "Racial, sexual and age inequalities in chronic dialysis," *Nephron*, 45: 257–63.

Kjellstrand, C. 1988. "Age, sex and race inequality in renal transplantation," Archives of Internal Medicine, 148:1305–9.

Laudicina, S. 1988. Medicaid Coverage and Payment Policies for Organ Transplants: Findings of a National Survey. Washington, D.C.: Intergovernmental Health Policy Project.

Monaco, A. 1989. "A Transplant Surgeon's Views on Social Factors in Organ Transplantation," *Transplantation Proceedings*, 21, 3: 3403–6.

Opelz, G. 1988. "The benefit of exchanging donor kidneys among transplant centers," *New England Journal of Medicine*, 318, 20: 1289–92.

Priester, R., and Caplan A. 1989. "Ethics, cost containment and the allocation of scarce resources," *Investigative Radiology*, 24, 11: 918–26.

Rescher, N. 1969. "The allocation of exotic medical lifesaving therapy," *Ethics*, 79: 173–86.

Salvatierra, O. 1988. "Optimal use of organs for transplantation," *New England Journal of Medicine*, 318, 20: 1329–31.

Siegler, M. 1984. "Should age be a criterion in health care?" *Hastings Center Report*, 14: 24–27.

Starzl, T., et al. 1989. "The Point System for Organ Distribution," *Transplantation Proceedings*, 21, 3: 3432–36.

Stevenson, L., Donohue, B., Tillisch, J., Schulman, B., Dracup, K., Laks, H., 1987. "Urgent priority transplantation: When should it be done?" *Journal of Heart Transplantation*, 6, 5: 267–72.

Transplant Lifelines. 1989. "Heart transplantation—a world experience," *Transplant Lifelines*, 3, 4: 3.

United Network for Organ Sharing. 1989. "Heart allocation policy," *UNOS Update*, 5, 1: 1–2.

Van Buren, C., Kerman, R., Lewis, R., and Kahan, B. 1989. "Exchanging donor kidneys," *New England Journal of Medicine*, 319, 16: 1092–3.

Van Thiel, D., Tarter, D., Gordon, R., et al., 1988. "Liver transplantation for alcoholic liver disease," *Journal of the American Medical Association.*

11.

Ethical issues raised by research involving xenografts

On October 26, 1984, Dr. Leonard Bailey and his associates at the Loma Linda University Medical Center in California implanted a heart from a 7-month-old baboon in a newborn human infant. The child, known publicly as Baby Fae, was afflicted with a fatal congenital abnormality of the heart known as hypoplastic left heart syndrome.[1]

The implant created an enormous controversy both within the medical community and among lay observers of the experiment. The questions it raised and continues to raise concern the competency of the child's mother to give informed consent to the procedure, the morality of killing an animal in order to attempt to save the life of a child, the adequacy of the scientific basis for undertaking this type of transplant in a young child, the competency of the medical team and medical center to undertake the experiment, the adequacy of existing review mechanisms governing human experimentation, the decision by the university not to disclose various documents pertaining to the implant (such as the informed consent form and research protocol), and the timeliness and accuracy of the information disclosed about the experiment by the university as it proceeded.[2-4]

The feasibility of using animals as a source of solid organs for transplantation is a subject that continues to provoke dispute within the medical community. The ongoing severe shortage of solid organs available to both adults and children suffering from renal, cardiac, or liver failure continues to focus the attention of Dr. Bailey and other physicians on the possibility of using animals as a source of solid organs. Given the continued interest of physicians at a number of medical centers in xenografting solid organs, it is important that the ethical questions raised by this highly experimental procedure be carefully examined in order that researchers, potential subjects and their families, policymakers, and the general public fully understand the complexities of the moral issues involved in this type of human experimentation.

The need for transplantable solid organs

Current research on xenografts is focused on three major organs: kidneys, livers, and hearts. Consideration has been given to the use of other organs such as bowel, pancreas, and lungs, but, for a variety of technical reasons, most physicians interested in xenografts have focused on kidneys, livers, and hearts. There is a demonstrable unmet need for each of these organs among both adults and children.

Kidneys

More than 100,000 persons are receiving dialytic therapy for renal failure in the United States. In 1984 another 6,730 received transplants of kidneys from either cadaver or living related donors.[5] While there is some dispute as to the number of dialysis patients who might benefit from a kidney transplant—partly due to the uncertain medical suitability of the members of this population for surgery, and partly due to uncertainty about the desires of dialysis patients themselves for transplants—there is little doubt that at least 10,000 persons would avail themselves of transplants if a sufficient supply of organs were available.[5] Some experts believe that the pool of potential kidney transplant recipients may be as large as 25,000 patients.[5]

It is difficult to obtain exact figures on the number of newborns and children who might benefit from kidney transplantation. The estimated incidence of end-stage renal disease in children younger than the age of 10 years is 0.3 to 0.4 per million per year.[6] More than 600 children in this age group have received transplants in the United States during the past 20 years.[6] Due to the unavailability of donors, very few of these have been infants or children younger than 1 year of age.

Livers

In 1984, 308 liver transplants were performed in the United States, primarily for children and adolescents suffering from congenital defects of this organ.[5] Since there is no means available at present to substitute artificially for the function of the liver, the number of persons actually awaiting transplants at any given time is relatively small—in the neighborhood of 300 individuals, most of whom are infants or children.

However, the need for livers for transplantation may expand rapidly as the technical dimensions of liver transplant surgery are perfected. There are hundreds of children and thousands of adults afflicted with various fatal diseases of the liver who might benefit from a liver transplant were the supply of organs available for this purpose increased.

Hearts

Approximately 400 heart transplants were performed in the United States in 1984.[5] However, the number of centers capable of attempting this procedure has increased dramatically. Moreover, the appearance of mechanical hearts that can act as temporary bridges until an organ can be found may significantly increase the number of persons who might benefit from cardiac transplant surgery.

At present, there are at least 100 individuals awaiting cardiac transplants at various medical centers around the United States. Recent studies have estimated that at least 12,000 adults might benefit from cardiac transplantation were a sufficient supply of organs available.[7]

There are also approximately 25,000 infants born each year in the United States with congenital heart disease. Approximately 7,500 of these infants' conditions are considered life threatening. Hypoplastic left heart syndrome, the condition that afflicted Baby Fae, is the fourth most common congenital heart problem, affecting approximately 500 infants each year.[8] The deaths of these infants account for nearly one fourth of all cardiac-related mortality occurring during the first week of life.

Supply of transplantable solid organs

There are approximately 100,000 fatal accidents in the United States each year. Of this number, most organ procurement specialists believe that between 12,000 and 27,000 might serve as a source of solid organs for transplant.[9,10] The lower estimate is based on the number of brain deaths occurring among those who range in age from 5 to 55 years of age. The higher estimate includes all those suffering brain death from birth to age 65 years.

Stricter suitability criteria (i.e., age and comorbidity) are utilized with respect to cardiac and liver donors than are applied to kidney donors. Recent studies indicate that fewer than 1,000 viable donor hearts are available from cadaver sources under existing medical and social policies.[7] A much larger number of those suffering brain death would be suitable donors of kidneys.

The prevailing system for procuring organs, which is based upon voluntary donation by means of written directives in the form of driver's license checkoffs or donor cards or as a result of consent by next of kin when no documentation exists, yields between 10 percent and 15 percent of the available cadaver donor pool for kidneys. Between 2,000 and 2,500 persons served as a donor of one or more solid organs in 1984.[11] Approximately one third of all kidneys transplanted in the United States are obtained from living related donors.

The system for obtaining organs from cadaver sources is not marked by a high degree of efficiency. This is particularly true of donations from infants and children. Very few infants who are born anencephalic, or brain dead, are utilized as cadaver donors.

There can be no doubt that a shortfall exists between the

available supply of kidneys, livers, and hearts from cadaver sources and the number of persons awaiting transplants of these organs. Moreover, even if the current system of procuring organs from cadaver sources were modified so as to increase the efficiency of cadaver organ procurement, there would still exist a significant shortfall in the number of kidneys, livers, and hearts available for transplantation to children and adults.

The scientific status of xenografts

Clinical trials

Most clinical studies of xenografts were conducted in the early 1960s. These involved attempts to transplant kidneys from chimpanzees or baboons to adults using the then-available forms of immunosuppressive therapy. The vast majority of these grafts failed within two months after surgery.

Three attempts were made during the late 1960s in the United States to transplant livers from animals to human beings. All involved attempts to transplant livers from chimpanzees to young children afflicted with biliary atresia. All three grafts failed within two weeks after the initial surgery.[12,13]

Four attempts have been made to use animal hearts as a means of cardiac substitution. The first involved the transplant of a chimpanzee heart to a 68-year-old man at the University of Mississippi Medical Center in 1964. Two other attempts were made in the late 1970s in South Africa. In these experiments, baboon hearts were used with the intent of facilitating the return of left ventricular function in patients suffering from cardiogenic shock. Both subjects died within four days of the surgery.[14,15]

The fourth case was that of Baby Fae.[1] A baboon heart was used whose blood type did not match that of the recipient (*New York Times,* Oct. 17, 1985, p. B11). The researchers felt that the ABO barrier would prove surmountable as a result of the recipient's immature immune system when subjected to the newly available immunosuppressive drug cyclosporine. The graft functioned for 20 days.

Animal trials

A relatively small number of researchers have attempted cross-species transplants in various animals over the past twenty years.[16-19] These studies suggest that xenograft rejection resembles allograft rejection with respect to both cellular and humoral factors. There appears to be a powerful correlation between the degree of genetic difference between donor and recipient and the speed with which a xenograft is rejected. A few recent trials involving cyclosporine show improved graft survival in various species.[20-22] Little research has been done to determine which immuno-suppressive regimen provides maximal graft survival. Nor has there been much published research involving newborn or very young animals.

The scientific status of xenografts

The animal and clinical experience obtained to date with respect to the use of animals as a source of solid organs for the replacement or supplementation of the function of human hearts, livers, and kidneys makes it clear that xenografting is a poorly understood, relatively untested, and therefore highly experimental procedure in both children and adults. The research done thus far involving xenografts in human beings might best be understood as approximating the earliest stages in the testing of new cytotoxic drugs.

In clinical pharmacology, phase 1 trials describe the initial introduction of a drug into human beings.[23] Usually, healthy volunteers are used, after extensive animal testing, in an effort to determine the pharmacological activity of new agents and their levels of toxicity. These initial tests involving human subjects are aimed solely at assessing the biological effects of a drug in human beings.

Occasionally, phase 1 trials are undertaken with cytotoxic drugs in terminally ill subjects for whom conventional treatment has failed or does not exist, and when animal studies indicate that a new drug may possess useful therapeutic properties. Such experimentation is permitted only with the full, informed consent of subjects and after the development of a well-designed research protocol that has been closely reviewed by both the National Cancer Institute and the Food and Drug Administration.[23,24]

If human experimentation involving xenografts is closely analogous to phase 1 trials of cytotoxic drugs, then such experimentation must meet the highest ethical and legal standards for the following reasons: (1) The data available concerning clinical trials of xenografts are extremely limited and the outcomes of these trials have been poor. Moreover, the majority of the trials were conducted under scientific and technical circumstances drastically dissimilar to those that now prevail in the field of transplantation, making any generalization from the available data problematic. (2) The amount of data available in the published, peer-reviewed literature on cross-species transplants among animals, while somewhat promising, is relatively slight. (3) The experience obtained to date with cadaver and living related transplants from human sources indicates that significant problems involving graft rejection, graft-*versus*-host disease, and other adverse outcomes still exist. (4) Any human subjects involved in future trials would be terminally ill and therefore highly vulnerable. This vulnerable status is particularly apt in describing the status of infants and young children.

The technical, scientific, and psychosocial complexities involved in xenografting hearts, livers, and kidneys to adult human beings are still enormous. The power of newly available immunosuppressive drugs (such as cyclosporine) to counteract graft rejection is poorly understood. Tissue matching capabilities between primates and humans, while much improved in recent years, are still far from perfect.

These problems are, if anything, more daunting where children and infants are concerned. The ability of infants and children to sustain xenografts is a subject of much controversy and dispute among pediatric surgeons.[25] Nor is it known whether or for what period of time animal organs will grow and support normal or near-normal development in newborns and young children.

The obvious questions that arise in considering the ethics of human experimentation involving xenografting are these: (1) Should further research involving xenografts in human subjects be permitted? (2) If so, what ethical standards, regulations, and public policies ought to govern such research?

The ethics of initiating further research involving human subjects at the present time

A number of factors must be weighed in evaluating the case for continuing research involving xenografts in human subjects. Does the demonstrable need for an increase in the supply of organs justify ongoing research involving human beings? Have the medical profession and public officials done everything within reason to maximize the supply of organs that is available to those currently or soon to be in need? What alternatives to xenografts currently exist and what alternatives are likely to exist in the near and long-term future? Are the data available from animal and clinical trials suggestive enough to support further efforts involving human subjects at present?

There can be little doubt that a real need exists for developing a viable form of therapy for those persons afflicted with life-threatening forms of organ failure. Many critics of human experimentation involving organ replacement, via both mechanical substitutes and transplants from animal and human sources, note that a greater emphasis should be placed upon research that might eventuate in strategies for modifying behaviors known to produce irreversible organ failure, such as smoking and alcohol abuse (*Time,* Dec. 10, 1984, pp. 70–73; *Washington Post,* Nov. 14, 1984, p. D7). Such strategies could lead to greater decreases in morbidity and mortality at lower cost than might be possible through the development of techniques permitting organ replacements.

But the development of such strategies will do nothing to help those now afflicted or soon to be afflicted with end-stage organ failure. Moreover, preventive measures will do little to benefit those born with congenital defects and dysfunctions of life-sustaining organs. While research on preventive health measures intended to produce modifications in unhealthy life-styles is critical to the reduction of morbidity and mortality in the American population, it offers little hope to those currently or soon to be afflicted with life-threatening organ failure. Nor can those who advocate greater research into public health measures aimed at modifying risk-creating life-styles or unhealthy behaviors guarantee the successful outcome of such inquiries.

It is also true that national public policy has not fully addressed existing deficits in the current system for procuring solid organs from cadaver sources.[11] While it is indisputably true that those in need of transplants are far more likely to receive therapeutic benefit from the receipt of human as opposed to animal organs, it is uncertain whether the general public and its elected representatives are willing to examine carefully the flaws and faults of a system that obtains donations from less than 20 percent of suitable adult donors and almost none from newborn and infant donors.

The reality facing those now or soon to be afflicted with irreversible end-stage organ failure, their physicians, and the general public is that modifications in public policies to alleviate the shortage in human cadaver organs for transplantation are not in the immediate offing. Nor are changes in the setting of basic research priorities, which might lead to reductions in the prevalence of organ failure in the general population as a result of modifications in behavior and lifestyles known to produce life-threatening organ failure. Most importantly, even if organ procurement from human cadaver sources were to become significantly more efficient, there would still remain a gap between the available supply of human organs and the need for them.

End-stage organ failure of the heart, kidney, and liver will continue to take a toll of lives among infants, children, and adults for the foreseeable future. With the exception of end-stage kidney failure, no form of artificial organ replacement is likely to become available in the near future that might serve as a permanent therapeutic option.

At the same time, scientific and technical understanding of the biology and immunology of xenografting is, at best, primitive. A great deal of research must be done on cellular and animal models in order to advance present scientific understanding of this procedure.

There would appear to exist a pool of terminally ill persons, both children and adults, for whom no therapeutic alternatives exist or are likely to exist in the near future. Many of these individuals are faced with the prospect of inevitable death or, for some renal patients, a quality of life maintained by artificial means that is lower than they desire and are willing to tolerate.

Given these realities, it would appear ethically defensible to allow research involving xenografting in human subjects to proceed in those areas where no reasonable alternative therapy exists. The plight of those in need, the lack of viable therapeutic options, the low probability that public policy will be modified to enhance access to cadaver organs, and the fact that end-stage organ failure is likely to continue to be a pressing health care problem are factors that would appear to weigh heavily against prohibitions, bans, or moratoriums on clinical trials of xenografts at this time. While there are no scientific data that justify the recruitment of potential subjects for the purposes of therapy, the plight of those dying of end-stage organ failure would appear to justify allowing their participation in further clinical trials to advance scientific understanding of the feasibility of xenografting when appropriate ethical and scientific requirements have been met.

Killing animals for research involving xenografts

One factor that might weigh against the continuation of research involving the use of animals as a source of solid organs for humans afflicted with end-stage organ failure is the need to kill animals for this purpose. While it is true that prevailing public policy in the United States allows animals to be killed for a variety of reasons, including general medical research, education, safety and efficacy testing for drugs and commercial products, recreation, and eating, it is also the case that killing animals for the explicit purpose of research intended to develop therapeutic options—which would require the further killing of animals in order to benefit the terminally ill—may raise ethical problems that are unique or specific to xenografting.

In recent years a great deal of effort has been devoted by some members of the general public, the philosophic community, and even the medical and scientific communities to draw attention to questionable practices involving the use and handling of animals for scientific purposes. Some critics of animal experimentation have argued that such practices violate the rights of animal subjects, particularly when they involve significant amounts of pain and suffering for the animals involved.[26]

If viable methods existed for generating a sufficient increase in the supply of organs from cadaver donors, or for making available other therapeutic options for those faced with life-threatening illness or disabilities, then certainly it would be wrong to capture, breed, and kill animals systemically for purposes that might be served in some other manner. Unfortunately, for both scientific and practical reasons, the development of options to benefit those in need is not likely at the present time.

This is not to say that our society is under no obligation to develop such alternatives. Rather, the immediate nonavailability of such options, when combined with a moral point of view that accords greater value to an individual human life than an individual animal life, other things being equal, would appear to justify, at least for the time being, killing animals for the purposes of further research involving xenografts. However, in the long run, serious attention must be given to the morality of killing animals for this purpose if therapeutic alternatives are possible.

The regulation of xenograft research involving human subjects

Despite the uncertainty and ignorance that cloud current understanding of the feasibility of using animal organs as transplants for human beings, continued research on cellular, animal, and human subjects would appear to be morally justified. However, the lack of empirical knowledge concerning both biological and psychosocial aspects of this surgery would appear to require that all such research, whether publicly funded or not, be conducted in accordance with strict conformity to existing federal, state, and professional society regulations concerning human experimentation.

Indeed, the vulnerability of the human subjects who might be asked to serve in further clinical trials, particularly those who are infants or children, is so compelling as to demand unusual efforts on the part of researchers and institutional review boards to respect the autonomy, rights, and dignity of potential subjects.[27]

The vulnerability of both healthy and terminally ill human subjects involved in the earliest stages of drug testing has led the federal government to enact strict standards for monitoring research in this area. A similar system of review and monitoring would appear to be appropriate for the regulation of any further attempts involving xenografts. While the Food and Drug Administration has no mandate to extend its regulatory oversight to medical procedures that do not involve drugs or medical devices, it would seem appropriate that such a mandate be granted before further clinical trials are undertaken.

Researchers and the members of institutional review boards are under a strong obligation to make clear to potential subjects, or their surrogates in the case of children or mentally incompetent subjects, the highly experimental nature of all forms of xenografting. Potential subjects or their surrogates must have complete and comprehensible information about the limits of scientific understanding concerning the efficacy of the surgery, their right to terminate participation in the experiment at any time, any other experimental procedures that will be undertaken as part of xenograft surgery, and any and all alternatives to xenografting that are available.[23,24] Researchers interested in pursuing human trials would also appear to be under a strict obligation to inform potential subjects or their surrogates that *nothing* is known as to the long-term viability of xenografts in human beings.

Only those researchers and institutions willing to subject their research protocols and human subject protections to public scrutiny ought to undertake clinical trials of xenografts. Peer review of the competency of researchers and the scientific basis for their research is a sine qua non where terminally ill subjects are concerned. While subject confidentiality and privacy must be fully honored and protected, researchers, institutional review boards, and institutional officials must understand that their primary duty is to protect the autonomy and interests of subjects who are extremely vulnerable to coercion, misunderstandings, and a failure to comprehend the rationale for undertaking a clinical trial. Subjects or their surrogates must understand that the primary goal of research involving xenografts at the present time is to demonstrate the feasibility of such surgery. Only when it is clear to the medical community, regulatory bodies at the local and federal levels, and the general public that both researchers and their subjects or surrogates fully understand that clinical trials involving xenografts have as their primary goal the acquisition of generalizable knowledge should further research be undertaken.

References

1. Bailey LL, Nehlsen-Cannarella SL, Concepcion W, et al: Baboon-to-human cardiac xeno-transplantation in a neonate. *JAMA* 1985; 254:3321–3329.

2. Caplan AL: Good intentions are not enough: The case of Baby Fae. *Transplant Today* 1985; 2:4–7.

3. Annas GJ: Baby Fae: The 'anything goes' school of human experimentation. *Hastings Cent Rep* 1985;15:15–17.

4. Sheldon R: The IRB's responsibility to itself. *Hastings Cent Rep* 1985;15:11–13.

5. *An Update on Organ and Tissue Donation and Transplantation in the United States Today.* Washington, DC, American Council on Transplantation, 1984.

6. Lum CT, Fryd DS, Polta TA, et al: Results of kidney transplantation in the young child. *Transplantation* 1982;34:167–171.

7. Evans RW, Manninen DL, Overcast TD, et al: *The National Heart Transplantation Study: Final Report.* Seattle, Battelle Human Affairs Research Centers, 1984.

8. Vinocur B: Bailey's answers only provoke more questions. *Med World News,* in press.

9. Guttman FM: Organ transplantation in children. *Pediatr Ann* 1982;11:910–915.

10. Bart KJ, Macon EJ, Humphries AL Jr, et al: Increasing the supply of cadaveric kidneys for transplantation. *Transplantation* 1981;31:383–387.

11. Caplan AL: Organ procurement: It's not in the cards. *Hastings Cent Rep* 1984;14:6–9.

12. Starzl TE: Orthotopic heterotransplantation, in *Experience in Hepatic Transplantation.* Philadelphia, WB Saunders Co, 1969, pp 408–421.

13. Starzl TE, Ishikawa M, Putnam CW, et al: Progress in and deterrents to orthotopic liver transplantation, with special reference to survival, resistance to hyperacute rejection, and biliary duct reconstruction. *Transplant Proc* 1974;6:129–139.

14. Hardy JD, Chavez CM: The first heart transplant in man. *Am J Cardiol* 1968;22:772–781.

15. Barnard CN, Wolpowitz A, Losman JG, et al: Heterotopic cardiac transplantation with a xenograft for assistance of the left heart in cardiogenic shock after cardiopulmonary bypass. *S Afr Med J* 1977;52:1035–1038.

16. Reemtsma K: Heterotransplantation-theoretical considerations. *Transplant Proc* 1971;3:49–57.

17. Perper RJ: Renal heterotransplant rejection. *Transplantation* 1971;12:519–523.

18. Shons AR, Najarian JS: Xenograft rejection in human beings. *Rev Surg* 1975;32:70–91.

19. Chartrand C, et al: Delayed rejection of cardiac xenografts in C6-deficient rabbits. *Immunology* 1979;38:245–249.

20. Danko I, Gebhard C, Scholz S, et al: Transplant aspiration cytology for monitoring of kidney xenograft under cyclosporin-A treatment. *Eur Surg Res* 1983;15:276–283.

21. Hammer C, Chaussy C, Welter H, et al: Exceptionally long survival time in xenogeneic organ transplantation. *Transplant Proc* 1981;13:881–884.

22. Harbin S, Heneghan JB: Growth of dog intestinal mucosa xenografts in nude mice. *Prog Clin Biol Res* 1985;181:467–471.

23. Levine RJ: *Ethics and Regulation of Clinical Research.* Baltimore, Urban & Schwarzenberg, 1981.

24. Barber B: *Informed Consent in Medical Therapy and Research.* New Brunswick, NJ, Rutgers University Press, 1980.

25. Breo DL: Is 'Baby Fae' transplant worth it? Experts mixed. *Am Med News* 1984;27:41–43.

26. Regan T: *A Case for Animal Rights.* Berkeley, University of California Press, 1983.

27. Ackerman TF: Moral duties of investigators toward sick children. *IRB* 1981;3:1–5.

Part V

Aging, chronic illness, and rehabilitation

12.

Is aging a disease?

Normality, naturalness, and disease

The belief that aging is a normal and natural part of human existence is commonplace in the practice of medicine. For example, no mention is made in most textbooks in the areas of medicine and pathology of aging as abnormal, unnatural, or indicative of disease. It is true that such texts often contain a chapter or two on the related subject of diseases commonly associated with aging or found in the elderly. But it is these diseases frequently encountered in the elderly—such as pneumonia, cancer, or atherosclerosis—rather than the aging process itself, that serve as the focus of description and analysis.

Why should this situation exist? What is so different about the physiological changes and deteriorations of the aging process that these events are considered to be unremarkable natural processes, while apparently similar processes in a young person are deemed to be diseases constituting health crises of the first order? Surely it cannot simply be the life-threatening aspects of diseases such as cancer or atherosclerosis that distinguish them from aging. For while it may be true that hardly anyone manages to avoid contracting a terminal disease at some point in life, aging itself produces the same ultimate consequence as these diseases. Nor can it be the familiarity and universality of aging that inure medical science to its unnatural aspects. Malignant neoplasms, viral infections, and hypertension are ubiquitous phenomena. Yet medicine maintains a stance toward these physical processes that is radically different from that which it holds toward the so-called "natural" changes that occur during aging.

What seems to differentiate aging from other processes or states traditionally classified as diseases is the fact that aging is perceived as a natural or normal process. Medicine has traditionally viewed its role as that of ameliorating or combating the abnormal, either through therapeutic interventions or preventive, prophylactic regimens. The natural and the normal, while not outside the sphere of medicine, are concepts that play key roles in licensing the intervention of the medical practitioner. For it is in response to or in anticipation of abnormality that physicians' activities are legitimated. As E. A. Murphy, among many other clinicians, has noted, "The clinician has tended to regard disease as that state in which the limits of the normal have been transgressed."[1] Naturalness and normality have, historically, been used as baselines to determine the presence of disease and the necessity of medical activity.

In light of the powerful belief that the abnormal and unnatural are indicative of medicine's range of interest, it is easy to see why many biological processes are not thought to be the proper subject of medical intervention or therapy. Puberty, growth, and maturation *as processes in themselves* all appear to stand outside the sphere of medical concern since they are normal and natural occurrences among human beings. Similarly, it seems odd to think of sexuality or fertilization as possible disease states precisely because these states are commonly thought to be natural and normal components of the human condition.

Nonetheless, it is true that certain biological processes, such as conception, pregnancy, and fertility, have been the subject in recent years of heated debates as to their standing as possible disease states. The notions that it is natural and normal for only men and women to have sexual intercourse or for women to undergo menopause have been challenged in many quarters. The question arises as to whether the process of aging in and of itself can be classified as abnormal and unnatural in a way that will open the door for the reclassification of aging as a disease process and, thus, a proper subject of medical attention, concern, and control.

Aging and medical intervention

The status of aging and dying as natural processes looms especially large in current discussions about the "right to die" and "death with dignity." Often those who debate the degree to which the medical profession should intervene in the process of dying disagree about the naturalness of the phenomena of aging and dying. If the alleged right to die is to be built on a conception of the naturalness of aging and dying, then the conceptual status of these terms vis-à-vis "naturalness" must be thoroughly examined. The question of the naturalness of aging, senescence, and death should be kept in mind in complex debates concerning the rights and obligations of patients and health professionals.

As noted earlier, the perception of biological events or processes as natural or unnatural is frequently decisive in determining whether physicians treat certain states or processes as diseases.[2] One need only think of the controversies that swirl around allegations concerning the biological naturalness of homosexuality or schizophrenia to see that this is so. This claim is further borne out by an argument that is frequently made by older physicians to new medical students. Medical students often find it difficult to interact with or examine elderly patients. They may feel powerless when confronted with the seemingly irreversible debilities of old age. To overcome this reluctance, older physicians are likely to point out that aging is a process that happens to everyone, even young medical students. Aging is simply part of the human condition; it should hold no terror for a young doctor. Students are told that aging is natural and that, while there may be nothing they can do to alter the inevitable course of this process, they must learn to help patients cope with their aging as best they can. It is as if teaching physicians feel obligated to label the obviously debilitative and disease-like states of old age as natural in order to discourage the student's inclination to treat the elderly as sick or diseased.

What is aging?

Why do we think of aging as a natural process? The reason that comes immediately to mind is that aging is a common and normal process. It occurs with a statistical frequency of one hundred percent.

Inevitably and uniformly bones become brittle, vision dims, joints stiffen, and muscles lose their tone. The obvious question that arises is whether commonality, familiarity, and inevitability are sufficient conditions for describing certain biological states as natural. To answer this question, it is necessary first to draw a distinction between aging and chronological age.

In a trivial sense, given the existence of a chronological device, all bodies that exist can be said to age relative to the measurements provided by that device. But since physicians have little practical interest in making philosophical statements about the time-bound nature of existence, or empirical claims about the relativity of space and time, it is evident that they do not have this chronological sense in mind in speaking about the familiarity and inevitability of aging.

In speaking of aging, physicians are interested in a particular set of biological changes that occur with respect to time. These changes occur at a variety of levels in human beings. At the molecular level, extensive research has shown substantial changes in enzyme activity among the elderly. At the cellular level, increase in age is correlated with increases in the length of the cell cycle during mitosis. At the level of organs and tissues, aging is correlated with deterioration in various joints, a decline in body potassium, wrinkled skin, thickening of the lens of the eye, a decline in immune function, and a decline in lung capacity.

There is a distinct set of psychological changes that constitute the aging process as well. For example, long-term memory tends to decline with age. Perceptual abilities such as visual acuity, depth perception, color discrimination, taste sensitivity, and pitch discrimination tend to decline as one becomes older. There are general declines in many intellectual abilities, particularly those involving speed of response in nonverbal, manipulative skills.

These types of cellular, organic, and psychological changes constitute the aging process. They do not occur at the same rate in all persons and do not proceed at the same rate within any particular individual. It is this set of biological and psychological changes[3]—not the mere passage of time—that constitutes the phenomena of aging.

Studies on animals show that similar patterns of change can be found occurring at different rates in a wide variety of mammals. The genetic disease progeria, which afflicts young children, presents many of the same biological and psychological changes associated with the aging process. Variations among normal human beings in the degree to which the signs of aging occur, and the fact that some young humans can be afflicted with the signs of aging, reveal that age and aging must be understood as distinct, although related, phenomena.

Naturalness, design, and function

While it is true that aging occurs at different rates in different people, such changes are universal and eventually inevitable. Universality and inevitability do not, however, seem to be sufficient conditions for referring to a process as natural. Coronary atherosclerosis, neoplasms, high blood pressure, sore throats, colds, tooth decay, and depression are all nearly universal in their distribution, and are seemingly inevitable phenomena. Yet it seems awkward to call these phenomena natural processes or states. The inevitablility of infection by micro-organisms among all humans does not cause the physician to dismiss these infections as natural occurrences of no particular medical interest. The physician may not intervene, nor even attempt to prevent such diseases, but such behavior is a result of a decision concerning an unnatural disease, not a natural process.

If universality and inevitability are not adequate criteria for defining naturalness, are any other criteria available by which naturalness can be assessed and used to drive a wedge between aging and disease? There is another sense of "natural"[4] that may prove helpful in trying to understand why physicians are reluctant to label aging a disease, preferring to think of it as a natural process.

This sense of naturalness is rooted in the notions of design, purpose, and function. Axes are designed to serve as tools for cutting trees. Scalpels are meant to be used in cutting human tissue. It would seem most unnatural to use axes for surgery and scalpels for lumberjacking. In some sense, although a skillful surgeon might, in fact, be able to perform surgery with an axe, it would be unnatural to do so. Similarly, many bodily organs—the liver, spleen, blood vessels, kidneys, and many glands—can perform a variety of functions. They can even compensate for the functions of organic tissues that are damaged. But these are not the purposes or functions they were "designed" to perform. While the arteries of many organisms are capable of constricting to maintain blood pressure and reduce the flow of blood during hemorrhage-induced shock, one essential function of the arteries is not to constrict in response to such circumstances. The presence of vasoconstriction in arteries is, in fact, an unnatural state that signals to the physician that something has gone seriously awry in the body. It may be that much of our willingness to accept aging as a natural process is dependent upon some sense of "natural" function.

Two answers are commonly given to the question: What is the function of aging? The first is a theological explanation. God, in punishment for the sins of our ancestors in the (proverbial) garden of Eden, caused humans to age and die. According to this view, people age because the Creator saw fit to design them that way for retribution or punishment. Aging serves as a reminder of our moral fallibility and weakness.

The second view, which is particularly widespread in scientific circles, is that the purpose or function of aging is to clear away the old to make way for the new for evolutionary reasons. This theory was first advanced by the German cytologist and evolutionary biologist August Weismann at the turn of the century.[5] Weismann argued that aging and debilitation must be viewed as adaptational responses on the part of organisms to allow for new mutational and adaptive responses to fluctuating environments. Aging benefits the population by removing the superannuated to make room for the young. The function of aging is to ensure the death of organisms to allow evolutionary change and new adaptation to occur.

In both of these views aging has an intended purpose or function. And it is from this quasi-Aristotelian attribution of a design that the "naturalness" of aging is often thought to arise.

The concept of biological function

Rooting the source of the naturalness of biological processes in ideas of function or purpose has its drawbacks, the primary one being that philosophers have by no means reached anything even vaguely resembling a consensus about the meaning of such terms as "function" or "purpose."

Fortunately, it is possible to avoid becoming bogged down in an analysis of functional or purposive statements in analyzing the function of aging. The only distinction required for understanding the function of aging is that between the aim of explaining the existence of a particular state, organ, or process and the aim of explaining how a state, organ, or process works in a particular system or organism. Functional or purposive statements are sometimes used to explain the existence of a trait or process historically. At other times, such statements are used mechanistically to explain how something works or operates. If we ask what the function, or role, or purpose of the spleen in the human body is, the question can be interpreted in two ways: How does the spleen work—what does it do in the body? Or, why does the spleen exist in its present state in the human body—what, historically, explains why persons have spleens?[6]

It is this latter sense of function, the historical sense, that is relevant to the determination of the naturalness or unnaturalness of aging as a biological process. For while there is no shortage of theories purporting to explain how aging works or functions, these theories are not relevant to the historically motivated question about the function of aging. The determination of the naturalness of aging, if it is to be rooted in biology, will depend not on how the process of aging actually operates, but rather on the explanation one gives for the existence or presence of aging in humans.[7]

Does aging have a function?

Two purported explanations—one theological, one scientific—of the function or purpose of aging have been given. Both are flawed. While the theological explanation of aging may carry great weight for numerous individuals, it will simply not do as a scientific explanation of why aging occurs in humans. Medical professionals may have to cope with their patients' advocacy of this explanation and their own religious feelings on the subject. But, from a scientific perspective, it will hardly do to claim that aging, as a result of God's vindictiveness, is a natural biological process, and hence not a disease worthy of treatment.

More surprisingly, the scientific explanation of aging as serving an evolutionary role or purpose is also inadequate. It is simply not true that aging exists to serve any sort of evolutionary purpose or function. The claim that aging exists or occurs in individuals because it has a wider role or function in the evolutionary scheme of things rests on faulty evolutionary analysis. The analysis incorrectly assumes that it is possible for biological processes to exist that directly benefit or advance the evolutionary success of a species or population.

Evolutionary selection rarely acts to advance the prospects of an entire species or population. Selection acts on individual organisms and their phenotypic traits and properties. Some traits or properties confer advantages in certain environments on the organisms that possess them and this fact increases the likelihood that the genes responsible for producing these traits will be passed on to future organisms.

Given that selective forces act on individuals and their genotypes and not species, it makes no sense to speak of aging as serving an evolutionary function or purpose to benefit the species. How then do evolutionary biologists explain the existence of aging?[8] Briefly, the explanation is that features, traits, or properties in individual organisms will be selected for if they confer a relative reproductive advantage on the individual or his or her close kin. Any variation that increases inclusive reproductive fitness has a very high probability of being selected and maintained in the gene pool of a species. Selection, however, cannot look ahead to foresee the possible consequences of favoring certain traits at a given time; the environment selects for those traits and features that give an immediate return. An increased metabolic rate, for example, may prove advantageous early in life in that it may provide more energy for seeking mates and avoiding predators; it may also result in early deterioration of the organism due to an increased accumulation of toxic wastes in the body of an individual thus endowed. Natural selection cannot foresee such delayed debilitating consequences.

Aging exists, then, as a consequence of a lack of evolutionary foresight; it is simply a by-product of selective forces which increase the chances of reproductive success in the life of an organism. Senescence has no function; it is simply the inadvertent subversion of organic function, later in life, in favor of maximizing reproductive advantage, early in life.

The common belief that aging serves a function or purpose is based on a misunderstanding of evolutionary processes. It would further seem that the common belief that aging is a natural process, as a consequence of the function or purpose it serves in the life of the species, is also mistaken. Consequently, unless it is possible to motivate the description on other grounds, aging cannot be understood as a natural process. And if that is true, and if it is actually the case that what goes on during the aging process closely parallels the changes that occur during paradigmatic examples of disease,[9] then it would be unreasonable not to consider aging as a disease.

Theories of aging and the concept of disease

A consideration of the changes that constitute aging in human beings reinforces the similarities between aging and clear-cut examples of somatic diseases. There is a set of external manifestations or symptoms: greying hair, increased susceptibility to infection, wrinkling skin, loss of muscular tone, and, frequently, loss of some mental ability. These manifestations seem to be causally linked to a series of internal cellular and subcellular changes. The presence of symptoms and an underlying etiology closely parallel the standard paradigmatic examples of disease. If the analogy is pushed a bit further, the case for considering aging a disease appears to become even stronger.

There are many theories as to what causes the changes, at the cellular and subcellular level, that produce the signs and symptoms associated with aging.[10] One view argues that aging is caused by an increase in the number of cross-linkages in protein and nucleic acid molecules. Cross-linkages lower the biochemical efficiency and dependability of certain macromolecules involved in metabolism and other chemical reactions. Free radical by-products of metabolism are thought to accumulate in cells, thus allowing for an increase in available linkage sites for replicating nucleic acid strands and activating histone elements. This sort of cross-linkage is thought to be particularly important in the aging of collagen, the substance responsible for most of the overt symptoms we commonly associate with aging, such as wrinkled skin and loss of muscular flexibility.

Another view holds that aging results from an accumulation of genetic mutations in the chromosomes of cells in the body. The idea underlying this theory is that chromosomes are exposed over time to a steady stream of radiation and other mutagenic agents. The accumulation of mutational hits on the genes lying on the chromosomes results in the progressive inactivation of these genes. The evidence of a higher incidence of chromosomal breaks and aberrations in the aged is consistent with this mutational theory of aging.

Along with the cross-linkage and mutational theories, there is one other important hypothesis concerning the causes of aging. The auto-immune theory holds that, as time passes and the chromosomes of cells in the human body accumulate more mutations, certain key tissues begin to synthesize antibodies that can no longer distinguish between self and foreign material. Thus, a number of auto-immune reactions occur in the body as the immunological system begins to turn against the individual it was "designed" to protect. Certain types of arthritis and pernicious anemia are examples of debilities resulting from the malfunction of the immunological system. While this theory is closely allied to the mutation theory, the auto-immune view of aging holds that accumulated mutations do not simply result in deterioration of cellular activity but, rather, produce lethal cellular end products that consume and destroy healthy tissue.

It would be rash to hold that any of the three hypotheses cited—the cross-linkage, mutational, or auto-immune hypotheses—will, in the end, turn out to be *the* correct explanation of aging. All three views are, in fact, closely related in that cross-linkages can result from periodic exposure to mutagenic agents and can, in turn, produce genetic aberrations which eventuate in cellular dysfunction or even auto-immune reactions. What is important, however, is not whether *one* of these theories is in fact *the* correct theory of aging, but that all of the current plausible theories postulate mechanisms that are closely analogous to those mechanisms cited by clinicians when describing other disease processes in the body.

The concept of disease is, without doubt, a slippery and evasive notion in medicine.[11] Once one moves away from what can be termed "paradigmatic" examples of disease, such as tuberculosis and diphtheria, toward more nebulous examples, such as acne or jittery nerves, it becomes difficult to say exactly what the criteria requisite for labeling a condition a somatic disease are. However, even though it is notoriously difficult to concoct a set of necessary and sufficient conditions for employing the term "organic disease," it is possible to cite a list of general criteria that seem relevant in attempting to decide whether a bodily state or process is appropriately labeled a disease.

One criterion is that the state or process produces discomfort or suffering. A second is that the process or state can be traced back to a specific cause, event, or circumstance. A third is that there is a set of clear-cut structural changes, both macroscopic and microscopic, that follow in a uniform, sequential manner subsequent to the initial precipitating or causal event. A fourth is that there is a set of clinical symptoms or manifestations (headache, pain in the chest, rapid pulse, shortness of breath) commonly associated with the observed physiological alterations in structure. Finally,[12] there is usually some sort of functional impairment in the abilities, behavior, or activity of a person thought to be diseased. Not all diseases will satisfy all or any of these criteria. One need only consider the arguments surrounding the proper classification of astigmatism, alcoholism, drug addiction, gambling, and hyperactivity to realize the limited resolving power of these criteria. Nevertheless, advocates of all persuasions regarding controversial states and processes commonly resort to considerations of causation, clinical manifestations, etiology, functional impairment, and suffering in arguing the merits of their various views concerning the disease status of controversial cases.

With respect to the conceptual ambiguity surrounding the notion of disease, it is important to remember that medicine is by no means unique in being saddled with what might be termed "fuzzy-edged" concepts. One need only consider the status of terms such as "species," "adaptation," and "mutation" in biology, or "stimulus," "behavior," or "instinct" in psychology to realize that medicine is not alone in the ambiguity of its key terms. It is also true that, just as the biologist is able to use biological theory to aid in the determination of relevant criteria and their fulfillment for a concept, the physician—as many writers have noted—is able to use his or her knowledge of the structure, design, and function of the body to decide upon relevant criteria for the determination of disease.

If one accepts the relevance of the five suggested criteria, then aging, as a biological process, is seen to possess all the key properties of a disease. Unlike alcoholism or nervousness, aging possesses a definitive group of clinical manisfestations or symptoms; a clear-cut etiology of structural changes at both the macroscopic and microscopic levels; a significant measure of impairment, discomfort, and suffering; and, if we are willing to grant the same tolerance to current theories of aging as we grant to theories in other domains of medicine, an explicit set of precipitating factors. Aging has all the relevant markings of a disease process. And if my earlier argument is sound, even if an additional criterion of unnaturalness is added to these five, aging will still meet all the requirements thought relevant to the classification of a process or state as indicative of disease.

Some ethical arguments against treating aging as a disease

What consequences hinge on the decision to refer to a process or state such as aging with the word "disease" rather than with some other term? Obviously, a great deal. Medical attention, medical support, medical treatment, and medical research are devoted to the treatment, care, amelioration, and prevention of disease. While it is possible to view the activation of this vast professional machine either as a positive good or as a serious evil, an array of implications surrounds the decision of the medical profession to consider a phenomenon worthy of its attention. Some groups have actively proselytized for the acceptance of certain conditions, such as alcoholism or gambling, as diseases. Other groups have worked to remove the label of disease from behavior such as homosexuality, masturbation, and schizophrenia. A number of motives and concerns underlie these arguments. The question is, what value considerations should be considered relevant to the determination of whether a particular state, process, or condition is a disease?

I do not propose to try to identify the relevant nonorganic criteria affecting the choice of the disease label. Rather, I want to consider three specific arguments that might be raised against calling aging a disease—a classification that, of necessity, keeps the aged in touch with the medical profession.

The first counterargument is that the decision to call aging a disease would be pointless, since doctors cannot at present intervene to treat or cure aging. This argument does not stand up to critical scrutiny. There are many diseases in existence today for which no cure is known, but no one proposes that these disorders are any less diseases as a consequence. Furthermore, the emphasis on treatment and cure implicit in this argument ignores the equally vital components of medical care involving understanding, education, and research. The interest of the patient and of the medical profession in the healing function of medicine might make it difficult for physicians to accept aging as a disease, but the difficulty in achieving such acceptance does not provide a reason for rejecting the view.

The second argument is that to call aging a disease would involve the stigmatization of a large segment of the population; to view the aged as sick or diseased would only increase the burdens already borne by this much-abused segment of society. The problem with this argument is that it tends to blur public perceptions of disease in general with the particular problem of seeing aging as a disease and the ensuing undesirable connotations. To deny that aging is a disease may simply be an easy way to avoid the more difficult problem of educating the medical profession and the lay public toward a better understanding of the threatening and nonthreatening aspects of disease. Contagiousness, death, disability, and neglect may be the real objects of concern in stigmatizing disease, not disease in itself.

Finally, it might be claimed that there would be a tremendous social and economic cost to calling aging a disease. The claim is perhaps the most unconvincing of the three that I have offered. One factor especially relevant to the determination or diagnosis of disease would seem to be that the physician confine his or her concerns to the physical and mental state of the individual patient; social and economic considerations would appear to be quite out of place. Genetic and psychological diseases place a large burden on society; dialysis machines and tomography units are tremendously expensive. But these facts do not in any way change the disease status of schizophrenia, kidney failure, or cancer. It may be the case that the government might decide not to spend one cent on research into aging or the treatment of aging. But such a decision should be consequent on, not prior to, a determination of whether aging is a disease. This argument simply confounds the value questions relevant to a decision as to whether something is a disease with value questions relevant to deciding what to do about something after it has been decided that it is a disease.

I have suggested a number of possible value issues and social problems that may enter into the decision of the medical profession to label a state or process a disease.[13] I have also suggested that none of these issues and problems would seem to rule out a consideration of aging as a disease. The determination of disease status and the question of how physicians and society should react to disease are distinct issues. Considerations of the latter variety ought not to be allowed to color our decisions about what does and what does not constitute a disease.

Most persons in our society would be loath to see aging classified and treated as a disease. Much of the resistance to such a classification derives from the view that aging is a natural process and that, like other natural processes, it ought not, in itself, be the subject of medical intervention and therapeutic control. I have tried to show that much of the reasoning that tacitly underlies the categorization of aging as a natural or normal process rests on faulty biological analysis. Aging is not the goal or aim of the evolutionary process. Rather it is an accidental by-product of that process. Accordingly, it is incorrect to root a belief in the naturalness of aging in some sort of perceived biological design or purpose since aging serves no such end. It may be that good arguments can be adduced for excluding aging from the purview of medicine. However, if such arguments can be made, they must draw on considerations other than that of the naturalness of aging.[14] Given the parallels that exist between aging and other paradigmatic cases of disease, there would appear to be no reason not to classify aging as a disease.

Notes

1. E. A. Murphy, *The Logic of Medicine* (Baltimore: Johns Hopkins University Press, 1976), p. 122. See also E. A. Murphy, "A Scientific Viewpoint on Normalcy," *Perspectives in Biology and Medicine*; and G. B. Risse, "Health and Disease: History of the Concepts," in *Encyclopedia of Bioethics*, W. T. Reich, ed. (New York: The Free Press, 1978), pp. 579–585.

2. S. Goldberg, "What is 'Normal'?: Logical Aspects of the Question of Homosexual Behavior," *Psychiatry* 38 (1975):227–242; Charles Socarites, "Homosexuality and Medicine," *Journal of the American Medical Association* 212 (1970):1199–1202; and I. Illich, "The Political Uses of Natural Death," *Hastings Center Studies* 2 (1974): 3–20.

3. See E. Palmore, "United States of America" in E. Palmore (ed.), *International Handbook on Aging* (Westport, CN: Greenwood Press, 1980), pp. 434–454, for further discussion of the nature of aging.

4. See D. B. Hausman, cf., "What Is Natural?," *Perspectives in Biology and Medicine* 19 (1975):92–101, for an illuminating discussion of the concept.

5. A. Weismann, *Essays Upon Heredity and Kindred Biological Problems*, 2d ed. (Oxford: Clarendon Press, 1891).

6. For a sample of the extant explications of the concept of function, see L. Wright, "Functions," *Philosophical Review* 82 (1973):139–168; R. Cummins, "Functional Analysis," *Journal of Philosophy* 72 (1975):741–765; and M. A. Boden, *Purposive Explanation in Psychology*, Cambridge: Harvard (1972). See also E. Nagel, *Teleology Revisited*, New York: Columbia, (1979).

7. Further discussion of the distinction between explaining the opera-

tion of a trait or feature and explaining the origin and presence of a trait or feature can be found in A. L. Caplan, "Evolution, Ethics and the Milk of Human Kindness," *Hastings Center Report* 6:2 (1976), pp. 20–26.

8. G. C. Williams, *Adaptation and Natural Selection* (Princeton: Princeton University Press, 1966); and M. T. Ghiselin, *The Economy of Nature and the Evolution of Sex* (Berkeley: University of California Press, 1974).

9. For an interesting attempt to analyze the concepts of illness and disease, see C. Boorse, "On the Distinction Between Illness and Disease," *Philosophy and Public Affairs* 5:1 (1975), pp. 49–68.

10. A. Comfort, "Biological Theories of Aging," *Human Development* 13 (1970): 127–39; L. Hayflick, "The Biology of Human Aging," *American Journal of Medical Sciences* 265:6 (1973), pp. 433–45; A. Comfort, *Aging: The Biology of Senescence* (New York: Holt, Rinehart and Winston, 1964).

11. R. M. Veatch, "The Medical Model: Its Nature and Problems," *Hastings Center Studies* 1:3 (1973), pp. 59–76.

12. Boorse, "On the Distinction Between Illness and Disease."

13. The role played by values in explicating the concepts of health and disease is notoriously controversial. See, for example, J. Margolis, "The Concept of Disease," *Journal of Medicine and Philosophy* 1 (1976):238–255. I do not wish to enter this debate here. Rather, I am simply making the point that if aging is to avoid the label of disease, it must be on valuational grounds alone.

14. Certainly arguments can be made against ageism regardless of the disease status of aging. See D. H. Fischer, "Putting Our Heads to the 'Problem' of Old Age," in R. Gross, B. Gross, and S. Seidman (eds.), *The New Old: Struggling For Decent Aging* (Garden City, NY: Anchor, 1978), pp. 58–63.

13.

Let wisdom find a way
The concept of
competency in the care of
the elderly

Few concepts play a more central role in determining the care of elderly patients than the concept of competency. The presence or absence of competency determines the degree to which patients have control over their medical care. If it is true that informed consent is the ethical linchpin of the professional/patient relationship, then the determination of competency is an essential element of patient care.

When a patient is manifestly competent, final authority over all decisions pertaining to health care rests, legally and ethically, with the patient (Donagan, 1977). When, on the other hand, competency is plainly absent (as is the case with very young infants, the severely retarded, or the comatose), responsibility for medical decisions necessarily moves into the hands of other parties—health care providers, family members, friends, guardians, or, in some cases, the courts.

A certain amount of consensus has emerged in our legal system during the past decade as to the steps that health care professionals should take when decisions must be made for a manifestly incompetent patient (Robertson, 1983). Society has slowly moved toward the creation of mechanisms, such as the assignment of guardians and the creation of ethics committees. These allow third parties to take control when patients cannot make decisions for themselves.

Unfortunately, clarity in the law about the responsibilities and duties owed to patients who are plainly incompetent does not eliminate the problems that competency raises on a day-to-day basis for health care providers and families. There are many patients, particularly among the elderly, whose abilities to make decisions regarding their medical treatment are difficult to determine.

Vulnerability

Changes in the demographics of the population of the United States as well as major advances in the efficacy of medical intervention in treating acute medical problems (Verbrugge, 1984) have created a large and growing class of older patients with more chronic illness. The competency of many of these people, particularly those who are in hospitals or nursing homes, is impaired or diminished in significant ways. However, many are not so severely impaired as to make it self-evident that they ought to be viewed as entirely incompetent to make any or all decisions related to their health. Many of these patients fall into the category of, in Bernice Neugarten's (1974) felicitous phrase, the "old-old."

Some of the patients who fall into this conceptual gray zone possess variable levels of competency depending upon the setting in which they live, the time of day, or the degree to which they are under the influence of various psychoactive drugs. Other patients are afflicted with a degree of impairment of either their cognitive or emotional abilities that does not render them obviously unable to participate in all decisions concerning their care.

While we should avoid stereotyping elderly persons, it is nonetheless true that the sick elderly are, as a class, more prone than are other segments of the population to illnesses that can result in impaired competency. Those elders who are receiving care in hospitals or nursing homes are often afflicted with biological disorders that can limit their mental functioning. Certain diseases—such as Alzheimer's disease, stroke, or depression—are more likely to afflict older persons. Various physiological changes involved in the process of senescence itself may also produce decreases in certain cognitive and emotional capacities (Palmore, 1980).

Biological disorders are not the only source of impaired competency. Older persons with medical problems are more likely to be institutionalized than are other patients, and their institutionalization lasts for longer periods of time. As numerous studies have convincingly shown (Altman, 1975; Dohrenwend, 1975), institutionalization can itself have an adverse impact on competency.

The sick and institutionalized elderly often lack the economic and social resources requisite for zealously advocating their interests. As a result, they are more likely to fall prey to attempts to override their choices. The sick elderly and the old-old are often excluded from decisions regarding their own health care for no other reason than that they have a hard time being heard in institutional settings. In highly bureaucratized health care institutions, those who do not speak loudly and forcefully are either not heard or simply ignored.

Complexities of competency

Few concepts have occasioned as much dispute and controversy as the definition of competency. A review of some of the most popular definitions will give a sense of the lack of consensus that prevails.

The President's Commission for the Study of Ethical Problems in Medicine and Biomedical and Behavioral Research (1982) viewed competency as consisting of three elements: "(1) possession of a set of values and goals; (2) the ability to communicate and understand information; and (3) the ability to reason and to deliberate about one's choices."

Roth et al. (1977) suggest that to be considered competent an individual "must be able to comprehend the nature of the particular conduct in question and to understand its quality and its consequences." And Abernathy and Lundin (1980), after providing a useful review of the legal and cultural aspects of competency, conclude that "any competency calculus should include consideration of the patient's ability to receive, process and produce information, the patient's history and general social setting, and consideration of the patient's behavior."

A variety of state legislatures have also attempted to grapple with defining competency. Most have attempted to define incompetence since the law presumes competency to be present unless it can be proven otherwise. A typical example is the Illinois statute, which defines incompetence as "any person who because of insanity, mental illness, mental retardation, old age, physical incapacity or imperfection or deterioration of mentality is incapable of managing his person or estate and any person who because of gambling, idleness, debauchery or the excessive use of intoxicants or drugs, so spends or wastes his estate as to expose himself or his family to want or suffering" (Ill. Stat. Ann. 1976).

Another state statute utilizes the following definition: "an incompetent is a person incapable by reasons of insanity, mental illness, imbecility, idiocy, senility or other mental incapacity, of either managing his property or caring for himself or both" (Wash. Rev. Cod. Ann., 1967).

While numerous court cases review the rights of patients to refuse treatment (particularly for religious reasons), there are surprisingly few attempts at definitions of competency in US court cases. Two of the most important cases where an attempt has been made to provide a standard are *Grannum* v. *Berard* and *Schiller*. In *Grannum*, the court argued that, ". . . the test being whether the person in question . . . possessed sufficient mind or reason to enable him to understand the nature, the terms, and the effects of the transaction" (422 P.2d at 812, Wash. 1967). And, in *Schiller*, the standard adduced was, ". . . the test may be stated as: does the patient have sufficient mind to reasonably understand the condition, the nature and the effect of the proposed treatment, attendant risks in pursuing the treatment and not pursuing the treatment" (In the Matter of Schiller, 372 A.2d 360, N.J. Super, 1977).

Perhaps the best that the medical professional can hope to gather from these varied efforts at definition is that there are at least two distinct senses of competency—legal and medical. The legal sense of the term concerns itself primarily with a person's ability to responsibly manage property and finances. The medical sense attempts to pinpoint those elements of physical, emotional, and cognitive ability requisite for participation in decisions concerning one's own medical care. While the legal status of competency serves a variety of important social and economic functions, it is of little help to clinicians who must decide the degree to which their patients ought to be involved in determining the course of their treatment.

While it may not be impossible to arrive at an exact definition of competency, in the medical sense of the term, it is surely not a simple task. The lack of consensus as to the precise definition of competency may mean that the best that philosophical analysis can hope to provide is a set of criteria to help outline the major dimensions of competency.

Clinical standards

An alternative approach to the medical meaning of competency is to see what standards clinicians actually apply in medical settings. Determinations of competency are often based on one or more of the following considerations:

1. Compliance with medical opinion.
2. Membership in a particular class or category, e.g., "elderly," "violent," "poorly motivated."
3. Orientation as to time, place, and person.
4. Ability to pass a mental status examination.
5. The presence of inappropriate behavior, such as delusional thinking, sexual forwardness, or a loss of inhibition.
6. Affective stability.
7. The ability to show integrative thinking (Gutheil and Applebaum, 1982; Sherlock, 1983).

It is important to note that the first two criteria on this list are very different from the others. Using compliance or noncompliance with medical opinion might be termed, following the President's Commission (1982), as an "outcome" approach to the analysis of competency. It is not the process by which a patient reaches a decision but, rather, the actual content of the decision that, on this standard, shows competency.

The second criterion, assignment to a pre-existing category, might be termed the "membership" approach. Everyone, regardless of their particular capacities, is viewed as incompetent if they are accurately classified as members of a category that is generally seen as incompetent.

Neither of these approaches has much to recommend it. The

outcome approach is obviously suspect because it relies only on professional judgments about what counts as an acceptable decision. Such judgments are rarely explicitly articulated and even more rarely justified. The primary aim of a competency assessment is to determine whether a patient should be allowed to determine the course of his or her care. Using compliance with medical opinion or community standards of reasonableness defines in advance that only those who agree with these standards will be judged competent. All others lose their autonomous right to choose.

Similarly, there is sufficient empirical evidence for important variations in the capacities of individual patients within the category of elderly to make the membership approach entirely suspect (Stanley et al., 1984). Simply being old or institutionalized is not sufficient proof of incompetency!

The remaining clinical standards on the list represent efforts to make particular judgments about a specific patient's reasoning abilities and level of comprehension, as well as about the magnitude of the consequences of various decisions. These are all examples of what might be termed "functional" assessments of competency.

The functional approach to competency determination would seem far preferable to the alternatives that are sometimes used. It is true that no unanimity of opinion exists about the accuracy of various measures of cognitive and emotional stability, integrative thinking, and the like. Nevertheless, a functional approach to competency determination holds out the greatest chance of assessing individual decision-making capacity against a backdrop of professional disagreement, cultural pluralism, and societal uncertainty.

It's not so dismal

What are most disputes about competency really about? Where does this review of the philosophical, legal, and practical standards of competency leave us? Perhaps we are not in so dismal a situation as might be feared.

It is certainly the case that attempts to pinpoint *the* meaning of competency in clinical settings are motivated by the desire to obtain some understanding of the degree to which patients can be and should be involved in directing their own care. It is also true that the varied references to ability, appropriateness, and comprehension evident in clinical practice represent efforts to struggle with the properties that, empirically speaking, ought to be present for the patient's full or partial participation. The fact that concerns about appropriate behavior, harm, and compliance are so pervasive in clinical practice shows that assessments of competency are often motivated by a concern for the values that ought to take priority in decisions about patient care.

Frequently in medicine the desire to respect autonomy clashes with another important value, the desire to do good or, as it is sometimes called, the duty of benevolence. Physicians, nurses, and social workers want to use their knowledge and skills to advance the well-being of those in their care. The problem is that all too often the desire to do good conflicts with the obligation to respect autonomy. Patients may have preferences that conflict with professional judgments about what interventions would be in their best interest.

Two key moral principles must be considered in deciding what role to accord the patient in determining the course of medical intervention. The standard used by some courts and favored by many health professionals is that of "best interest." According to this norm, those charged with decision-making for patients with diminished or absent competency should undertake those medical interventions that they believe will be in the patient's best interests in terms of health and welfare. Other courts and commentators have argued for a standard of "substituted judgment" in which clinicians should attempt to decide about the acceptability of medical interventions as the patient would have decided had he or she been fully competent (Robertson, 1985).

There is a very real and powerful tension between the desire to be benevolent and the desire to respect autonomy. When doubts about competency exist, the "best interest" standard looks toward patient health and welfare as the controlling values; the "substituted judgment" standard gives individual autonomy priority.

These clashes of moral principle are not easy to resolve. In general, our society has tended to place greater priority on autonomy. For example, our legal system does not recognize any obligation on the part of physicians to treat persons who might benefit from their skills but who cannot pay. Nor does it recognize any obligation to donate life-saving tissues and organs or to participate in medical experimentation that might benefit those who are sick or dying. Autonomy usually trumps benevolence when these values conflict.

But this is not always the case. Sometimes physicians are encouraged by the law, or at least by medical tradition, to override autonomy in the interests of benevolence. Physicians and nurses routinely ignore the requests of burn patients and those suffering from paralyzing injuries to be allowed to die in the hope that these patients will accommodate themselves to the realities of their circumstances.

Clashes between respect for autonomy and the desire to be benevolent are often at the heart of disputes about the proper course of medical intervention for elderly patients. However, these ethical disagreements often masquerade as disputes about competency. When clinicians call upon psychiatrists to make a competency determination for a difficult patient, or when physicians in an acute care system label an elderly patient who is refusing life-saving surgery "confused," it is usually because they want to give more weight to the principle of benevolence than to the principle of respect for autonomy. The need to formulate a definition of competency may abate if it is understood that often what is really at issue is not what criteria are indicative of competency but rather which moral principle ought to govern the care of the elderly—respect for autonomy or benevolence.

Wisdom

Most of the contemporary efforts to resolve issues pertaining to competency in the literature of philosophy, law, and medicine involve attempts to locate a single criterion of competency that can serve as a universal standard for assessment. But matters are not so simple, particularly for older patients, where competency can be a function of setting, resources, and social contact. Competency may wax and wane depending on mood, time of day, and physiological health. However, many elderly patients suffering from diminished competency once were in a position to competently make choices about the nature of their medical treatment. This has direct implications for the answer that ought be given in attempting to cope with the conflict between benevolence and autonomy.

If any group can be said to have established authentic values, preferences, and goals concerning the kind of medical treatment they desire, surely it is the elderly (Dworkin, 1976). It may be impossible to decide what an infant or retarded person would want in the way of medical care. These people may not have attained sufficient levels of mental functioning to establish preferences, much less to think through choices about health care. But this is hardly true of the elderly.

A person who has lived a full life, who has acquired the wisdom that only experience can bring, is surely not akin to an infant or a retarded person with respect to the articulation of personal values about health care. The fact that the elderly have the wisdom that only age can bring would seem to require that thorough efforts be made to identify their preferences and choices and that special weight be accorded their autonomy.

If serious efforts are made to establish the values of elderly patients early on in the course of medical treatment, it should be possible to establish a baseline of patient desires that can guide care should impairments of competency arise. Those with chronic health problems can be informed about the kinds of decisions that may eventually arise with respect to matters such as the provision or withdrawal of artificial means of life-support or the initiation of aggressive efforts at resuscitation. If these issues are addressed and discussed in an open and frank manner early on in the course of an elderly patient's treatment, the patient will then be in a position to make informed, reflective choices about the course and direction of care should impairments of competency arise.

It is often possible to establish early on in the medical care of elderly patients the exact nature of their preferences, desires, and values. Health care providers who deal with this group therefore have an obligation to discuss with elderly patients all aspects of their present and possible future medical treatment. While competent elderly patients may not understand all of the options and all of the rationales concerning various forms of medical care, there is no reason to assume that they cannot be informed about them. Once informed, they can deliberate about the values and goals that they would like to guide the decisions of their health care providers should their competency diminish in any way.

In situations where elderly patients have had an opportunity to deliberate about and formulate reflective choices regarding the course of their medical care, then, should they suffer from impairments to their competency, a doctrine of substituted judgment should be followed insofar as is possible. Authentic patient desires can and should be used to guide treatment decisions.

Moreover, whenever possible, family members should be encouraged to take an active role in discussing the desires of their loved ones. While it has become popular in recent years to diminish the role families play in decisions about medical care, families are often in the best position to articulate the values that ought to guide care when competency is diminished or absent.

If health care providers make a sustained effort to involve family members early on in discussions with elderly patients about their care, then family members will be in a better position to act, not as surrogate decision-makers, but as what might be termed "proxy amplifiers." For those elderly who suffer from diminished or variable competency, loved ones may be able to act as amplifiers of authentic patient desires rather than simply as usurpers of patient autonomy and authority. When competency is manifestly present in an elderly patient, every effort should be made by health care professionals to assure that the wisdom of age is acknowledged and preserved should situations arise where it may be difficult to articulate or assert.

There are, of course, many situations in which little or nothing is known about the choices and values an elderly patient might have made regarding his or her care. In such circumstances, health care providers must of necessity follow a "best interest" standard in making judgments about the direction and course of care. Best interest is a moral principle that is useful in direct proportion to the degree of irremediable uncertainty or ignorance that exists regarding patient values, choices, and preferences.

Some may argue that a policy of substituted judgment cannot adequately protect patient autonomy since it is hard to know with certainty what a patient would have wanted, or because competent elderly patients sometimes change their wishes about medical treatment after surviving an episode of acute illness.

But are such worries really a sufficient basis for diminishing the importance of autonomy? No group is better qualified to formulate authentic and well-grounded value choices than the elderly. This fact in and of itself places a strong obligation on family and providers to respect the legacy of a competent choice in situations where competence is suspect or obviously diminished.

It is true that choices and values evolve. As a result, family members and health care providers must realize that respect for autonomy is a process, not an event. It is only by taking seriously the need to talk with and educate elderly patients about the choices that they must face with respect to health care that the elderly will be allowed to exercise the wisdom that accrues only to those who have had the opportunity to acquire it. Once it is realized that disputes about competency are in reality often disputes about whether benevolence or respect for autonomy ought to guide medical practice, the definition of competency may become less important for those who care for the elderly.

References

Abernathy, V. and Lundin, K., 1980. "Competency and the Right to Refuse Medical Treatment," In V. Abernathy, ed., *Frontiers in Medical Ethics.* Cambridge, MA: Ballinger.

Altman, I., 1975. *The Environment and Social Behavior.* Monterey, CA: Brooks-Cole.

Dohrenwend, B., 1975. "Sociocultural and Social-Psychological Factors in the Genesis of Mental Illness." *Journal of Health and Social Behavior* 16:365–392.

Donagan, A. 1977. "Informed Consent in Therapy and Experimentation." *Journal of Medicine and Philosophy* 2(4):310–27.

Dworkin, G., 1976. "Autonomy and Behavior Control." *Hastings Center Report* 6(1):23–28.

Gutheil, T. and Applebaum, P., 1982. *Clinical Handbook of Psychiatry and the Law.* New York: McGraw-Hill.

Neugarten, B., 1974. "Age Groups in American Society and the Rise of the Young-Old." *Annals of the American Academy of Political and Social Science* 415:187–97.

Palmore, E., 1980. *International Handbook on Aging.* Westport, CT: Greenwood Press.

President's Commission for the Study of Ethical Problems in Medicine and Biomedical and Behavioral Research, 1982. *Making Health Care Decisions.* Washington, DC: USGPO.

Robertson, J., 1983. "Procreative Liberty and the Control of Conception, Pregnancy and Childbirth." *Virginia Law Review* 69(405):55–80.

Robertson, J., 1985. "The Geography of Competency." *Social Research.*

Roth, L. et al, 1977. "Tests of Competency to Consent to Treatment." *American Journal of Psychiatry* 134:182.

Sherlock, R., 1983 "Competency to Consent to Medical Care: Toward a General View." *General Hospital Psychiatry* 5:2–7.

Stanley, R. et al, 1984. "The Elderly Patient and Informed Consent." *Journal of the American Medical Association* September 14:1135–37.

Verbrugge, Lois M., 1984. "Longer Life by Worsening Health? Trends in Health and Mortality of Middle-aged and Older Persons." *Milbank Memorial Fund Quarterly/Health and Society* 62(3).

14.

Is medical care the right prescription for chronic illness?

Chronic illness and disability are much-discussed topics in the world of health policy. Arguments rage as to whether the nation's population is growing sicker as it grows older.[1] It certainly seems that more people who in previous decades would have died from congenital conditions, injuries, or severe illnesses are now being kept alive but with varying degrees of impairment and morbidity. It is commonly noted that the price of successful acute care medical interventions is a population that will live longer but be sicker.

Economists, politicians, and the occasional physician seem to take a perverse delight in proffering Cassandra-like forecasts of an America overwhelmed by the demands of the aged, the diseased, and the disabled. The practitioners of the dismal science are living up to their name by engaging in a somewhat unseemly competition to see who can issue the most doleful assessment, the direst warning about the imminent insolvency of Medicare, social security, and special federal programs such as the Veterans Administration hospital system. Professional wisdom has it that these programs will soon be awash in a torrent of chronically ill and disabled persons who will in turn drown them in a sea of red ink.[2]

In the context of these hotly contested political and policy debates, it might seem naive if not downright stupid to suggest that the issues raised by chronic illness and disability require ethical rather than economic analysis for their resolution. Nonetheless, I believe that this is so. Answers to the questions of how much should be spent on the chronically ill and disabled, what priority ought to be accorded policies aimed at helping those who are chronically ill or disabled, and what goals should guide health care interventions directed at these populations depend on the ethical weight that is accorded chronic illness and disability.

Perhaps the major question requiring critical reflection is whether chronic illness ought be understood as a category or type of illness in itself. Do disability and chronic illness bear important similarities to acute illness? If not, they may require different responses from patients, health care providers, and policy makers.

If chronic illness does not require the same response from society as acute illness and if the services sought and needed are different, then the consequences for social policy and fiscal solvency may be different as well. Only if chronic illness and disability fit—or are forced to fit—into the prevailing conceptual framework for treating and paying for acute disease do increases in the proportion of chronically ill and disabled need to keep so many of those charged with balancing local, state, and federal budgets awake at night.

What is the relationship between acute and chronic conditions?

If chronic illness and disability differ in no important respects from acute illness or injury and are merely diseases that afflict a person over an extended period of time, then deciding how much should be spent to help the chronically ill and disabled will add nothing to the debates about equity and justice in the domain of health care. Chronic illness and injuries, as well as genetic anomalies capable of producing long-term impairment or dysfunction, while differing in degree from acute illness, would not be different in kind.

Those who have disabling pain, chronic arthritis, or chronic emphysema would gain or lose little in their efforts to secure a share of the resources available for health care by noting that their afflictions are permanent and incurable. The fact that a medical problem persists over time might increase the needs of the chronically ill and disabled relative to those of others with medical problems, but it would mean nothing in terms of the moral weight assigned to the needs of those with chronic or incurable disabling conditions.

If the chronically ill and disabled are concerned with securing a greater share of the nation's health care resources, they might indeed by happy to have their conditions treated as possessing the same moral weight as bacterial meningitis, a myocardial infarction, a sudden severe depression, a gunshot wound, or other dramatic examples of acute injury and illness. The treatment of acute illness and injury dominates the organization of our health care system, the educational orientation of our academic medical centers, the norms that guide interventions by health care professionals in hospital and other institutional settings, and the regulatory and reimbursement schemes that have evolved for treating illness and disease.[3] Simply viewing chronic illness and disability as a subcategory of illness and disease generally, therefore, would require a drastic revision in both clinical and societal policies concerning the allocation of health care resources to the chronically ill and disabled.

Advocates of the chronically ill and disabled are well aware of this fact. A great deal of the political advocacy on behalf of the chronically ill and disabled focuses on the similarity of their needs to the needs of those with acute illnesses. The language of equal rights is much in evidence when advocates for the disabled and the chronically ill present their case in Washington or in the various state capitals.[4]

The case for lumping disabilities and chronic conditions in with acute and emergency medical problems is based on the premise that our society seems willing to recognize the moral claim generated by the needs of those with life-threatening illnesses. The push to create a program of insurance to cover the costs of catastrophic illness within the Medicare program illustrates the moral power of acute medical problems in commanding scarce federal dollars. Since needs for acute medical care can generate societal obligations to satisfy these needs in the context of a hospital emergency room, as many have observed,[5] it would seem to be the most effective political strategy for those trying to secure resources for the chronically ill and disabled to draw analogies between these conditions and acute, life-threatening diseases.

This strategy might, in fact, be practical for obtaining more resources than are now being allotted for the needs of the chronically ill and disabled. Chronic illnesses and disabilities have not evoked the same degree of concern as acute, life-threatening illnesses. On first inspection, therefore, there might appear to be no benefit in distinguishing between acute and chronic medical problems.

The inadvisability of drawing any sharp distinctions between acute and chronic health care needs is further reinforced by the well-known aversion of insurance companies, the federal government, and other third parties to paying for the treatment of chronic medical problems. Such attitudes are not unique to reimbursement programs. Prepaid health plans such as health maintenance organizations (HMOs) and preferred provider organizations (PPOs) are notoriously reluctant to assume the financial costs of chronic illness and disability. Our financing schemes for reimbursing the costs of illness are oriented toward acute episodes of disease, precise categories of diagnosis and treatment (exemplified in the diagnosis-related group—DRG—system used in Medicare's prospective payment scheme), and measurable outcomes of progress and cure. Chronic illness and disability do not fare well under these criteria.

The reason for the relative underfunding of services and institutions aimed at helping those with chronic illnesses and disabilities is also well known. There is a fear that if third-party payers were to cover the costs of disability and chronic conditions they would soon go broke. If chronic illness and disability were treated on a conceptual par with acute illness, it seems that there would be a very real threat that the chronically ill and disabled—because of their complicated and continuing medical needs—would simply "hijack" all the resources made available for health care or for any other social purpose.[6] The fiscal burden that might be created by more generous reimbursement policies for chronic conditions is illustrated by Medicare's only attempt to reimburse the costs of chronic illness—the end-stage renal disease program for those with chronic renal failure.

In 1972 Congress created a special program to cover the costs of dialysis for all who suffered from kidney failure. At the time, the program was expected to cost $200–300 billion and to extend benefits to approximately 20,000 people. Today, the end-stage renal disease program pays more than $3 billion to cover the costs of dialysis for more than 100,000 patients.[7] Experts predict increases in both the number of eligible claimants and the amount of money spent for at least another ten years.

The costs of treating chronic renal failure left a searing impression on the minds of policy makers. Avoiding the creation of another program like that for end-stage renal disease has become dogma among many legislators and bureaucrats in Washington.

The threat of injustice in the distribution of resources is the most important political reason for distinguishing between acute and chronic illness. The projected costs of covering nursing home care, outpatient medications, the provision of therapies in the home, and comprehensive care of the handicapped and mentally ill are so large as to make it difficult for politicians to allow disability and chronic illnesses to be considered as deserving as acute illness.

But cost is not the only reason for drawing a distinction between acute and chronic medical problems, nor is it obviously a morally sound reason. If the only thing special about chronic illness and disability is that they are expensive to treat, this in itself is not a particularly impressive basis for drawing sharp distinctions between what we feel obligated to pay for in health care and what we do not. There is another reason to hesitate before arguing that chronic illness and disability merit the same societal concern and fiscal outlays that acute medical problems and emergencies currently receive: possible loss of personal autonomy.

Professional authority and individual autonomy

Acute illness is the province of medicine. Physicians have almost complete sovereignty over diagnosis, treatment, palliation, and rehabilitation where acute illness is concerned.

If those concerned with securing a greater share of society's resources for chronic medical problems try to do so by arguing that these problems are nothing more than a subspecies of the general class of disease, chronic illness and disability will be subject to the same models, standards, evaluative criteria, and professional control as acute illness. The resulting threat to independence and autonomy posed by dependency on the medical system and medical professionals may be a higher price than the chronically ill and disabled ought to be willing to pay.

Time and again newspaper and television broadcasts show how difficult it is for the acutely ill to retain control over their own medical care.[8] Decisions are often made with little or no consultation with competent patients. And when competent patients issue clear directives about the nature and course of their care, be they Jehovah's Witnesses or members of the Hemlock Society, physicians and hospital administrators sometimes pay little attention. All too often the only way of retaining autonomy over health care decisions concerning one's own body is to threaten a lawsuit or media campaign.

A very real danger of extending the medical model to chronic illness is the potential loss of personal freedom and autonomy to professionals. Thus, calls to extend acute care models of medical practice to settings such as nursing homes must be viewed with caution. While turning a nursing home into a hospital or a private home into an intensive care unit may improve the quality of care for the elderly who reside in it, personal autonomy may yield to the kind of professional authority that characterizes the practice of acute care medicine. This is little time for talk in the increasingly impersonal and technological world of acute care medicine.[9]

Are we obligated to help the sick?

Americans, despite their aversion to chiselers, malingerers, and sluggards, do acknowledge a moral obligation to help those who cannot help themselves. Those with acute illnesses have been able to secure a share of public funds obtained by compulsory taxation primarily on the ethical ground that each citizen has an obligation to help meet the health needs of those who are unable to meet their own needs.

The citizens of the United States like to believe that people with heart attacks or broken bones will not be left to fend for themselves just because they lack the means to pay for treatment. Our public philosophy seems to be that those who become acutely ill or who suffer acute injuries are entitled to receive government assistance as long as they can demonstrate clear-cut need. The existence of a need is seen as necessary to create an obligation on the part of society.

Recent interest in making transplants available without regard to the ability of the recipient to pay and in providing catastrophic health insurance coverage reflects precisely this degree of perceived moral obligation on the part of the public. In health care, unlike other areas of life, a need for life-saving medical treatment is held by most citizens to be a sufficient moral ground for requiring others to help pay for its provision, assuming that the needy cannot afford to pay out of their own pockets.

Why should this be so? Why is it that in a society that tolerates enormous differences in access to housing, education, and employment opportunities, health needs occupy a position of special moral standing?

To understand why health care needs elicit a degree of compassion that other needs do not, it is necessary to consider the moral foundations of beneficence in American society. Nearly every moral theory that has any currency in our society posits a duty of beneficence, a duty to aid when the following conditions are met:[10]

1. A need is obvious, serious, and life-threatening.

2. Assistance rendered must stand some chance of meeting or alleviating the need.

3. Those requiring assistance from others must not have any reasonable alternative sources of aid.

4. Providing assistance must not create undue burdens on or risks to those giving the help.

These conditions say nothing about the liability or culpability of those who are in need. At least when lives hang in the balance, our society has remained relatively indifferent to the cause of a person's need in determining a general obligation of beneficence. People who do not wear seat belts or whose drinking leads to the need for a liver transplant may receive aid from publicly funded sources if the conditions outlined above are met. We do not, at least in theory, make allocation decisions based on the worthiness of patients or their social status.[11]

If the major moral outlooks current in our society, both religious and secular, countenance at least a minimal duty of beneficence—an obligation to help others or to meet the needs of others when the conditions outlined above are met—then it is easy to see why life-threatening medical needs have generated so much concern in American health policy. People who have heart attacks or sudden renal failure have clear-cut, life-threatening needs and are not in a position to help themselves. Since in most cases it does not cost very much to pay for the services required to help each individual, and since health care professionals know how to treat heart or kidney failure, it would seem that we have a duty to provide resources or to tolerate a degree of taxation sufficient to enable those who cannot pay for the requisite services to have access to them.

But clarifying the moral underpinnings of this obligation of beneficence reveals why those with chronic medical problems may continue to find it difficult to tap into the same vein of moral concern—even in a society as enamored of independence and personal autonomy as the United States. Chronic conditions and disability do not tap the same reservoir of beneficence as acute illness and injury.

Chronic conditions, although they can be severely limiting and can cause serious dysfunction, often lack the obvious need for assistance associated with acute illness. Those in chronic pain with hypertension, diabetes, or arthritis may not be visibly in need of help. Those with disabling injuries or suffering the after-effects of a mild stroke, while surely in need of assistance, are nevertheless still able to perform many of the activities of day-to-day living.

Chronic conditions and disability not only permit disagreement and uncertainty about a person's level of need, but also have not been demonstrated to be as responsive to treatments as most acute medical problems.

In general, physicians and nurses know how to help those with acute medical problems. Although organ transplants sometimes fail and not every heart attack victim can be saved, the vast array of everyday health problems admit of a course of treatment that is both routine and likely to work.

It is generally not clear, however, and it is far from scientifically proved what kinds of assistance would help those with chronic conditions to gain relief. Whether it be for low back pain or rehabilitation after a massive stroke, the efficacy of standard treatments for chronic conditions is not well established.

If more were known about the effectiveness of attempts to rehabilitate persons with spinal cord injuries or coping with chronic pain, perhaps more money would be made available to ensure that persons with these conditions had access to care. But with so little known about whether medical intervention does any good in such cases, it is hard to command a greater share of public resources when so many other claims are being made on them for acute and emergency medical services and for other types of social goods (education, defense, public works, and so on).

Matters are made worse by the emphasis our society places on autonomy and free choice. One way to view curing is to see it as restoring a person to a state of autonomy and free choice, unimpaired by illness or disease.[12] But the chronically ill and disabled often are left in permanent states of dependency by their conditions—not an especially popular status in our culture.

The obligation to help the chronically ill and disabled is also weakened by the belief that, whereas only physicians and trained medical personnel can help the acutely ill, many other people— spouses, children, relatives, friends, members of religious and fraternal organizations—are capable of providing the kind of aid that is in fact most useful for those with chronic medical problems. No one believes that a husband has a special duty to relieve a case of bacterial meningitis that his wife might contract. But many people believe that it is his duty to provide for her should she become blind, wheelchair bound, demented, arthritic, or diabetic. The possibility of family assistance undercuts the moral pressure felt by others to provide for those with chronic medical needs.

The provision of aid to those with acute illness and injury seems not to entail undue risks or burdens (or at least did not seem to do so until health care costs began escalating rapidly). But chronic conditions demand aid that is burdensome, both financially and in the ways it affects the lives of those giving it. Society views it very differently when a person is asking for help to pay for having a gall bladder removed than when that person requests assistance for spina bifida, Alzheimer's disease, or cystic fibrosis. The needs are great in all cases, but the burden of providing help seems much more onerous and, to put the point baldly, endless in the case of chronic conditions.[13]

One final reason for the moral asymmetry between the provision of public funds for acute and chronic medical problems is confusion about whether chronic medical problems or disabilities really are diseases. Uncertainty about the categorization of chronic medical problems condemns those with such impairments and disorders to a kind of conceptual limbo, in which lines of responsibility among those with disabling conditions, their families, health care professionals, social welfare agencies, and other social institutions are not clearly drawn.

Chronic illness, disability, and the medical model

The dominant philosophical outlook on chronic illness in the United States is that it does not require any special ethical status. Although we are willing to acknowledge the possibility that mental illness differs in important and significant respects from physical illness as a category or type of disease, there is little inclination to consider chronic diseases as constituting a significantly different class from acute conditions.

There are many articles about the limits of the medical model in understanding and treating mental illness, but there are no analogous discussions where chronic disease is concerned. With the possible exception of mental disorders, modern medicine views disease as a single category or, in more philosophical terms, as a natural "kind," with acute and chronic disease just variants on a single theme.

But is this classification valid? Should chronic disease and disability be lumped together with acute illnesses and injuries? Or are there differences significant enough to place them in two separate categories of disease? And if so, do they require different methods of care and different responses from those responsible for creating health policies?

What is the medical model?

In the medical model the goal of health care is to cure disease.[14] Disease is defined as any dysfunction of an organ, organ system, or structure,[15] and health is understood as the absence of disease. Those who subscribe to these definitions see little need to make value judgments about whether or not a person is sick; one merely measures the appropriate physiological variables, and the answer is obvious to anyone with the proper training. The medical model presumes that all diseases have quantifiable physiological causes with definite onsets and, if left untreated, predictable outcomes.

Some may protest that this description of the medical model is a straw man, that health care providers know better than to treat patients simply as vessels containing dysfunctional kidneys, bladders, or thyroids. But despite recent efforts to broaden the goals of medical care beyond the narrow aim of restoring normal function, for many kinds of hospital-based medical care this account is accurate.[16] It is certainly a model that dominates many textbooks of surgery, immunology, pathology, infectious disease, and, increasingly, psychiatry.

The sick role

One of the most important contributions made by those studying the sociology of medicine has been to show how different the perception of illness by patients and society is from that of professionals within the medical system. Perhaps the best-known exposition of the cultural and social dimensions of disease is Talcott Parsons's definition of what he termed the "sick role."[17]

Parsons noted that health and disease have a special status in American society. He observed that in our achievement-oriented society health is given an especially high priority because it is a prerequisite for being able to work, which is a critical capacity in a competitive free-market society.

The social construction of disease, according to Parsons and those who have extended his analyses, is a far cry from the professional understanding of disease as defined by the medical model.[18] Our ordinary understanding of disease—what Parsons termed the sick role, or what might usefully be termed the illness model—is based on four conditions that cause us to recognize someone as ill: a person is incapable of curing himself; is exempt from usual roles and duties; wants to get better; and wants to seek help from experts and to receive treatment.

Disease, chronic illness, and disability— a poor fit

What is interesting about the analysis of disease in the medical model and the more expansive analysis in the illness model is that chronic illness and disability do not fit well into either model. Chronic illness and disability are remarkable for the fact that they often lack a clear-cut physiological cause, onset, or outcome. The disabled and the chronically ill cannot have function restored. Part of the very definition of a chronic condition is that it is incurable. Moreover, many of the problems of the chronically ill have as much to do with sociology and politics as with physiology.

Those with chronic conditions obviously would like medicine to cure or alleviate their disabilities. But in lieu of cures, access to buildings, jobs, housing, and education are of greater concern than what neurology, rehabilitation medicine, or psychiatry has to offer.

Even at the social level, though, the chronically ill and disabled are in trouble even under the illness model. To some extent health care professionals in particular and society in general hold the chronically ill responsible for their own cures.

Motivation and compliance are the virtues expected of the chronically ill and disabled in health care settings. Patients seen to have "motivational problems" risk fast abandonment by their health care professionals. Society has equally high expectations, at least to the extent to which the media celebrate those who have stopped "whining" about their ailments and gotten on with their lives.

The chronically ill and disabled, while exempt from some social roles and duties, are often capable of doing what everyone else does—if society will let them. They face a peculiar Catch-22 dilemma, though: they want to carry out the roles and duties that they are capable of, but they must depend on society's recognition that they cannot and should not be expected to carry out *all* the usual roles.

As noted earlier, a key ethical requirement for feeling a duty of beneficence to another is that the recipient be truly in need of help. Yet a critical precondition for receiving respect from others in our society is that a person not be perceived as dependent, needy, or receiving aid. The acutely ill can face this dilemma with the knowledge that their state is temporary. The disabled and the chronically ill have a much harder time of it, since their needs are seemingly endless.

The chronically ill and disabled often encounter medical problems that require professional help. But, unlike those who require only brief, episodic interactions with the world of medicine to cope with acute or emergency medical problems, they do not want to spend their entire lives dependent on health care institutions and professionals. Thus, they do and yet do not want to seek out medical expertise, another tension that tends to delegitimate the authenticity of their needs and claims.

On strictly medical grounds, chronic illness and disability do not fit the model of disease that prevails within our medical system.[19] Nevertheless, there are many reasons for those who are chronically ill and disabled to conform to the requirements of that model, both to gain access to the medical system and to gain legitimacy for their conditions in a society disinclined to be tolerant of anyone who will not pull his or her own economic weight.

The wisdom of securing resources or the sympathy of the public by squeezing chronic illness and disability into the medical model, however, is disputable, as some health policy commentators have cogently observed.[20] The goals of the chronically ill and the disabled are not necessarily those of the acute care patient. If chronic illness and disability are not readily subsumed under the standard definition of disease and illness, meeting the needs of the chronically ill and disabled may require a redefinition of their problems as well as a reassessment of the kinds of services that can best meet their needs.

Reclassifying chronic illness and disease

To a great extent, recent policy debates about chronic illness focus on whether it is worthwhile for society to invest resources in medical care that results in large numbers of persons living longer but being sicker.[21] As the pressure to contain health care costs escalates, policy options are framed as requiring a choice between paying for acute medical care needs of the many and providing exotic care for the unusual medical care needs of the few.[22] The needs of children, the mentally ill, the elderly, the disabled, the dying, and the chronically ill are seen as competing against one another for a finite and diminishing pool of resources.

Is it necessary, however, to see health policy as constrained by the need to make hard choices among the competing claims of those with various types of disorders and diseases? Is it true that what constitutes optimal care for one group will necessarily be the same for others?

As we have already seen, there are significant differences between the definitions of acute and chronic diseases. These differences significantly weaken attempts to fit chronic illness under the rubric of acute disease or to draw upon the kinds of arguments for beneficence that have been persuasive in pushing our society to meet the acute and emergency medical needs of its poor and elderly.

The solution to helping those with chronic diseases and disabilities may not require government officials and physicians to perform health care triage. Rather, the prospects of governmental fiscal insolvency occasioned by the provision of public funds for chronic illness and disability might be lessened if they could be removed from the domain of the medical model of disease and placed in a separate category. Such a redefinition might contribute to a more precise understanding of both chronic illness and disability while appealing to the beneficent impulses of the American public to help those who cannot meet their own needs, either for want of economic means or for lack of willing helpers.

The chronically ill and disabled are not diseased

The solution to the public policy dilemma of how to afford the costs associated with chronic illness and disability is very much a function of the classification or conceptualization of these conditions. We have seen that chronic illness and disability do not meet the requirements of the traditional medical model of disease. Surprisingly, they do not conform to the criteria of a more inclusive illness model either. And perhaps most surprisingly, they do not meet the requirements for eliciting a duty of beneficence on the part of others as this obligation is understood under most theories of ethics.

Two strategies might be chosen in light of these findings. One approach would be to broaden either the standard medical model of disease or the illness model to incorporate chronic illness and disability. In doing so, it may be possible to appeal to the same principle of beneficence that has proved so effective in securing resources for those with acute or catastrophic diseases.

The other strategy would be simply to admit that chronic conditions and disability, while often having their roots in disease or illness, are conceptually distinct from these categories. Although those who are disabled or chronically ill often endure medical crises just as other members of society do, it may be conceptually confusing—and may deprive them of their autonomy—to lump them under a medical or illness model of disease.

Numerous advocacy groups for the disabled and the chronically ill have objected to the notion that those with chronic impairments or disabilities ought to be viewed as permanently sick. Such a classification, while commanding great moral force for securing resources from the health care system under the principle of beneficence, comes at a high price. It means that the chronically ill and disabled will be seen by both health care professionals and society as permanent patients meriting assistance, but also meriting paternalistic charitable aid. In a society that treasures independence and autonomy, assuming the role of permanent patient is not likely to ensure the dignity and equality of those in constant need of medical treatment.

"Demedicalizing" chronic illness and disability

In listening to what those with disabilities or chronic impairments say they want, it becomes plain that we need to abandon the attempt to squeeze them into the framework of disease or illness or to make them the recipients of societal beneficence by expanding their access to models of care inspired by acute care medicine. Those with impairments or disabilities that are not immediately life-threatening do not want constant access to medical care and the ministrations of health care professionals; they want to be given the same opportunities other Americans enjoy to maximize their abilities and capacities.

The disabled seek equality of opportunity with respect to housing, education, employment, and recreation. They wish to be seen as ordinary citizens who may require social interventions or accommodations to allow them to participate as fully as possible in the ordinary activities of daily life. Consequently, efforts to expand the medical system to absorb more of the chronically ill and disabled, while well motivated, are misguided. Of course, the medical needs of the chronically ill and disabled ought to be met, but on the same moral grounds that our society recognizes as appropriate for guaranteeing access to health care for any citizen, disabled, impaired, or not.

To argue that we need more medical specialists in chronic illness or disability, more hospitals and long-term care facilities for the chronically ill and disabled, and a greater emphasis on the provisions of medical therapies for the disabled is to miss the point. What many of those with chronic illnesses or disabilities need is equal opportunity, not beneficence or charity. The acutely ill or those facing catastrophic health care emergencies require our beneficence and charity, but those with chronic illness or disabilities who are not facing an acute medical crisis deserve something radically different—the right to equality of opportunity.

The key to sound public policy with respect to chronic illness and disability is not the creation of more teaching nursing homes in academic medical centers or a greater emphasis on chronic illness in our schools of nursing or medicine. Medical professionals need to understand the nature of acute illness in a person with impairments or disabilities to the extent that such illness is different or more likely when disabilities are present. But those with chronic illness or impairments need from society less emphasis on the medical aspects of chronic disease and more emphasis on the social adjustments necessary to assist them in becoming full participants in society.

In other words, the disabled and chronically ill have a right to expect the "demedicalization" of chronic disease in favor of the provision of social services, educational programs, vocational training, and the removal of architectural barriers. We need social policies aimed at restoring and enhancing the autonomy of persons whose impairments or disorders cannot be cured.

The moral foundation for access to such services is different from that for claiming access to medical services that are beyond a person's financial means. Those with disabilities or chronic impairments can lay claim to requisite social services for themselves or those with whom they live on the grounds that, while they may be no more entitled to equality of outcome than any other citizen, they are entitled to equality of opportunity. Those with non–life-threatening chronic impairments cannot be cured, but they can require social policies that maximize their opportunities for choice and freedom.

To say that those with chronic illnesses or impairments do not require access to health care is not to say that they need little or no contact with physicians, nurses, and other health care providers. Obviously, many aspects of chronic illness or disability are amenable to some forms of medical intervention, either for the palliation of symptoms or because people with chronic conditions may be more vulnerable to acute or emergency medical problems than other members of society are.

To say that the social or public policy response to chronic illness is better formulated under the rubric of opportunity than of beneficence is to say that access to health care should not be the major preoccupation of public policy. This is not because it would be expensive to attempt to help those with chronic impairments or disorders in this way, although in fact it would be. It is because treating chronic illness and disability strictly as medical problems requiring medical responses "disenfranchises" a large segment of society by making them permanent objects of social beneficence, a status that few if any members of our society would wish to occupy.

If the chronically ill and disabled can be weaned from the medical system, they may be able to reach their full potential at less cost. Moreover, every individual's enjoyment of autonomy and independence may be enriched.

Chronic illness and disability have a remarkable power. Those who endure a disability must think long and hard about the nature of their own identity and about what it is that they want to be and become. The onset of a chronic illness or disabling condition may actually enhance autonomy by forcing direct decisions about goals, personal plans, values, and life-style choices, which are all too often pushed aside by the able-bodied or healthy as too frightening.

Perhaps it is easier to fit chronic illness and disability into a medical or illness model because doing so avoids the challenge that impairment and disability pose to our sense of personal identity and responsibility. The impaired and the disabled become persons worthy of charity, not of choices.

Chronic illness and disability remind us all not only of our technological or scientific limits but also of how difficult it is to be truly independent or autonomous. While we pay much lip service to these lofty notions in our political rhetoric, the prospect of confronting choices about who we are and who we really want to be is simply too terrifying for many of us. Disability is a reminder that to be truly autonomous one must be willing to reflect consciously on one's identity and aspirations. If that is so, the appropriate public policy response is not to figure out how our society can afford to pay for access to medical technology or health care professionals for those with chronic illness or disability. Rather, it is to confront, openly and honestly, the challenge of creating social policies that are necessary to enhance the opportunities of those who lack certain abilities or capacities. Reflection on the ways our society can maximize opportunities for those with impairments and permanent disabilities will inevitably enhance the freedom and autonomy of everyone, disabled or not.

Notes

1. James F. Fries, "Aging, Natural Death, and the Compression of Morbidity," *New England Journal of Medicine*, vol. 303 (1980), pp. 130–35; E. Schneider and J. Brody, "Aging, Natural Death, and the Compression of Morbidity: Another View," *New England Journal of Medicine*, vol. 309, no. 14 (1983), pp. 854–56; and Lois Verbrugge, "Longer Life but Worsening Health?" *Milbank Memorial Fund Quarterly*, vol. 62, no. 3 (1984), pp. 475–519.

2. Henry Aaron and William Schwartz, *The Painful Prescription* (Washington, D.C.: Brookings Institution, 1984); Jerry Avorn, "Benefit and Cost Analysis in Geriatric Care," *New England Journal of Medicine*, vol. 310 (1984), pp. 1294–1301; Joseph Califano, *America's Health Care Revolution* (New York: Random House, 1986); Roger W. Evans, "Healthcare Technology and Resource Allocation," *Journal of the American Medical Association*, vol. 249, no. 15 (1983), pp. 2047–53; Richard D. Lamm, *Megatraumas* (New York: Houghton Mifflin, 1985); and Richard D. Lamm, "We Can't Afford the Health Plan," *New York Times*, February 19, 1984, p. A31.

3. Irving Lewis and Cecil Sheps, *The Sick Citadel* (Boston: Oelgeschlager, Gunn and Hain, 1983); and Paul Starr, *The Social Transformation of American Medicine* (New York: Basic Books, 1983).

4. Gerben DeJong and R. Lifchez, "Physical Disability and Public Policy," *Scientific American*, vol. 248, no. 6 (1983), pp. 40–49.

5. Norman Daniels, *Just Health Care* (New York: Cambridge University Press, 1985).

6. Lamm, *Megatraumas*; and Lamm, "We Can't Afford the Health Plan."

7. Arthur Caplan, "Kidneys, Ethics, and Politics," *Journal of Health Politics, Policy, and Law*, vol. 6, no. 3 (1981), pp. 488–503.

8. George Annas, "Transferring the Ethical Hot Potato," *Hastings Center Report*, vol. 17, no. 1 (1987), pp. 20–21.

9. Jay Katz, *The Silent World of Doctor and Patient* (New York: Free Press, 1986).

10. Tom Beauchamp and James Childress, *Principles of Biomedical Ethics* (New York: Oxford University Press, 1979).

11. Arthur Caplan, "Equity in the Selection of Recipients for Cardiac Transplants," *Circulation*, vol. 75, no. 1 (1987), pp. 10–20.

12. Eric Cassell, *The Healer's Art* (Cambridge, Mass.: MIT Press, 1985).

13. C. Weiner et al., "What Price Chronic Illness?" *Society*, vol. 19, no. 2 (1982), pp. 22–30.

14. Arthur Caplan, "The Concepts of Health and Disease," in R. Veatch, ed., *Medical Ethics* (Boston: Jones & Bartlett, 1989), pp. 49–63.

15. Christopher Boorse, "On the Distinction between Disease and Illness," in Arthur Caplan et al., eds., *Concepts of Health and Disease* (Reading, Mass.: Addison-Wesley, 1981), pp. 545–60.

16. George Engel, "The Need for a New Medical Model," in Caplan et al., *Concepts of Health and Disease*, pp. 589–608.

17. Talcott Parsons, "Definitions of Health and Illness in the Light of

American Values and Social Structures," in Caplan et al., *Concepts of Health and Disease*, pp. 57–82.

18. David Mechanic, "Illness Behavior, Social Adaptation, and the Management of Illness," *Journal of Nervous and Mental Disease*, vol. 165, no. 2 (1977), p. 79–87.

19. Gerben DeJong, "Societal Duty and Resource Allocation," *Journal of Head Trauma Rehabilitation*, vol. 4, no. 1 (1989): 1–12.

20. Muriel Gillick, "Is the Care of the Chronically Ill a Medical Prerogative?" *New England Journal of Medicine*, vol. 310, no. 3 (1984), pp. 190–93; and Anne Somers, "Long-Term Care for the Elderly and Disabled—A New Health Priority," *New England Journal of Medicine*, vol. 307, no. 4 (1982), pp. 221–26.

21. Verbrugge, "Longer Life but Worsening Health?"; and Bruce Vladek and J. Firman, "The Aging of the Population and Health Services," *Annals of the American Academy of Political and Social Sciences*, vol. 468 (July 1983), pp. 132–48.

22. Aaron and Schwartz, *The Painful Prescription*; Lamm, *Megatraumas*; and Lamm, "We Can't Afford."

15.

Informed consent and provider/patient relationships in rehabilitation medicine

Current views concerning the ethics of provider/patient relationships

The nature of the moral rules and principles that ought to govern relationships between health care providers and their patients is one that has received a great deal of attention in the literature of bioethics.[3,16,20,25] Yet, despite the attention given to understanding the rights, duties, and responsibilities of patients and health care providers, very few (if any) analyses have drawn upon rehabilitation medicine as a source of examples for understanding the moral foundations of provider/patient relationships.

The existing discussions of provider/patient relationships make a number of assumptions about the nature of those engaged in the relationship and about the goals of medical intervention, assumptions which are worthy of special note. First, the examples and paradigms discussed in most of the bioethics literature are drawn almost exclusively from the context of either emergency or acute medical care. Decisions to implant an artificial heart, terminate respiratory therapy, or administer resuscitation to those who have suffered cardiac or respiratory failure dominate the available analyses.

Second, discussions of the ethics of provider/patient relationships nearly always presume that the goal of providing medical treatment is clear—to cure the disease afflicting the patient. While there is a large and growing literature on the ethics of human experimentation, and while some commentators recognize that not all interventions in acute or emergency medicine are of established efficacy, the fact remains that discussions of the ethics of medical care almost always assume that both patients and providers understand that the treatment being offered is intended to do no less than cure the patient.[6]

A third distinctive attribute of the relevant literature is the usual assumption that the relationship is built around a specific, readily identifiable health care problem.[1] Should a Jehovah's Witness be compelled to accept a blood transfusion as a part of surgery? What should a physician say to a patient with breast cancer who must face the prospect of surgery? Does an elderly patient have the right to refuse amputation of a gangrenous leg even if death will likely result? Such examples, which are the stock and trade of the existing literature of medical ethics,[13] presume that medical relationships are discrete, finite, and episodic.

Fourth, while there is an enormous literature devoted to the kinds of protections that ought be given to those who by reason of age, mental incapacity, or emotional impairment are not competent to make decisions for themselves,[10] the baseline of nearly all discussions of patients' rights and professional obligations is that of a competent patient negotiating in good faith to obtain the services of a specific health care provider. It is assumed that patients are free to seek the services of any provider they wish, and providers are free not to accept patients if they do not wish to do so.

The foundational moral principle which has emerged from these discussions is that of respect for individual patient autonomy. Competent patients must be given the right to control what happens to their bodies in any medical encounter. While health care professionals may and should be committed to an ethic that requires them to try to benefit their patients while not harming them, competent patients must be given the opportunity to control the provision of medical care even if death or disability may result,[3,7]

Time and time again American courts have held that competent adults have the right to refuse necessary medical care on religious or other grounds.[1,15] Philosophers and legal theorists have stressed that moral priority ought to be accorded the principle of respect for autonomy rather than to any other moral principle, even that of beneficence (the desire to help patients through the use of medical expertise and skills). While controversy surrounds the definition of competency,[4,5] the choices of a patient who understands the risks and benefits of a proposed medical treatment and who has been given the requisite information to make a deliberative choice about medical care must be respected by physicians, nurses, and other health professionals.

Yet the moral claims which have emerged from legal and ethical reflection on the nature of provider/patient relationships may not be readily applied to the practice of rehabilitation medicine. In rehabilitation, patients often must deal with a team of health care providers rather than with a single individual medical practitioner. While patients in acute or emergency settings are more or less passive with respect to the interventions that are proposed by health care professionals,[16,22] this is not at all the case in rehabilitation. Rehabilitation patients are constantly urged and, indeed, expected to take an active role in their own care.

Perhaps the most important difference between the ethical norms thought to govern provider/patient relationships in acute or emergency treatment and rehabilitation is the emphasis placed on obtaining informed consent in acute care settings. While acute-care providers may give only pro forma attention to informed consent, the fact remains that they are often unwilling to undertake medical interventions without the express written permission of the patient.

Those admitted to rehabilitation programs are sometimes not given the opportunity to accept or reject specific forms of care. Occasionally, explicit refusals of care by seemingly incompetent patients are simply ignored or overridden. The fact that many professionals interact with a patient over the course of months or even years means that models of informed consent based upon episodic interactions with specific health care providers may be of little utility in understanding the moral framework within which care is provided to those with chronic impairments of one sort or another.

The traditional model: medical paternalism

Historically, the medical profession has articulated a number of codes of conduct intended to provide guidance as to physician responsibilities. The moral requirements reflected in documents such as the Hippocratic Oath and the American Medical Association's *Principles of Medical Ethics*[1] enjoin physicians to act only so as to "benefit" the patient and to "do no harm" or "keep patients from harm." They insist that physicians maintain the confidentiality and privacy of the doctor/patient relationship at all times. On this traditional model of physician/patient relationships, as long as treatment is efficacious, only the patient has a right to end the relationship. Anything less would constitute abandonment by the physician of the patient.

Existing professional codes cast the physician in the role of the zealous advocate of the patient's best interests. The codes also state that it is the physician who is in the best position, as a consequence of specialized knowledge, skills, and clinical experience, to determine which medical interventions are in a patient's best interest in particular situations.[8,18]

A number of critics of such codes,[3,12,16,22-24] both within and outside of medicine, have argued in recent years for a somewhat more egalitarian model of physician/patient relationships. They contend that moral principles such as those reflected in existing codes of medical conduct are based solely upon the principle of beneficence. Critics of this model argue that moral rules which leave the determination of interests only in the hands of physicians are far too paternalistic.[7,11,16,23-25] Such rules accord patients few if any rights to participate in the formulation of a care plan and fail to respect the autonomy of individual patients to decide whether they will or will not accept various medical interventions.

A variety of writers[8,9,25] have articulated an alternative model of physician/patient relationships. This model interprets rights, duties, and responsibilities in a manner which is closely analogous to a legal contract.

The contractual model

On the contractual model of doctor/patient relationships, physicians are morally responsible for providing care, but only such care as is desired or requested by patients. The desire to do good, to be beneficent in the provision of medical care must, on this model, always respect the autonomy of individual patients, even if patients choose to reject care known to be beneficial in diagnosing or treating the effects of disease or injury.

The doctrine which has emerged as the guarantee of individual patient autonomy on the contractual model is informed consent. Patients, on the contractual model of physician/patient relationships, have an absolute right to make informed choices about whether they wish to receive care and about the degree and intensity of the care that they will receive.[8,25]

Historically, many physicians in the United States and other Western nations did not recognize an obligation always to be truthful concerning either diagnosis or prognosis.[16,18] Until recently, the paternalistic model held sway in the practice of medicine. As recently as the 1950s, it was not unusual for physicians to withhold information from patients who were seriously or terminally ill on the grounds that the truth was not always in the best interest of the patient. Physicians maintained that patients did not always want to know the truth, could not always comprehend the truth, or might be harmed if they were presented with the harsh realities associated with a particularly hopeless diagnosis. Moreover, some physicians were skeptical that laypersons could make intelligent choices about the kind of care necessary for the treatment of a specific medical problem.[16]

As the contractual model has come to have greater sway in medicine, there has been a steady shift in clinical practice toward the recognition of a powerful duty to share information about diagnoses and prognoses with patients. If it is true that patients ought have the right to control their medical care, if respect for autonomy carries more moral weight than the obligation of beneficence when these moral principles come into conflict, then patients have a right to know and physicians a duty to tell the truth. In fact, as a number of surveys and studies have demonstrated, truthtelling has come to occupy a much more central place in medical practice than was the case in the 1950s and 1960s.[16,20]

Informed consent has come to be the dominant moral rule for guiding physician/patient interactions in recent years. While many commentators note serious problems in putting this doctrine into practice, there is no doubt that the desirability of informing patients about their diagnoses and proposed medical care has received wide recognition from those in ethics, law, and health care. It is presumed that if a patient is mentally competent—as reflected in an ability to understand information about the risks, benefits, and consequences of medical treatment or the failure to initiate treatment—then patients ought be accorded the right to make choices about each and every aspect of their medical care.

Most physicians, and certainly most lawyers and courts, now believe that patients should not be coerced or tricked into providing their consent. Consent must be voluntary and free—the product of deliberative reflection on all possible courses of action. If this ideal is to be achieved in the practice of medicine, then physicians have a moral duty to tell the truth, to refrain from deceiving patients in any way, to accord their patients the right to withdraw their consent for medical care at any time, and to present all options and possibilities for treatment in a balanced and accurate manner.

The contractual model assigns a high value to confidentiality and privacy. Behaviors or policies that weaken the confidentiality and privacy of medical relationships are seen as undesirable in that they weaken the trust patients have and must have, according to some physicians, in their doctors. Moreover, the protection of confidentiality and privacy is central to the doctor/patient relationship on the contractual model, since it is the patient who can and should decide who will have access, if anyone may, to personal information about his or her diagnosis and medical care.[18]

Does the contractual model apply in rehabilitation?

An interesting aspect of provider/patient relationships in the context of rehabilitation is that clinical practice sometimes involves deviations from the ideal of the contractual model as reflected in the doctrine of informed consent. Informed consent is problematic.

While providers in rehabilitation recognize the importance of informed consent, in practice they are sometimes less aggressive or thorough in obtaining consent than are practitioners in other areas of health care. Although patients may give written consent to treatment, they may never be asked to provide consent for interventions such as physical therapy, occupational therapy, or vocational counseling. Even if consent is obtained early in the course of a particular treatment regimen, care may extend over months or years with no attempts to reaffirm patient consent. In some cases, explicit refusals of care are ignored or overridden, as in instances in which patients who have become paraplegic as a result of traumatic injuries request that no further medical care be given.

If it is true that informed consent does not have the same moral force in rehabilitation that it has in other domains of health care, perhaps this should not come as a surprise. After all, many of the conditions and circumstances for which a contractual model of provider/patient relationships evolved do not obtain in rehabilitation settings.

Unique aspects of clinical care in rehabilitation

Patients rarely receive care from a single physician in rehabilitation. Rather, patients must interact on a daily basis with a large number of specialists, many of whom are not physicians. The contractual model of informed consent presumes a one-on-one relationship. But rehabilitation candidates must deal with a host of health care providers of differing backgrounds and expertise. It is not surprising that a contractual model and its linchpin, the doctrine of informed consent, encounter practical difficulties in the context of such a complex set of provider/patient relationships.

Rehabilitative care often extends over periods of months or years. It can be delivered in institutional or home settings. The length of time involved, and the diversity of settings in which care is delivered, pose practical problems for a model of provider/patient relationships that presumes episodic interactions between highly trained professionals and autonomous patients in hospital settings or medical offices.

The families of patients often must assume active roles in providing care if the efforts of rehabilitation specialists are to be maximally efficacious.[17] Provider/patient relationships often must, as a result, reflect the involvement of third parties—spouses, children, parents, friends, etc., whose roles are simply not acknowledged in the contractual view of provider/patient relationships. Issues of privacy and confidentiality are complicated by practical realities associated with the involvement of many parties, both medical and nonmedical.

Competency and autonomy in rehabilitation

Experienced health care providers in rehabilitation are sometimes skeptical about the degree of autonomy that patients actually possess upon entry into a rehabilitation setting.[21] While it would be easy enough to dismiss such attitudes as nothing more than examples of traditional medical paternalism, there are some patients who enter rehabilitation with severe levels of impairment and little hope of cure. There is a subpopulation of patients who pose special problems for understanding competency and presuming autonomy in rehabilitation—specifically, those patients who have suffered severe impairments as a result of unexpected and unanticipated disease or injury.

Can a person who has suddenly lost the use of limbs or who is suddenly unable to speak or to be understood truly be said to be the "same" person, much less a person who is competent to make important decisions as to the type of medical care that will be given? Those in rehabilitation must care for patients who may have had little time to adjust to the reality of severe impairment and who have little experience or familarity with disability.

Disability is not a subject that is widely discussed or understood by the average American. Consequently, even when patients retain the capacity to make decisions concerning their care, they may need time to be educated as to their options in learning to cope with dysfunction and permanent impairment.[14]

Rehabilitation professionals believe themselves to have a more accurate idea of the possibilities available for those with severe impairments than do many patients and their families. True, persons with congenital disabilities or long-standing impairments resulting from chronic illness are likely to understand the significance of impairment for their own lives and to possess a strong sense of personal identity. But those who find themselves suddenly and unexpectedly impaired lack this long-term experience. Rehabilitation specialists know that while such patients may be mentally competent to make decisions, they may also require time to adjust to the realities of impairment and to learn about the possibilities for adjusting to such impairments.[14]

Enhancing and restoring autonomy

In cases where a contractual model of provider/patient relationships might make more sense later in the course of care of those with sudden-onset, severe impairments, in the earliest stages of the rehabilitation process providers take, and ought to take, a more directive and tacitly paternalistic approach to those in their care than would be found ethically acceptable on the contractual model. While most theories of ethics require that persons respect the autonomy of others, these theories do recognize certain exceptions. One important exception concerns those instances in which a person's short-term autonomy may be enhanced by a paternalistic intervention intended to assure the possibility of long-term autonomy.

For example, if someone were to observe a man about to cross a bridge that had been weakened by a storm, it would be morally permissible to intervene to stop the man from crossing the bridge, even if he protested the interference. Assume the person about to cross is not aware that the bridge is weak and there is not time to inquire as to what he does or does not know. Interference would be justified on the grounds that the denial of free choice in the short run would be compensated for by the increase in free will and autonomous behavior conferred by saving a person from death.

In an analogous fashion, rehabilitation professionals may be justified in overriding or ignoring the wishes of patients upon entry to a specialized unit for treatment if there are reasons to believe that the person either has not adapted to the traumatic realities of impairment, or that the patient will require some time to fully appreciate the possibilities available for coping with and adapting to chronic impairment.

Many rehabilitation professionals believe that trust is an essential element of provider/patient relations for accomplishing treatment goals. In the earliest stage of rehabilitation, the notion of a contract, with its connotations of adversarial haggling between equals as to the goals of care, seems inappropriate as a model for provider/patient interactions. Patients may need to be motivated or encouraged, rather than merely having their options presented in a disinterested or neutral manner.

The contractual model exemplified in the emphasis on the importance of informed consent in physician/patient relationships presumes that the patient is both competent and willing to make rational decisions. But, rehabilitation professionals are often faced with the challenge of trying to restore or encourage autonomous behavior in patients who are depressed, disoriented, or demoralized by the severity of their impairments. The trauma of experiencing sudden, severe, and incurable disability leaves some patients emotionally unwilling to try to make decisions for themselves, even though they retain the cognitive capacities to do so.[17]

The capacity for free, voluntary choice may have to be recreated in patients, since it may be unrealistic to expect such capacities to be present in those who have suffered grievous and irreversible impairments.[2] The challenge frequently facing medical professionals in rehabilitation is not how to respect autonomy, or whether to obtain informed consent at every stage in the rehabilitative process, but to discover what steps and activities are morally permissible in the hope of restoring autonomy, and with what degree of persuasion, or even coercion.

A greater tolerance of paternalism may be justified when health care providers know from clinical experience that a process of accommodation and acceptance is necessary in order to allow patients to come to grips with the reality of irreversible impairments. Some patients do report retrospectively the importance of a "cooling off" period in adjusting to the reality of severe impairment.[17] If it is true that time is essential in allowing patients to accommodate to the reality of severe impairment, then this would seem to indicate some need to adjust the prevailing understanding of the ethics of professional/patient relationships, at least for some patients in some settings, to allow for the presence of paternalistic medical care.

Obviously, an argument to the effect that paternalism may be justified for some patients at some points in rehabilitation settings is not a license for paternalism in all areas of medical care. Provisions must be made for each patient for restoring autonomous control as soon as possible. How this can best be done is a matter for discussion and debate among rehabilitation professionals, their patients, and others. But in order for such discussions to occur, it must first be acknowledged that the realities of rehabilitation require that paternalistic actions be viewed to some extent as morally legitimate.

Decisions to terminate treatment

Another important inadequacy of the contractual model in the rehabilitation context concerns decisions to terminate treatment. Rehabilitation specialists are frequently confronted with the need to make hard choices as to the allocation of their resources among a variety of potential recipients. They may be forced to terminate care for one patient before mutually agreed upon goals are attained, in order to provide assistance to another for whom the benefits of initiating care are likely to be significantly greater.

The necessity of allocating increasingly scarce resources among those with different capacities for benefit means that providers may not always be as forthcoming about the reasons for terminating inpatient rehabilitation as they might want to be or ought to be. It also means that it is the team of providers rather than the patient or family who are much more likely to determine the timing of discharge. While the contractual model calls for the final decision about the termination of treatment to be vested in the patient, in rehabilitation a team of providers conferring with the family is likely to retain control over decisions as to who will continue to receive care and who will be transferred home or to other settings.

If this is so, then while a certain amount of paternalism may be justified for certain patients at the time of entry into a rehabilitation program, extra efforts must be made to insure the autonomous participation of patients when treatment is to end. Certainly, those patients who have undergone a course of treatment for a reasonable period of time are in a position to understand whether or not they wish to continue. While autonomy, or at least the will to exercise it, may be diminished at the beginning of treatment, every effort must be made to ensure that a model of provider/patient interactions is developed which fully acknowledges and respects autonomy as a key element in decisions to end care. Third-party payors also have an obligation to acknowledge and respect patient autonomy where decisions to end rehabilitative care are concerned.

The educational model

The contractual model does not appear to be a valid framework for articulating the ethical boundaries of provider/patient relationships for every patient at all times in rehabilitation. The contractual model is strongly linked to the provision of care at a specific time by a physician. The concreteness and time frame presumed within the model are not always valid within a rehabilitation context.

Provider/patient interactions in rehabilitation require a model of care that is sensitive to the evolving capacities and adaptations that take place between providers and patients over long periods of time. Such a model must also recognize the necessity of involving many parties, some of whom are physicians and some not. It must also remain sensitive to the disparities of control and power that exist in institutional settings, where much of medical rehabilitation is delivered. It must also recognize the fact that rehabilitation professionals must sometimes undertake interventions aimed at restoring or maximizing autonomy rather than simply presuming its existence, as is the case in the contractual model of care.

What might be termed an educational model is, perhaps, more appropriate to the rehabilitation setting. On such a model, health care providers are allowed more leeway in the initial phases of care to act in a paternalistic manner toward their patients. They have the option of ignoring or overriding patient choices concerning the course of care if and only if they can justify such a decision in the name of either enhancing or restoring autonomy.

An educational model would still require health care providers to endeavor to obtain the consent of patients for specific medical interventions. And no invasive or potentially life-threatening intervention could be undertaken without the express approval of a patient. But greater latitude would be given to physicians, nurses, and other specialists to attempt to persuade their patients of the desirability of undertaking and actively participating in a plan of rehabilitation. In the earliest stages of care which follow the onset of unexpected, irreversible, and severe impairment, the health care team has an obligation to act in ways that encourage patients to participate in their own care, not simply to present options.

This means that the initial stages of rehabilitation will be characterized by more paternalistic types of interventions than would normally be viewed as ethically acceptable in other arenas of health care. At the same time, such a model requires that mechanisms be created for monitoring the capacities and abilities of patients to make autonomous choices and for restoring autonomous control to patients once they have had the opportunity to accommodate themselves to the realities of chronic impairment.

One such mechanism might consist of regularly scheduled meetings between patients, families, and team members in order to assure constant feedback between professional points of view and patient perspectives. Another might be the creation of an independent committee to review the course of care for every patient in a rehabilitation setting in order to assure that confidentiality, privacy, and autonomy are respected to a degree consistent with maximal accommodation to chronic impairment, and that full and complete autonomy is restored to patients as soon as they have been given a reasonable opportunity to undertake a course of therapy.

An educational model will require health care professionals to state clearly to patients upon acceptance into a rehabilitation program that they will be dealing with a diverse team of health care professionals for a long period of time. Patients and their families must understand exactly who is responsible for the efficient performance of the team and who holds ultimate responsibility for team management. While team approaches require the full participation of a diverse range of professionals, such a model should not be allowed to generate uncertainty in the patient's mind about the nature of authority and responsibility in the provision of treatment.

Patients should be told that they have the right to request changes in the composition of the team to the extent that is practically possible in light of constraints on resources and the needs of other patients. Patients should also be told from the start of a rehabilitation program that others, including family members, will have access to information about their diagnosis and prognosis. Agreement should be reached on the degree to which family members will be given a say in the direction of treatment plans and the rationale for such involvement. Patients must also understand that confidentiality and privacy will be protected, but the realities of a team approach require that more persons have access to patient diagnoses and records than would normally be the case in acute care contexts.

Team members must be clear that decisions concerning the termination of care will be based on criteria and evidence available to both patients and team members. Decisions will be sensitive to the needs of other patients. Patients should understand as soon as they are capable of doing so that their continuation in a treatment program depends in part on factors that go beyond the question of whether further benefits can be obtained. They should also be told about the nature of their rights to request continuation of care and the options that are available to them to seek care from other providers in other settings.

The model proposed here is one that attempts to recognize the evolving nature of the relationship between providers and patients in rehabilitation. Its earliest stages are characterized by assigning a higher priority to beneficence than is given to the respect for autonomy. The model requires, however, that efforts to identify and assess levels of competency and autonomy be ongoing and zealous, and that once it is clear that patients have had an opportunity to accommodate to the realities of their functional impairments, their right to control the direction and composition of their rehabilitative care will be restored.

The educational model of provider/patient relations in rehabilitation does grant more leeway to professional values in caring for certain types of patients. But it also requires a rigorous effort on the part of health care professionals to quickly involve patients in all aspects of decisions to terminate care. If it is true that autonomy may be diminished by the onset of severe impairment, it is also the case that patients are in the best position, having had the experience of both impairment and efforts to provide strategies of accommodation for impairment, to make decisions about the termination of their care.

An educational model is not appropriate for every patient seeking or requiring rehabilitative care. Nor is it clear that such a model can be carried out in an environment where financial considerations are playing an increasingly important role in determining access to and discharge from rehabilitation settings. However, unless efforts are made to articulate a range of provider/patient models that can adequately capture the rights, duties, and obligations of a wide range of patients and providers, no progress will be possible toward making reforms in either the institutional or economic factors which play important roles in determining the way in which rehabilitation services are delivered to those who can benefit from them.

References

1. Beauchamp T, Childress J: *Principles of Biomedical Ethics*. Ed 2. Oxford, Oxford University Press, pp 90–96

2. Brody B, Engelhardt HT: *Bioethics*. Englewood Cliffs, New Jersey, Prentice-Hall, 1987

3. Buchanan A: "Medical paternalism," *Philosophy and Public Affairs*. 7:370–390, 1978

4. Caplan A: "Informed consent," *Lancet* 8516:1160, 1986

5. Caplan A: "Let wisdom find a way," *Generations* 10:10–14, 1985

6. Caplan A, Engelhardt HT (eds): *Concepts of Health and Disease*. Reading, MA, Addison-Wesley, 1981

7. Englehardt HT: *The Foundations of Bioethics*. New York, Oxford, 1986

8. Faden RR, Beauchamp TL: *A History and Theory of Informed Consent*. New York, Oxford, 1986

9. Freedman B: "A meta-ethics for professional morality," *Ethics* 89:1–19, 1976

10. Gaylin W, Macklin R: *Who Speaks for the Child?* New York, Plenum, 1982

11. Gert B, Culver CM: "The justification of paternalism," *Ethics* 89:199–210, 1979

12. Gillon R: "Autonomy and consent." *In* Lockwood M (ed): *Moral Dilemmas in Modern Medicine*. Oxford, Oxford University Press, 1985

13. Gorovitz S, Jameton A, Macklin R, Sherwin S, O'Connor J: (eds): *Moral Problems in Medicine*. Englewood Cliffs, NJ, Prentice-Hall, 1976

14. Hughes F: "Reaction to loss: coping with disability and death." *In* Marinelli RP, Dell Orto AE (eds): *The Psychological and Social Impact of Physical Disability*. Ed 2. New York, Springer, 1984, pp 131–136

15. Humber J, Almeder R: *Biomedical Ethics Reviews*. Clifton, NJ, Humana Press, 1983

16. Katz J: *The Silent World of Doctor and Patient*. New York, The Free Press, 1984

17. Kerson TA, Kerson LA: *Understanding Chronic Illness*. New York, The Free Press, 1985

18. Mappes TA, Zembaty JS: *Biomedical Ethics*. New York, McGraw-Hill, 1981.

19. May W: "Code, covenant, contract or philanthropy," *Hastings Center Report* 5:29–38, 1975

20. President's Commission for the Study of Ethical Problems in Medi-

cine and Biomedical and Behavioral Research: *Making Health Care Decisions.* Washington DC, Government Printing Office, 1982

21. Shontz FC: "Psychological adjustment to physical disability: trends in theories." *In* Marinelli RP, Dell Orto AE (eds):*The Psychological and Social Impact of Physical Disability.* Ed 2. New York, Springer, 1984, pp. 119–126

22. Szasz T, Hollender MH: "Basic models of doctor-patient relationship," *Arch Int Med* 97:585–592, 1956

23. Veatch R: *Death, Dying and the Biological Revolution.* New Haven, Yale University Press, 1976

24. Veatch R: "Models for ethical medicine in a revolutionary age," *Hastings Center Report* 2:5–7, 1972

25. Veatch R: *A Theory of Medical Ethics.* New York, Basic Books, 1981

16.

Can autonomy be saved?

I. The preeminence of autonomy

Respect for autonomy is the dominant value prescribed by bioethicists and legal scholars for mediating provider/patient interactions (Beauchamp and Childress, 1979; Childress, 1982; Engelhardt, 1986). The competent individual's right to control medical care is seen as valuable both for its own sake and instrumentally in the promotion of other values. A host of writers within and outside the health professions have insisted that self-determination in medical matters must be paramount since it is a fundamental good to be in control of what others can and cannot do to you. Autonomy is also assigned great weight since it is widely believed, especially in our pluralistic society, that the best means for assuring the interests and welfare of each citizen is to respect his or her autonomy.

The preeminence of autonomy reflects the fact that there is no broad consensus as to what constitutes good or bad with respect to the aims of health care (see Callahan, 1987, 1989; Caplan and Engelhardt, 1981; Engelhardt, 1986; Caplan, 1989). As Engelhardt (1986) and many other moral philosophers and bioethicists have insisted in their recent writings, it is not for want of trying that no consensus exists about the nature of the goods that best promote patient, client, or resident welfare. The absence of consensus is simply a reflection of incommensurable and unbridgeable differences between what individuals consider good for themselves or in their best interest.

If no obvious consensus exists as to what is good and what is bad in health care, since people come from so many different religious, ethnic and cultural traditions, since even so simple a procedure as a blood transfusion to save a life can become the subject of heated controversy between doctor and patient, the best strategy to pursue when patient meets provider is to respect autonomy. In the absence of a societal consensus about what is good, individual autonomy is, many bioethicists believe, the best available guide for deciding what doctors, nurses, and other health-care providers should do.

The celebration of autonomy in American medical ethics is not only a response to disagreement over what is good. It reflects the fact that Americans view autonomy as an essential prerequisite for moral action. Impair or destroy the potential for autonomous action and the possibility of morality is impaired or destroyed as well.

While there is much debate about the requisite conditions for autonomy to exist, with arguments raging over the relative importance of information, knowledge of alternatives, comprehension, voluntariness, and authenticity (Collopy, 1988; Kapp and Bigot, 1985), there are relatively few bioethicists who argue that respect for autonomy is not the preeminent value governing the actions of health-care providers. Insofar as a person is competent, respect for self-determination is a necessity (Annas, 1986; Kapp and Bigot, 1985).

Much of the writing about the autonomy of the elderly in bioethics focuses on treatment decisions that must be made for persons who are both incompetent and dying. The paradigmatic bioethics case involving an elderly person is that of a very old man or woman, demented, comatose, or vegetative, who is having one or more major organ systems sustained by a technological intervention in an acute-care setting. Moral debates swirl around what to do when patients such as these have come to the end of the acute-care road. How can the last embers of their autonomy be used to guide decision-making?

Questions of personal autonomy are difficult to see in these dire circumstances insofar are as they are nested within layers of debate about the moral duty of providers not to kill, the medical status and efficacy of interventions such as feeding tubes, and the proper role to accord to family members, courts, and ethics committees (Caplan, 1988, 1989). But severely impaired, dying persons hardly constitute the average or even a representative sub-sample of the elderly who use health services in the United States. The vast majority of elderly persons who use health-care services in hospitals, nursing homes, homecare programs, or who visit doctors' offices are neither demented nor dying (Kapp and Bigot, 1985). They have as much capacity, or, arguably, a greater capacity for autonomous action than any other group or class of persons.

The likelihood that older persons have a greater capacity for autonomy is based upon the realization that the older people are the more likely it is that they know with certainty their own values, beliefs, and preferences (Caplan, 1985, 1988, 1989). The presumption made in many cultures and among many ethnic groups that wisdom is a function of age is based on the belief that experience gives more opportunity for deliberation and choice. If that is so and if the capacity for autonomy is enhanced when people have more time to consider the options available to them, then age may be an advantage where autonomy is concerned.

II. Steps to protect and enhance the autonomy of the elderly in health care

The most visible manifestation of the desire to respect the autonomy of older Americans who utilize health-care services is the movement to enact state and federal legislation recognizing living wills. These laws recognize the right of competent persons to write legally binding advance directives to control the course of their medical care even if they become unable to communicate or incompetent to do so. Forty-one states and the District of Columbia have enacted such legislation (McCarrick, 1990). Congress has enacted a law, the Patient Self Determination Act of 1989 (S. 1766), which requires hospitals to give out information about living wills to every patient.

Living-will legislation is not the only example where legislative or regulatory efforts have been made to acknowledge the primacy of autonomy with respect to decisions about medical care. Twenty-five states and the District of Columbia have enacted durable power of attorney statutes which explicitly allow persons to designate surrogate decision makers who can control medical-care decisions in case of a loss of competency or the ability to communicate (McCarrick, 1990). Some states, such as Minnesota and New Jersey, include a recognition of durable power of attorney provisions in their living-will statutes.

Many other states and a large number of hospitals, medical systems, and federal health-care programs (such as the Veterans Hospital system) have issued regulations requiring hospital personnel to obtain written consent to DNR and DNI orders (Annas, 1986). Hospital ethics committees have been created, in Maryland by state law, at least in part to help assure that individual autonomy is protected from the beneficent as well as the malevolent intentions of health-care providers, family members, and friends.

Courts have been concerned with the protection of the rights of patients to control both their person and property. In every state, there is a system requiring a formal declaration of incompetency before decision-making power over medical decisions can be taken away from persons (Annas, 1986). Conservators and guardians are often appointed to protect the interests of persons who have been deemed incompetent to govern their own affairs, but only when there has been a court-reviewed demonstration of incompetency (Kapp and Bigot, 1985). These protections reflect a strong societal commitment to the preeminence of autonomy with respect to matters of both health and property (Caplan, 1985).

Autonomy also stands supreme in most of the literature of health-care ethics. Kind words for paternalism are few and far between (Childress, 1982). Sympathetic comments concerning a standard of disclosure that is anything other than what the reasonable person would want to know or what the particular person would want to know are even scarcer. The Freddy Kruger of bioethics for the better part of two decades has been the doctor who pushes his or her values onto the patient (Engelhardt, 1986; Faden and Beauchamp, 1986; Veatch, 1981). This devil has been completely exorcised and a large part of contemporary bioethics scholarship seems to be devoted to the task of assuring that the paternalistic doctor stays dead and buried (Doukas and McCullough, 1988). Autonomy is firmly rooted at the foundation of the contemporary bioethical canon (Beauchamp and Childress, 1979; Callahan, 1987; Faden and Beauchamp, 1986; Veatch, 1981).

A large number of influential writers in the literature of both bioethics and health care have stressed a model of provider/patient interactions that views the relationship as one of contract between mutually consenting parties (Faden and Beauchamp, 1986; Veatch, 1981; Veatch, 1989). Respect for autonomy and the exercise of autonomy are the linchpins holding the contractual model together.

Courts also have been very concerned with respect for autonomy. In the many cases which have come to trial concerning the rights of competent patients to govern the course of their health care, state courts and even the Supreme Court, have been clear in asserting the absolute right of competent persons to control their care (Annas, 1990; Cruzan, 1990). Even where disputes have existed about the treatment of incompetent adults who once were competent, state and local courts in nearly every jurisdiction have strained mightily to accord respect to the value of autonomy. The only exceptions appear to be court opinions in New York and Missouri, and these opinions are notable primarily because they require high standards of evidence to be met before according respect to the prior wishes of once competent patients, not because they ignore the importance of autonomy (Annas et al., 1990).

Autonomy is the value given the highest priority in ethics and law. Competency is seen as the necessary condition for the capacity to be autonomous to exist. At least in theory, older Americans are seen as having the same right to self-governance with respect to decisions about their health care as any other members of society. Yet, despite all the academic, legislative, judicial, and professional attention paid to autonomy, many older Americans and many health-care providers are worried that the existing health-care system does not afford adequate protection to those who wish to act in an autonomous manner with respect to their health care. There is a great deal of concern in both academic and lay discussions of health care that the system still robs people of their ability to act autonomously when they desire to do so (Collopy, 1988; Kane and Caplan, 1990). Why is this so?

III. The failure to adequately protect autonomy

There is much support for the importance of autonomy in clinical settings. Doctors and nurses report in survey after survey that they support the concept of advance directives, an endless parade of religious authorities endorse them, politicians bless them, and public-opinion polls show strong support for them (Emanuel and Emanuel, 1989). Yet, the living will, and its close relative, the durable power of attorney, must, to date, be counted as abject failures with respect to the protection of autonomy. No more than 10 percent of the population has either a living will or a durable power of attorney (Emanuel and Emanuel, 1989). Physicians and nurses report that living wills are rarely used in clinical practice (Shapiro et al., 1986). And there are tremendous problems making sure that the living wills which do exist are tracked and found as patients move through the health care system (Miles, 1987).

Similarly dismal statistics are reported for the practices surrounding the issuance of DNR (do-not-resuscitate), DNI (do-not-intubate), and DNT (do-not-treat) orders in hospitals and nursing homes (Finucane and Denman, 1989). One study (Stolman, 1989) reports that only 20 percent of patients participated in the issuance of DNR orders. Even in studies analyzing the situation of only patients who had been deemed competent by their health-care providers at the time orders were written, only 43 percent of patients had participated in any way in the issuance of these orders (Stolman, 1989).

Part of the reason for the relative ineffectiveness of living wills is that clinicians, despite their support for the concept of living wills and other forms of advance directives, are deeply skeptical that such documents can really be effective in guiding the course of health care. In the words of one experienced geriatrician, "Physicians who are at the bedside . . . when [ethical] dilemmas arise . . . generally recognize that specific decisions applicable to all nursing home residents cannot be mandated" (Ouslander, 1989, p. 2586). Doctors and nurses think that living wills and advance directives, even when they do exist, are too vague and lack sufficient specificity to provide much guidance concerning the clinical management of patient care (Annas, 1986; Emanuel and Emanuel, 1989).

Other reasons frequently cited for the failure of living wills and other existing forms of advance directives to assure autonomy in health care include clinicians' dislike for documents they perceive as blurring the line between controlling care and accelerating death, and the fact that many who sign living wills fail to tell their physicians that they have done so (Emanuel and Emanuel, 1989). Even when patients tell their physicians that they have a living will, they may fail to discuss the document, leading to a situation where the physician feels dissatisfied with the document because he or she has had no input in its creation. Finally, physicians and nurses are not very good judges of what patients would have wanted when they have not specifically communicated their wishes (Uhlmann, Pearlman, and Cain, 1989).

All of these reasons are important factors to consider in attempting to establish procedures, practices, and public policies that will create an environment in which autonomy can flourish. Many ethicists (and, indeed, many lay people) agree that, in lieu of a broad societal consensus about the aims and goods toward which health care ought to strive, autonomy is the only plausible response. It is, therefore, imperative that effective mechanisms exist for assuring the opportunity to exercise autonomy for every person receiving care in the health care system. Can any form of written advance directive serve to protect autonomy? There are reasons to think not.

IV. The failure of donor cards in organ procurement: a case study in the limits of advance directives

The dismal record to date regarding the ability of living wills to either assure autonomy or be useful in shaping clinical practice should come as no surprise. An earlier effort with advance directives in a related area of health care has not proven to be especially effective at protecting autonomy.

In the late 1960s, every state in the United States enacted laws—with the support of health-care providers, public opinion polls, and hosannas from religious authorities—to create organ-donor cards. The motivation for these legislative efforts was not to obtain organs (Caplan, 1984) but to protect the autonomy of every American with respect to decisions regarding the disposition of bodily remains. Yet, despite nearly twenty-five years of efforts to educate the public about the importance of donor cards, this mini social experiment in advance directives has been a failure. It is an illustrative failure for those who see living wills or other forms of written advance directive as solutions to the protection of autonomy.

Specialists in organ and tissue procurement readily admit that few of the organs and tissues obtained from cadaver sources in the

United States are procured on the basis of a donor card or directive written by the deceased. The reasons for this are critically important for understanding why living wills have not proven effective in enhancing the autonomy of those in the health-care system and will not be effective in the future.

First, few Americans have signed donor cards. This is so despite the fact that public-opinion polls taken over the past twenty years consistently indicate that the majority of Americans say they support transplantation and are willing to be organ and tissue donors (Caplan, 1984). The directive permitting organ donation appears on the back of driver's licenses in nearly every state, yet no more than 20 percent of all Americans have signed it. The best explanation of why this is so would appear to be that most Americans find the subject of death distasteful, frightening, or both. They are no more inclined to think about organ donation than they are to buy life insurance, make a will, or purchase a funeral plot—all areas where behavioral avoidance is hardly unknown.

In addition to a strong desire to duck the subject, there is evidence that Americans do not sign donor cards because they do not trust their doctors and health-care providers. Specifically, many Americans seem to fear that if they sign a donor card they may not receive aggressive, life-saving care if they wind up in a hospital emergency room. The fear is especially marked among minorities and the poor.

Similar obstacles to those responsible for the low rate of participation in signing donor cards exist for living wills and other forms of written advance directives. Most Americans will not sign them because they prefer to avoid the subject of how to manage their own dying. Some simply will dump their autonomy and rely on their families to make sound decisions. Since the same distrust that is in evidence with respect to cadaveric tissue and organ donation is likely to be at work in the realm of living wills, many will not sign advance directives of any sort for fear that their medical care may be adversely effected.

V. Fear, loathing, and living wills

Living-will legislation is relatively new—the first state law was enacted in California in 1977. Still, the fact that so few Americans have signed living wills or other forms of advance directives indicates that it is likely that Americans are leery of such documents. Aside from the distasteful nature of the subject, trust is the key ingredient that will fuel the public's enthusiasm for advance directives.

Many Americans no longer have a personal physician or family health-care provider, either because they lack health insurance or because they receive care in institutional or practice settings where doctors and nurses are assigned to them on a rotating basis (Priester, 1990). They have little reason or opportunity to form relationships in which they grow to trust those giving them care. Where matters of life and death are concerned, trust (as the organ donor card experience makes clear) is essential. If, for whatever reason, health care is perceived as an encounter between strangers, few people will be willing to leave directions about the care they wish to receive, for implementation by people they do not know.

Moreover, at a time when many people are worried about the move to ration health care, especially among the elderly (Califano, 1987; Callahan, 1987, 1989), some will see a living will or advance directive as a means, not to assure autonomy but as a gimmick to save the government or private payors money by allowing less than comprehensive care to be delivered to those who have signed advance directives. If the rates of malpractice insurance prevailing in the United States are any measure, distrust of the health-care system is rampant. Distrust is a poor climate in which to foster enthusiastic participation in the preparation of advance directives, especially for persons who worry that their lives may be disvalued because of their age.

The failure of donor cards in matters pertaining to the disposition of bodily remains is not due exclusively to low rates of public participation in filling them out. A significant obstacle to the utility of donor cards in assuring autonomy is that doctors, nurses, and administrators do not trust the documents. Whenever someone dies, the first reaction of hospital personnel in matters of organ donation is to obtain the permission of family members, regardless of whether a donor card exists (Caplan, 1984; Caplan and Virnig, 1990). Families are given almost total control over matters pertaining to donation.

The practice of according family members veto power over the autonomy of the deceased has many sources. Hospitals fear conflicts and lawsuits from families if they act against their wishes. The dead do not sue, so, even if a signed, valid donor card exists giving permission for organ harvesting, no hospital or doctor will do anything unless family permission is also obtained. Doctors and nurses are also respectful of families because they see dying as a family matter. They try to meet the needs of the family as well as the patient when someone is dying.

There is every reason to think that the same concerns will prevail with respect to living wills and other forms of written directives. If all that is available is a living will and the family is not aware of or did not support the contents of the document at the time it was created, it is highly unlikely that health-care providers will go against family wishes. The dead do not complain and do not litigate. Families do. Families will be heard at the bedside regardless of whether or not a living will exists.

Finally, one of the greatest problems facing the practice of organ-donor cards as a vehicle for guaranteeing autonomy is that no autonomy can be respected if no one asks about organ donation. When someone dies, hospital personnel must raise the subject of organ donation and inquire whether a donor card exists. Recent studies indicate that despite the enactment of legislation in forty-four states requiring requests to be made of family members about organ and tissue donation when someone dies in a hospital setting, more than a third of all hospitals never do so, and an even larger number do so only sporadically (Caplan and Virnig, 1990; Caplan and Welvang, 1989).

These problems will arise with respect to living wills. Even when a living will exists, it is entirely predictable that health-care personnel will not discover the document in time for it to do any good or that it will be lost as patients are transferred around the various component elements of our increasingly intricate health-care system (Miles, 1987).

Living wills, like donor cards, are useful documents. Not as guarantees of autonomy, but because they provide evidence to families of the preferences and choices of someone who is no longer able to communicate. No form of advance written directives is likely to be effective in protecting or enhancing autonomy unless the issues highlighted by the donor-card experience—avoidance, trust, respect for family interests, and failure of hospitals to discover documents—are adequately addressed.

VI. The inadequate scope of living wills

The experience with a living-will system in the United States in the domain of organ and tissue donation does not bode well for the ability of public policies (or hospital and nursing-home protocols) that depend upon living wills, to assure or enhance patient autonomy. But the difficulties with living wills do not end there. Another grave problem with living wills is their limited scope.

Many states have enacted living-will laws that make explicit provisions that the document cannot be activated unless a person has been diagnosed as terminally ill or imminently dying (e.g., California, Minnesota, and North Dakota have this sort of triggering language). The goal of such legislation is to ensure the welfare of those who are not dying from undertreatment. There are obviously difficult decisions that must be faced by persons whose ability to communicate may be impaired or absent but who are not terminally ill or dying. And physicians are notoriously poor at predicting mortality for many types of disease and injury.

The model language suggested in many state statutes and by many patient-advocacy groups and health-care professionals (Emanuel and Emanuel, 1989; McCarrick, 1990) focuses almost exclusively on decisions about life-prolonging, high-technology interventions. References abound to "artificial" technology and "heroic measures." But many decisions facing those who are not competent to decide for themselves do not concern high-technology interventions (Kane and (Caplan, 1990).

Even a cursory look at the residents of nursing homes (Kane and Caplan, 1990) makes it clear that a good number of residents are capable of autonomous behavior. Few of the manifestly competent residents of nursing homes seem especially concerned about assuring that their autonomy will be protected when it comes to life-saving medical care. Insofar as their autonomy is concerned, they are very concerned about the content of their daily lives and those activities and practices that can enhance the quality of their lives.

Elderly Americans, like other members of our society, do not spend their waking hours thinking of themselves as potential candidates for the surgical or medical intensive-care unit. They will worry about what happens there if and when they get there. In the here and now, they are concerned with the same mundane, ordinary elements of daily living—sleep, food, shelter, clothing, recreation, sex, entertainment, mobility, friends, family, comfort, money, and work—that occupy the time and attention of other persons.

But it is precisely with respect to the ordinary and the mundane that our medical institutions perform most poorly in respecting autonomy. We struggle mightily to figure out how to respect the autonomy of those who are comatose or vegetative but devote almost no attention to the problem of respecting the autonomy of those who are quite intact, mentally and physically. In acute care hospitals, long term care facilities, home care programs and even, to some extent, in hospices, routine tends to predominate over individuality. Those who are dependent on others for care and assistance in daily living often find their autonomy ignored, not only about matters of life and death but also in matters of daily living (Kane and Caplan, 1990).

Living wills rarely grapple with issues of autonomy in health care settings that exist outside the realm of terminally illness and the incompetent. Their focus is so driven by concerns about the control of life-saving technologies that even if they were an effective vehicle for assuring and enhancing autonomy in those settings, which they probably are not, their scope would rarely overlap with what many elderly patients believe to be critical areas of autonomy.

VII. Supplementing living wills

A number of commentators have written about the problems surrounding living wills. A very few have tried to suggest improvements, emendations, or alternatives to this approach to the protection of autonomy for impaired persons receiving critical care (Johnson and Justin, 1988; Doukas and McCullough, 1988, 1991; Gibson, 1989).

Medical directives

One of the most interesting suggestions comes from Linda and Ezekiel Emanuel (1989). They call for the creation of a new form of advance directive, "the medical directive," to replace living wills. Their proposed directive consists of five parts, "(1) an introduction, (2) a section containing four paradigmatic scenarios of illness in which preferences for medical care are given, (3) a section for the designation of a proxy decision maker, (4) a section for organ donation, and (5) a personal statement" (1989, p. 3289).

The introduction is basically a description of what advance directives are. Commendably, the Emanuels note that, to be effective, an advance directive must be given to one's physician and family. They recognize that health-care providers will take family wishes and needs seriously even if law and social policy do not. The donor card section is fairly straightforward, as is the designation of a proxy decision maker. Proxies are to be guided by the other sections of the medical directive.

The innovative parts of the medical directive are the sections discussing paradigmatic illness scenarios and the personal statement. Four scenarios are presented so as to elicit the preferences of the person making out the directive concerning medical care. These include falling into a permanent vegetative state (PVS) without being terminally ill, becoming comatose with little chance of recovery, suffering brain damage and becoming terminally ill, or suffering brain damage but not becoming terminally ill. Obviously the key thrust of this section of the document is to allow for greater specificity in eliciting autonomous choices from competent persons regarding their wishes if they become incompetent to control their medical care in situations of serious disability or terminal illness.

The personal statement covers "personal values concerning the limits of treatment" under the four scenarios. But no guidance is given as to how such values ought to be elicited from the person making out the document or what style of presentation should guide the preparation of the personal statement to maximize its utility.

The Emanuels' document is an improvement over the language frequently used in living-will legislation or model living wills. But the medical directive is focused exclusively on the acute hospital setting and the use or withdrawal of high-technology interventions. The scenarios add specificity in the content of the directives given, but there are many, many situations—even in the context of critical care—which are not addressed. In many ways the medical directive is more attentive to the anxieties of health-care providers who may be uncertain how to proceed with the withdrawal or forgoing of medical interventions than it is to the concerns and interests of persons who are dying or of those who are not dying but who may nonetheless be unable to communicate their wishes.

The medical directive does not address many people's reluctance to discuss the kinds of dismal scenarios proposed as paradigmatic in the document. Nor is there any reason, especially in light of the long-ineffectual experience with donor cards, to presume that the personal statement which is requested will have any bearing on how surrogates or health-care providers interpret the document. And, while the document is to be shared with family members, no attention is given to the issue of what to do should families attempt to override or veto an advance directive or when surrogate decision-makers fail to agree. The medical directive may enhance autonomy for the comatose, PVS, or brain-damaged person receiving high-technology acute care, but the members of these groups are the least able to appreciate whatever autonomy benefits the document provides them.

The values history

An alternative approach to the problem of assuring and enhancing autonomy in acute-care settings is the compilation of a "values history." This is the approach suggested by Doukas, McCullough, and Lipson in a number of recent articles (McCullough and Lipson, 1989; Doukas and McCullough, 1988, 1989, 1991). These writers see the values history as a "useful supplement to the living will." The values history comes in two parts; a section which "invites the patient to identify which values and beliefs regarding terminal care are most important to him or her," and a second section which "invites the patient to make explicit decisions in advance, given those values and beliefs." The primary goal of the values history approach is, like the medical directive, to help decrease vagueness and a lack of specificity with respect to the administration of acute care and to diminish the prospects for medical paternalism.

The values-history section on "directives," while specific with respect to the kinds of options and alternatives that may be offered to a seriously ill person, is tightly focused on acute-care interventions such as CPR, ventilators, intubation, TPN (total parenteral nutrition—exclusively intravenous feeding), dialysis, intensive-care admissions, and the like. Specificity is desirable, but many clinicians are likely to feel that in the absence of a specific set of clinical facts and a specific prognosis the previously expressed preferences of patients concerning CPR, insulin, or a ventilator will not suffice for guiding care.

The more interesting element of the values history proposed by Doukas and McCullough is the section called "Values." This section of the values history requests information about attitudes concerning length of life and quality of life. The person making out the document is asked to select statements from a list of fourteen, which include "I want to maintain my capacity to think clearly," "I want to feel safe and secure," "I want to be treated in accord with my religious beliefs and traditions" in order to flesh out his or her views about the quality of life. The person filling out the form is then asked which of the three elements of quality of life is the most important relative to the others that may have elicited a positive response.

The advantage of this sort of information is that it provides a general framework against which family members and providers can assess the likely desirability of particular medical actions in specific clinical circumstances. Family members are much more likely to feel comfortable with language that is couched in value terms rather than in the technical arcana of health care.

The addition of a section on general values plays another crucial, if underappreciated, role in facilitating the evaluation of a written directive. By having a general discussion of values it becomes possible to detect inconsistencies that may exist between general values and the specific responses given to particular forms of medical care in acute-care settings. General values information becomes a valuable tool for assessing the authenticity of claims about the degree of medical care a person wishes should they become seriously ill, impaired, or both (Caplan, 1985, 1988).

The limits of the values history are that it does not address the problem of what to do about the natural reluctance of persons to prepare such a document. Nor does the document address the need for portability of written directives within the health-care system. The authors say little about where or how they derive the questions that they provide concerning the component elements of value which are meant to provide guidance about the quality of life sought by patients—a crucial omission with reference to so controversial a subject as the quality of life. Nor do they say how a health-care provider or family member ought to elicit responses to the proposed questions in order to maximize the chances that the choices made really do represent the person's deeply held, authentic values. There is no attention given to the question of the limits of autonomy. If a person says they desire any and all forms of care possible, no matter how marginal, must this care then be given?

The values history is, nevertheless, a major step forward in that it recognizes that the solution to the problem of specificity that has confounded living wills, and to the problem of possible familial disagreement, is to have available more information about personal values. The major failings of this version of the values history are that it does not give much guidance on certain crucial matters: (1) how to obtain adequate responses from those to whom the document is offered, (2) how to convince people to respond to the document when they want to avoid it in the first place and may not completely trust those asking the questions, and (3) what presumptions or empirical evidence underlie the questions used to elicit statements about basic values and quality of life considerations.

Values history form

Another recent effort to improve upon the living will in the form enacted in state and federal law is the values history form developed by a group under the direction of Joan Gibson at the University of New Mexico. The values history form has a number of advantages for enhancing the autonomy of the elderly.

First, it has a much broader scope than any other proposed advance directive. While the document inquires about the existence of written legal documents such as a living will or durable power of attorney, it seeks to elicit information on values and preferences about a broad range of medical interventions, some pertaining to critical care and some to routine or ordinary support.

Second, the values history form asks those filling out the document to provide information about their attitudes toward their doctors and other caregivers. The matter of distrust is addressed head on by asking those who fill out the form to state their likes and dislikes regarding those giving them care.

Third, the document also explicitly requests information about the relationship the person has with his or her family. The danger that some family members may not agree with the wishes or choices expressed in the document, or may compete to be the proxy decision-maker, is anticipated in advance.

Lastly, the values history form asks those who fill it out to comment on their overall attitudes toward life and their religious backgrounds and beliefs. Specific questions—such as "What activities do you enjoy?" "What makes you laugh/cry?" "What do you fear most?"—actually appear in print! It should be obvious that these questions are intended to provide information in a general way that can be used to guide not only acute medical care but the routine care of persons who may be unable to communicate or who have their autonomy partially impaired.

This general information can serve as a check in order to determine the authenticity of someone's statements or preferences on other parts of the form. Inconsistencies are likely to be obvious when questions are asked not only about dialysis or CPR but also about a person's fears, hopes, and sources of joy.

The major weakness of the values history form is that its authors say little as to how the specific questions used in the values history form were arrived at. In matters as sensitive as ascertaining personal values, it is surely reasonable to expect some rationale or justification as to why anyone should believe there is a connection between the questions asked, the responses that are made to them, and a person's most cherished values. Furthermore, there is no direction available for persons administering the form about how to do so, leaving the door open for both flexibility and idiosyncrasy.

The values history form is much less specific than either the medical directive or the values history about the details of critical care. The complaints of providers about the lack of specificity regarding particular interventions are not likely to be met by a form that only solicits input on dialysis, organ donation (no tissue donation is mentioned), CPR, respirators, nutrition, and fluids in the most general of terms.

But a real virtue of this document is its willingness to address head on the issue of trust. Information is solicited about trust both in providers and in family members.

VII. The values baseline

None of the new generation of modified advance written directives is a panacea. They all face problems of scope, specificity, validity, and replicability. However, some of the problems faced by written directives have nothing to do with the directive. They are the products of our society's unwillingness to address issues that cannot be solved simply by obtaining written evidence of autonomous choice in advance of impairment or disability.

The primary problem facing nearly all of the newer generation of advance directives is that they are heavily oriented toward the solution of problems in acute-care settings faced by providers and families rather than by patients. Autonomy is one of the last concerns of someone who is in the final stages of dying or in a permanent coma. The primary concern of most people is either not to wind up in such a state or, if they do, to make it as short and as comfortable as possible.

It is families and care-givers who need help deciding how to make autonomous decisions when acute illness robs a person of autonomy. The previously expressed autonomous wishes of a permanently non-autonomous agent are a somewhat odd place to turn for answers. Personal choice cannot always provide answers to the problems that trouble health-care professionals and families in the most difficult and hopeless situations in acute-care medicine. Despite the skepticism of many bioethicists about the possibility of any consensus, society and the professions must strive to formulate some answers, some boundaries, some common goals for managing the care of the terminally ill and the severely mentally impaired.

If one wants autonomy to be taken seriously, despite the needs and interests of families, then, to be meaningful, the pursuit of autonomy must start long before the crisis setting of the intensive-care unit or emergency room. Respect for autonomy requires a knowledge of an individual's values, lifestyle, and commitments. Health-care providers must begin to routinely compile values baselines as assiduously and aggressively as they now monitor blood gasses and BUN (blood urea nitrogen) levels if autonomy is to flourish. At a time when many housestaff officers do not know the religion of their patients or whether or not the patient has a living relative, there is room for improvement.

Who is responsible for autonomy?

A major problem with advance directives, be they the standard living will (as now mandated in legislation) or more sophisticated forms (such as the medical directive, values history, or values history form), is that providers must rely upon individuals to seek out a form and complete it. Autonomy is treated as the responsibility of the patient or client, not the provider. But this view of who has responsibility for assuring autonomy is wrong.

The provision of good health care—acute, preventative, rehabilitative, or palliative—regardless of who is providing the care and what the setting is, requires that the provider be reasonably acquainted with the wishes, desires, goals, and lifestyle of the patient or client. The recipients of care need to be informed so that they can cooperate with the prescriptions of their health-care providers. The information necessary to maintain and enhance autonomy, especially for older patients who may have more reason to worry that their autonomy is less likely to be accorded respect, cannot be treated as optional. Nor can it be treated solely as the patient or client's responsibility. Respect for autonomy entails not only trying to comply with what patients want but making a reasonable effort to insure that people will have access to a health-care provider that they feel comfortable enough with to trust to tell what it is that they want.

All health-care institutions and providers must make sure that a maximal effort is made to collect and retain this information in a form that can be readily transferred from setting to setting. The burden of collecting and maintaining such information is not the patient's but the provider's. Whatever sort of written directive is used, it should be used by all providers whenever a new health-care relationship is formed between a provider and an institution. Of course patients are free to withhold information—coercing autonomy is a very tricky business in health care—but the primary duty to make a good faith effort to collect information requisite to permit autonomy to be maintained and enhanced belongs to providers.

In order to achieve this end it may make more sense to view the compilation of information pertaining to autonomy not as the completion of a precisely constructed written instrument but rather as an ordinary, routine aspect of compiling a patient or client history. That is to say, all providers should strive to obtain information about a patient's values just as they try to collect information about general health, medications used, sexual history, genetic history, and other aspects of physical and mental well-being.

While special forms administered at special times are now all the rage, routinization of the collection of relevant information in a situation of trust is likely to provide the greatest boost to personal autonomy. If the collection of information about preferences, wishes, choices, and desires were to be seen as an ordinary (not extraordinary) component of the provision of all forms of health care, autonomy would have a better chance of flourishing in the hospital, hospice, or nursing home. A special form or document attended by special ceremonies and signatures may be necessary to satisfy legal or bureaucratic requirements; it may make the health-care professionals feel at ease about how they will direct the care of an acutely ill patient, but it is not likely to do much for patient autonomy. What is required is that patients have health-care providers to whom they feel they can entrust their wishes and goals, and institutions which require providers to routinely and vigorously collect information that will enable them to have at least a rough idea of what their patients' autonomous wishes, desires, preferences, and goals might be.

The collection of information should not be fraught with high drama and anxiety. It should be a matter of routine in order to generate the kind of trust that will allow for the honest disclosure and exchange of information about deeply personal matters.

The excuses that there is no time, that values cannot be measured, or that reimbursement is inadequate where talking is concerned are totally unacceptable on moral grounds. If we mean what we say about the primacy of autonomy in our society, then it is a basic duty of government to see to it that each citizen has access to a health-care provider he or she can know and trust. Every health-care provider is obligated to obtain information bearing on autonomy and to do so every time a new health-care relationship is formed. Information about values should be constantly updated through chart notes and in patient records. The process of ascertaining patient values must begin long before terminal illness or incompetency if it is to do any good where patient autonomy is concerned.

Distrust is at the heart of the problem where autonomy is concerned. The only solutions to the problem are to guarantee access to health care for all and to emphasize the need for conversation—and lots of it (Katz, 1984). It is important that conversation not be confined to doctors and patients. Nurses, social workers, and other health professionals must feel the duty to collect information bearing on autonomy. A good values baseline will depend not only on what information is collected but on the atmosphere that surrounds the collection of information and who is present when it is obtained.

What information needs to be collected?

The greatest challenge in maintaining and enhancing autonomy for anyone receiving health care, be they elderly or not, is figuring out exactly what sorts of information would help identify their ends. This is where the existing forms of advance written directives are weakest. But this is through no fault of those who are trying to improve upon the earlier versions of living wills. It is merely a function of the fact that very little is known about how to detect information concerning autonomy and how to record and store it in a manner that will make it useful for the purposes of delivering care.

In lieu of a robust theory which can link autonomy to the elicitation of specific preferences, desires, attitudes, and wishes, there is a set of issues which seem prima facie to be of importance where autonomy is concerned. All patients or clients in the health-care system should be asked about their relationship with family and friends—if they have any, who they are, which ones they like, which they do not like and why. People need to be asked about their lifestyles and what they do that makes life interesting and worthwhile. They also need to be asked what makes them miserable or afraid, hopeful or despondent. Information about religious beliefs, while obviously necessary, is frequently never collected. Questions about hobbies, recreational pastimes, jobs, travel, and education seem appropriate. So too do questions about drug use, sex, companionship, desire for privacy, and attitudes toward health care and health-care providers. Even basic questions—Do you like TV or listening to the radio? Do you enjoy reading, going to the movies, playing chess, working puzzles, weaving potholders, or gardening?—ought to get on the list since a good deal of chronic and rehabilitative care pivots around these sorts of issues.

A shocking if simple truth is that, if providers need to know what kinds of information to collect about autonomy, one way to find out is to ask patients what sorts of things they consider important in their lives. Few efforts (Kane and Caplan, 1990) have been made to systematically survey elderly persons about their preferences or thoughts concerning the importance of various matters to them. The easiest way to make progress on this front is to simply go and ask elderly persons who live in various sorts of settings about their values. If this information is properly collected and verified, it could then begin to serve as the foundation for a "patient-centered" values baseline.

Another obvious issue in trying to collect information pertinent to values is who should do the collecting. The collection of information is an obligation of each and every health-care provider and institution. However, positing a general obligation does little to tell practitioners who want to discharge their obligation how best to do so.

It is not clear what kinds of training if any would help people compile a useful values baseline. But it is clear that, to collect large amounts of information in a format that is accessible and useful, some sort of standardized and uniform instrument must be developed. Standardization is particularly important for the elderly, who may be moved from one type of setting to another throughout the course of their health care and thus will have many different people searching for basic information regarding their autonomy. Standardization is also necessary so that people of different backgrounds and experience can be given an equal opportunity to articulate their values to a highly diverse set of health-care providers.

Can values be measured?

One of the sorest points of contention between social scientists and ethicists is the measurement of values. Most ethicists view efforts to measure values with a mixture of amusement, horror, and condescension. But the fact remains that uncertainty about the validity of normative or prescriptive beliefs should not be confused with the ability to ascertain and record information about values.

Two tactics seem useful in thinking about how to develop a standardized set of questions that could constitute the core of a values baseline. First, there ought to be a process by which information is collected from those whose autonomy is to be maintained. Second, information can also be solicited from experts in ethics, theology, and law since these disciplines have the closest contact with theories of autonomy and the analysis and explication of the concept. The two information streams could then be integrated and tried with various types of consensus panels to determine their validity. The general point is that a values baseline requires the collection of information in a manner that assures both an openness to new categories of information and some kind of reliability rating.

In measuring or ascertaining values it would seem useful and essential to give people an opportunity to indicate levels of comfort or discomfort with particular elements of a values baseline beyond a simple yes or no. This is not a feature much in evidence among those promoting the use of written advance directives. But it is not beyond the realm of existing measurement theory to permit people more discretion and shades of opinion than they are now being offered.

There have been efforts to use Likert-type scales to measure responses in a way that permits gradations of agreement or disagreement (Gortner, Hudes, Zyzanski, 1984). Of course providers may be more comfortable with blacks and whites rather than greys, but the pursuit of autonomy is for patients and clients, not for the peace of mind of providers.

VIII. Problems with a values baseline

The problems confronting the effort to "de-ghettoize" autonomy for the elderly, to move providers of care away from special forms—delivered at special moments under special circumstances, and whose scope is restricted to the most extraordinary circumstances: when patients are least able to give a damn about autonomy—are enormous. Little is known about what the elderly want, much less about how to measure and record the information. Even less is known about how best to train providers to collect such information and use it.

A huge problem confronting efforts to maintain and preserve autonomy by constructing a values baseline is the challenge the collection of such information poses for patient privacy and confidentiality. A woman may not want her husband to make decisions regarding her care should she become incompetent, but she may not want her husband to know. If information about sex and recreational habits are to be collected as prerequisites for ordinary forms of autonomy, there are ample opportunities available for embarrassment as well as autonomy. There are also many outside parties who would have a keen interest, for legal and financial reasons, in having access to personal information.

The timeliness of information is an obvious problem for the notion of a values baseline. A baseline established in a doctor's office may mean little when a critical-care nurse is trying to decide what to do concerning the use of morphine for the relief of pain seven years later in a hospital.

Some may even say that the idea of a values baseline is flawed because it is superfluous. All that the notion of a values baseline boils down to is the collection of a thorough patient history, which is something that providers do a poor job at now and are not likely to improve at merely because a new label is stuck onto an old obligation.

But the biggest problems facing the values baseline are the problems that have been cited for living wills. A lack of trust rooted in the growing impersonality of care (Priester, 1990), inadequate availability of care, a fear of the consequences of rationing, and worries about ageism are the biggest obstacles to autonomy. In addition, autonomy is jeopardized by the desire to avoid unpleasant subjects, the difficulties providers have in getting beyond the moral dilemmas of acute care to the mundane matters of autonomy that are of great concern to their patients (Kane and Caplan, 1990), the difficulty of collecting information in a way that guarantees it will be found, and assuring that third parties, including families, will pay any attention to it.

The concept of a values baseline has the advantage of making the protection of autonomy routine rather than extraordinary. It encourages persons to face the fragility of their autonomy by putting the onus of initiating discussion of the subject on the person who provides care. It also has the advantage of being a vehicle for the building of trust rather than providing an opportunity for the mere assertion of or demand for autonomy. In the end it does not matter so much what system of measurement is used and what format and training techniques evolve. Without an environment of trust, autonomy cannot survive.

References

Annas, G., 1986, "The right of elderly patients to refuse life-sustaining treatment," *Milbank Memorial Quarterly,* 64:95–162.

Annas, G., et al., 1990, "Bioethicist's Statement on the U.S. Supreme Court's Cruzan Decision," *New England Journal of Medicine,* 323, 10, September 6: 686.

Beauchamp, T., and Childress, J., 1979, *Principles of Biomedical Ethics,* New York: Oxford.

Califano, J., 1987, *America's Health Care Revolution*, New York: Random House.

Callahan, D., 1987, *Setting Limits*, New York: Simon and Schuster.

———, 1989, *What Kind of Life?*, New York: Simon and Schuster.

Caplan, A., 1984, "Organ procurement: it's not in the cards," *Hastings Center Report*, 14, 5, October: 6–9.

———, 1985, "Let Wisdom Find a Way," *Generations*, 10:10–14. Reprinted in the present volume.

———, 1988, "The Termination of Medical Interventions for the Elderly" in G. Maddox and E. Busse, eds., *Aging: The Universal Human Experience*, New York: Springer: 636–47.

———, 1989, "Ethical Issues in the Care of the Elderly," in R. Kane et al., eds., *Improving Health in Older People*, New York: Oxford: 667–81.

———, 1989, "The Concepts of Health and Disease," in R. Veatch, ed., *Medical Ethics*, Boston: Jones and Bartlett: 49–63.

———, Engelhardt, H., and McCartney, J., eds., 1981, *Concepts of Health and Disease*, Reading, MA: Addison-Wesley.

Caplan, A., and Welvang, P., 1989, "Are required request laws working?", *Clinical Transplantation*, 3, 3: 170–76.

Caplan, A., and Virnig, B., 1990, "Is altruism enough?", *Critical Care Clinics of North America*, 6, 4: 1007–1018.

Childress, J., 1982, *Who Should Decide?*, New York: Oxford.

Collopy, B., 1988, "Autonomy in Long Term Care: Some Crucial Distinctions," *The Gerontologist*, 28: 10–17.

Cruzan v. Director, Missouri Department of Health, 110 S.Ct. 2841 (1990).

Doukas, D., and McCullough, L., 1988, "Assessing the values history of the elderly patient regarding critical and chronic care," in J. Gallo, W. Reichel, and L. Anderson, eds., *Handbook of Geriatric Assessment*, Rockville, MD: Aspen: 111–24.

Doukas, D., and McCullough, L., 1991, "The Values History," *The Journal of Family Practice*, 32, 2, 1991: 145–53.

Emanuel, L., 1989, "Does the DNR Order Need Life Sustaining Intervention?" *The American Journal of Medicine*, 86: 87–90.

Emanuel, L., and Emanuel, E., 1989, "The Medical Directive," *JAMA*, 261: 3288–93.

Engelhardt, H.T., 1986, *The Foundations of Bioethics*, New York: Oxford.

Faden, R., and Beauchamp, T., 1986, *A History and Theory of Informed Consent*, New York: Oxford.

Finacune, T.E., and Denman, S.J., 1989, "Deciding about resuscitation in a nursing home," *Journal of the American Geriatric Society*, 37, 8: 684–88.

Gortner, S., Hudes, M., and Zyzanski, S., 1984, "Appraisal of Values in the Choice of Treatment," *Nursing Research*, 33: 319–24.

Johnson, R., and Justin, R., 1988, "Documenting Patients' End-of-life Decisions," *Nurse Practitioner*, 13: 44–52.

Kane, R. and Caplan, A., eds., 1990, *Everyday Ethics*, New York: Springer.

Kapp, M. and Bigot, A., 1985, *Geriatrics and the Law*, New York: Springer.

Katz, J., 1984, *The Silent World of Doctor and Patient*, New York: The Free Press.

McCarrick, P.M., 1990, "Living Wills and Durable Powers of Attorney: Advance Directive Legislation and Issues," *Scope Note 2, National Reference Center for Bioethics Literature*, Washington: Kennedy Institute of Ethics.

McCullough, L., and Lipson, S., 1989, "A framework for geriatric ethics" in

W. Reichel, ed. *Clinical Aspects of Aging,* Baltimore: Williams and Wilkins: 577–86.

Miles, S., 1987, "Advance Directives to Limit Treatment: The Need for Portability," *Journal of the American Geriatrics Society,* 35: 74–76.

Ouslander, J., 1989, "Medical Care in the Nursing home," *JAMA,* 262, 18: 2582–90.

Priester, R., 1990, *Rethinking Medical Morality,* Minneapolis: Center for Biomedical Ethics.

Shapiro, R., et al., 1986, "Living Will in Wisconsin," *Wisconsin Medical Journal,* 85: 17–23.

Stolman, C., J. Gregory, D. Dunn, and B. Ripley, 1989, "Evaluation of the Do Not Resuscitate orders at a community hospital," *Archives of Internal Medicine,* 149, August: 1851–56.

Uhlmann, R., Pearlman, R., and Cain, K., 1989, "Understanding of elderly patients' resuscitation preferences by physicians and nurses," *Western Journal of Medicine,* 150: 705–707.

Veatch, R., 1981, *A Theory of Medical Ethics,* New York: Basic.

———, 1989, *Medical Ethics,* Boston: Jones and Bartlett.

Part VI

Money, medicine, and morality

17.

The high cost of technological development
A caveat for policymakers

Causes of rising costs of health care

It is often said that the rapid escalation in the cost of health care in the United States since World War II is due to the rapid increase in various forms of diagnostic and therapeutic technology. With total national expenditures in 1990 of almost $600 billion, which is over 10 percent of the gross national product, health care has become the second largest industry in the United States.

Technology certainly is not the only suspect among the possible causes of this dramatic increase in costs. The years since World War II have seen a dramatic rise in access to health care services for the general population, primarily as a result of the institution of social programs such as Medicare and Medicaid and the expansion of the Veterans Administration hospital system. Better access has meant that a larger percentage of the total population can utilize medical services and has produced a corresponding increase in the costs of providing care.

There has also been a gradual but steady increase in the number

of persons living past age 65—a group known to be intensive consumers of health care services. As the U.S. population ages, as the
baby boom generation moves on through middle and, eventually, old
age, there is every reason to assume that greater demands will be
made for health services.

Nevertheless, there can be little doubt that the introduction of
new and expensive forms of medical technology is, at least in part,
to blame for rising costs. If medical technology is defined broadly,
following the lead of the Office of Technology Assessment and other
federal agencies, to include not only devices or medical apparatus
but also new drugs and medical and surgical procedures (Office of
Technology Assessment, 1982), then the number of new technologies that have entered the medical field in the postwar era is simply
staggering. The following is a partial list of the technology that has
been introduced into medical care since 1950 (Comroe and Dripps,
1976):

automated blood chemistries
fractionated blood products
radionucleotide imaging
ultrasound
CAT scanning
NMR scanning
artificial organs
organ transplants
respirators
pacemakers
angioplasty
open-heart surgery
cardiac resuscitation
oral diuretics
parenteral nutrition
intensive care units in neonatology, cardiology, and pulmonary
   medicine
laser surgery

One need only look at the costs associated with a few of these new
technologies to see that the introduction of a host of innovative medical technologies during the past forty years places a significant burden
on the national pocketbook.

While reliable numbers as to costs are unfortunately not available for all technologies, there are data available on the costs of at least some procedures. These statistics illustrate how the development and evolution of useful technologies pose ethical challenges in the allocation of medical resources, both as a matter of national policy and at the patient's bedside.

Consider the costs associated with these fairly common procedures as of 1983 (Office of Technology Assessment, 1984; Melton, 1982):

neonatal care	$2 billion
artificial joints	$2 billion
renal dialysis	over $2 billion
heart bypass surgery	$1.5 billion
kidney transplants	$250 million

The average costs associated with a number of well-publicized surgical procedures or with various diagnostic devices are also significant (Office of Technology Assessment, 1984; Massachusetts Task Force on Organ Transplantation, 1984):

kidney transplant	$35,000 (first year)
heart transplant	$150,000 (first year)
liver transplant	$230,000
cyclosporin for one year	$15,000
NMR scanner	$3 million (per unit)
artificial heart	$250,000
lithotriptor	$1 million (per device)
laser for surgery	$200,000

Add the additional costs of providing highly individualized care for David, the young boy with severe immune deficiency syndrome, who lived for twelve years in a plastic bubble at a cost that easily exceeded $1.5 million (Breo, 1984a), or for a 750 gram (under two pounds) premature newborn in a neonatal unit at a cost of roughly $250,000 (Budetti et al., 1981). It is easy to see why most experts believe that new technology in itself is responsible for nearly 50 percent of the total increase in the costs of medical care during the past thirty years.

Two recent theses about the costs of medical technology

The history of the introduction of new and innovative technologies into medical care since World War II has evoked two interesting claims about the nature of the cost problem. Some commentators argue that it is not the big-ticket items such as artificial hearts or organ transplants that are responsible for the big jump in costs but, rather, that it is the overutilization of little-ticket, less costly forms of technology that is the culprit behind cost escalation.

Proponents of this thesis (Collen, 1977; Moloney and Rogers, 1979; Fineberg, 1979) argue that if health care costs are to be brought under control, we ought to educate physicians not to overutilize technologies such as urinanalysis, blood gas tests, and X-rays. While none of these tests is expensive in and of itself on a per procedure basis, the cost burden placed on the total health care system by ordering thousands and thousands of such tests is, in the aggregate, huge.

Proponents of this view of the source of rising health care costs like to point to improved physician education concerning the use of tests as one way to decrease the overall cost of health care. Unfortunately, there is not much evidence that the diagnostic testing behavior of physicians has been modified by educating them to the need for and prices of the tests (Schroeder et al., 1984a).

The other and more provocative thesis that has recently come into vogue in health policy discussions is what might be termed the no-fat view of medical technology. This view (presented most persuasively in a book that has enjoyed tremendous attention in the world of health policy, *The Painful Prescription* (Schwartz and Aaron, 1984)), maintains that all of the technology that has entered medical practice in the past thirty years or so is basically useful and beneficial. While it may be possible to temporarily slow the increase in health care costs by correcting the overuse of diagnostic technology, the overall trend toward rapidly increasing costs will continue as long as the basic biomedical research this nation generously funded through the NIH in the 1950s and 1960s continues to produce useful discoveries and inventions.

Proponents of the no-fat thesis concerning medical technology argue that the only way to cope with technology is to batten down the hatches and immediately begin to ration access. They argue that various European countries such as the United Kingdom have already instituted systems, at least informally, for choosing who will receive scarce resources by using criteria such as age, prognosis, waiting periods, and regional availability; our society should be prepared to follow suit if it wants to remain financially solvent. The grim message of the no-fat school is that only by limiting access to medical technology can we ever hope to afford it (Ginsberg, 1984; Johnson, 1984; Breo, 1984a).

I am not certain whether advocates of the little-ticket theory of the escalation in health care costs are correct. However, given the present legal climate in health care, which amounts to a rampant paranoia about malpractice, the prospects for reforming physician behavior with respect to the use of diagnostic technology appear to be dim.

It is the second thesis—the no-fat-and-therefore-ration view—that I believe needs critical examination. Enthusiasm for the validity of this view has grown so much in the past few years that it has fundamentally altered the nature of ethical discussion concerning the allocation of health resources.

In the early 1970s, ethical debate was dominated by the question of whether the United States ought to institute some form of comprehensive national health insurance for all in need. Today this subject is viewed as an exercise in liberal utopianism of the most dangerous variety. Arguments about national health insurance have now been supplanted by demands that philosophers, theologians, and others with an interest in medical ethics begin formulating ethically acceptable criteria for rationing access to technology.

While there is surely a need for discussion of criteria that ought to be used when hard choices have to be made about who will and will not have access to a particular form of technology when not everyone can do so, the case has not been persuasively made that there is no fat, only muscle, in the plethora of technologies currently available within the health care system. I think a powerful case can be made for the view that there is a good deal of fat in our health care system and that those concerned with medical ethics should not be willing to provide the rationing criteria that are being requested until the system is made as efficient and fat-free as is possible.

The evolution of the artificial heart

On November 25, 1984, William J. Schroeder became the fourth living recipient of an artificial heart in the United States. All the publicity that surrounded this experiment and the earlier trial in December 1982 on Dr. Barney Clark somewhat obscured the fact that a number of previous implants had already been attempted prior to the Clark and Schroeder implants. The details of these previous clinical efforts are important, since they help to illustrate the kinds of problems that arise in controlling the evolution and dissemination of new technologies in health care when the technological imperative— what can be done must be done—is allowed free reign.

In 1969 Dr. Denton Cooley, then at the Baylor College of Medicine, implanted a heart in a forty-seven-year-old patient. The patient survived for sixty-five hours. In May 1981 surgeons at the Temple University Hospital implanted the devices for a few hours in three persons who had been declared brain dead (Shaw 1984). And on July 23, 1981, Cooley attempted a second implant at the Texas Heart Institute on a retired Dutch bus driver, Willebrodus Meuffels, who had been flown to Houston by the Dutch government in order to receive a heart transplant. When no suitable donor could be found, Cooley decided to maintain the dying Meuffels on the device in hope that a donor might be located. The patient was maintained by an artificial heart for fifty-four hours. He then received a heart transplant only to die eight days later from what a Heart Institute representative termed "other complications that simply overwhelmed him" (Caplan, 1982).

Serious ethical questions were raised about Cooley's two attempts to implant an artificial device. In 1969 many physicians, including the renowned heart specialist Dr. Michael DeBakey, Cooley's colleague at Baylor, criticized his behavior as constituting a premature effort to utilize a mechanical heart. They argued that the heart had not been adequately tested in animal models and that the quality of life the device could provide did not merit a trial in a human being, even in desperate medical circumstances. Ultimately, Cooley resigned his teaching position at Baylor, stating that he did not feel he could comply with the then current federal regulations governing human experimentation (Fox and Swazey, 1978).

Cooley also acted in defiance of federal law in making his second effort with Meuffels. Cooley had made no effort to clear the use of an artificial heart with the Food and Drug Administration, the federal agency with regulatory responsibility over the development of new drugs and medical devices. Despite the fact that he was lauded in the press as a "medical pioneer" who had broken new ground, Cooley had stretched the boundaries of existing regulations governing medical technology in implanting an artificial heart into Meuffels, relying on the so-called emergency therapeutic waiver provision of the medical devices provision of the Food and Drug Act, which governs the use of any new medical device in human beings.

After Meuffels died, Cooley explained to officials at the Food and Drug Administration that he had been forced to act quickly in a desperate attempt to save a man's life. The executive director of the Texas Heart Institute wrote to the head of the Food and Drug Administration's Bureau of Medical Devices that the surgery had been performed only when all conventional resuscitative measures had been exhausted.

The Food and Drug Administration did not agree with this attempt to circumvent the regulatory provision requiring prior review by an institutional review board. While their reaction to Cooley's behavior received little attention in either the popular press or in the professional literature, they moved quickly to censure Cooley and to caution him against any further efforts to implant an artificial heart. The director of the Bureau of Medical Devices at the Food and Drug Administration, Victor Zafra, wrote to Cooley in a letter dated September 21, 1981, that:

> FDA believes that this artificial heart was not intended or designed for implantation solely in a specific patient. It was fabricated in advance and would appear to be appropriate for any of a number of patients. It does not appear that this device was designed specifically for Dr. Cooley's use in his professional practice. The federal government, through the NIH, has supported the development of an artificial heart for many years. The purpose of the program in which the Texas Heart Institute participated is to develop a totally implantable total artificial heart for commercial distribution. Given NIH's program for the development of a total artificial heart and its plans for implantation of such a device, once fully developed, in potentially thousands of patients each year, FDA does not agree that this, or any, total artificial heart is a custom device. (Caplan 1982)

Zafra concluded his letter by noting that any further implants at the Texas Heart Institute would be viewed as violating federal laws.

The race for success in the implantation of an artificial heart has resulted in serious conflicts between those who want artificial heart research to proceed at a rapid pace and those who believe that the costs, both to society and the recipients, of developing the device require caution. While the federal government has instituted regulations requiring both informed consent and committee review whenever new medical devices are to be given to human subjects, these regulations have not always been supported or honored by experimenters. One has to wonder about the efficacy of a system of technology assessment that can be circumvented so easily by those who wish to accelerate the pace of technological development in health care.

Dr. William DeVries, the surgeon who implanted artificial hearts into Barney Clark, William Schroeder, Murray Hayden, and Jack Burcham, when asked how he felt about being upstaged by Dr. Cooley in the race to be the first to use an artificial heart, remarked, "Cooley was the first to do it and he was the second to do it. It would take someone like Cooley to stand up to the Review Board and the FDA" (*Life,* 1981:36). DeVries, like Cooley, viewed the FDA requirements for careful review as just so much "red tape."

These remarks illustrate the kinds of tensions that have continued to beset those responsible for regulating the development of new medical devices and surgical procedures. New drugs or devices are, according to law, to be tried only on those patients who have not responded to standard, available medical therapies. This means that researchers must experiment on those who are the most severely ill, such as a Meuffels, Clark, or Schroeder.

Yet those who are the sickest patients are often not ideal recipients from the point of view of researchers. The severity of the underlying disease (in the case of Clark and Schroeder, severe degenerative cardiomyopathy) can make it difficult to know whether any complications that arise are due to a new device or to the patient's underlying medical problems. Moreover, dying patients with multiple complications are not as likely as healthier patients to fare well when they receive experimental treatments. In situations where physicians are competing with one another to be "the first" or where alternative forms of devices or new treatments are under development, as is the case with the artificial heart, researchers are often tempted, as was Cooley, to proceed less cautiously. When the desire to help hopeless patients is mixed with a strongly competitive research environment, biases can easily appear in the views of researchers about the pace at which medical research on new technologies should proceed.

Public policy in the United States has attempted to buffer the natural desire of researchers to proceed rapidly in testing new drugs and devices by requiring careful review by independent committees and by obtaining thorough informed consent from potential subjects. But as the behavior of Cooley, the remarks of DeVries, the carnival-like publicity atmosphere surrounding the Clark and Schroeder implants, and the incredibly rushed attempt to use the so-called "Phoenix" artificial heart as a "bridge" device at the University of Arizona readily reveal, if a researcher can gain sufficient autonomy or publicity, it is possible to sidestep ethical protections and considerations of social cost in ways that can lead to questionable allocations of health care resources.

Are the existing methods of regulating technology adequate?

The artificial heart that the team at Humana Audubon implanted into William Schroeder's chest is not the device the National Institutes of Health envisioned when it undertook the financing of an artificial heart program in the mid-1960s. At that time urgency and optimism were the dominant values governing U.S. science policy.

U.S. legislators were persuaded that thousands of lives could be saved if a crash program could be mounted to produce an artificial heart. The development of the heart was treated as a national emergency that required immediate intervention by the federal government (Bernstein, 1984a).

The National Heart Institute, at the direct request of Congress, created a special artificial heart office. This office was directed to sign contracts for the development of an artificial heart in July of 1965. The office expected to see a fully implantable total artificial heart available for mass distribution early in 1970. In fact, the NIH fully expected to implant the first artificial heart by Valentine's Day 1970.

The biomedical and scientific community did little at the time to disabuse U.S. legislators of the reality of estimates for the development of a total artificial heart. One group of medical scientists and biologists wrote the director of the National Heart Institute saying that the development of an artificial heart "is difficult, but easily manageable within the framework of our present scientific knowledge and technical proficiency." Other scientists lobbied legislators for funds noting that the artificial heart was no more complicated than a "guided missile or a subsonic bomber." The heart, they observed, was nothing more than a simple pump and its functions could easily be duplicated by a mechanical device (Bernstein, 1984a).

Estimates of the demand for the artificial heart were, during these early days, equally optimistic. In 1965 the Heart Institute hired six firms (whose previous work had been in the aerospace industry) to undertake feasibility studies and determine the need for an artificial heart. One firm estimated the demand for artificial hearts to be in the neighborhood of 10,000 per year. Another firm estimated that approximately 250,000 patients would require an artificial heart each year if one were to become available. Incredibly, the Heart Institute simply split the difference in these estimates and used the figure of 137,500 needy recipients in its estimates to Congress (Bernstein, 1984b).

The cost estimates used by these same consultants were also heavily weighted with optimism about the feasibility of developing a total artificial heart. Cost estimates for the device itself were placed at between $3,000 and $5,000. The operation was seen as adding an additional $5,000. Since the costs for Barney Clark's implant were well over $250,000, not including the cost of the device and the fees of his surgeons, which were donated without charge, the original projections were greatly off the mark.

In part this was a result of the fact that the original cost estimates did not include any figures for failures, either of the operation or of the device. Clark encountered numerous difficulties during his operation, including a broken valve, nosebleeds, psychological problems, and pulmonary problems (Berenson and Grosser, 1984). Schroeder suffered a number of strokes and a bout of severe depression. Some members of Clark's family expressed strong reservations about the quality of life afforded Clark by the Utah experiment (Breo, 1984b).

As has been true of many other estimates of the costs of medical technology, such as renal dialysis and organ transplants, studies by biomedical and bioengineering experts frequently pay little attention to the costs of managing complications or failures of medical technology. The artificial heart was treated in the cost/benefit studies of the 1960s not as an experimental device that would have to undergo a long period of technological evolution but, rather, as a well-understood therapeutic device whose benefits could be made available both rapidly and cheaply as a result of U.S. industry's ability to mass produce medical products with large commercial markets.

The following twenty years proved how overly optimistic the original discussion of an artificial heart had been. For despite the fact that the U.S. government has spent over $200 million on artificial heart research, medicine is still a long way from developing what the original proponents promised would take only $40 million over a five-year period.

None of the devices that have been implanted into either human beings or animals, including the one received by Barney Clark, the Jarvik 7, meets the requirements of a totally implantable artificial heart. The Jarvik 7, for example, has a power source that is external to the body. The pump itself is pneumatically driven by an air-compressor that is also located outside the body. The heart is not capable of altering its rate or output to adjust to the various demands made on it by different bodily activities (Wooley, 1984). By 1984, nearly twenty years after the artificial heart program was initiated, biomedical scientists and engineers had only been able to produce a partially implantable artificial heart.

Even these devices leave much to be desired in terms of their therapeutic capacities. For example, the power console necessary for driving the Jarvik 7 requires that the patient be kept tethered to an air compression unit at all times. The recipient's mobility is further impaired by the fact that no source of power has been developed that would allow the recipient to leave a hospital room for anything other than short periods of time.

The biological effects of artificial hearts on other organ systems are not well understood. While the pump implanted into Barney Clark functioned for 112 days, Clark suffered a number of serious side effects from the device, including acute renal failure, fever, hemorrhage as a result of anticoagulant drugs, diarrhea, vomiting, and seizures. In the words of the surgical team, "the procedure is still highly experimental. Further experience, development, and discussion will be required before more general application of the device can be recommended" (DeVries et al., 1984).

Do commerce and research mix?

In August of 1984 Dr. DeVries announced that he was leaving the University of Utah to move his artificial heart program to Audubon Hospital in Louisville, Kentucky. Audubon is owned by the Humana Corporation, one of a new breed of aggressive for-profit corporations moving rapidly into the provision of health care in the United States.

DeVries gave two reasons for moving his research. First, the Humana Corporation promised to provide financing for up to 100 artificial heart implants. The University of Utah, a publicly owned university-based hospital, had found it difficult to raise money either to cover the costs of Clark's operation or to allow for further implantations on new patients.

Second, DeVries complained about bureaucratic "red tape" that in his view had delayed the progress of the artificial heart program at Utah (Altman, 1984). By moving to an institution in the private sector, DeVries apparently hoped to avoid the close and careful process of committee review that had prevailed at the University of Utah.

What DeVries did not point out was that both he and the Humana Corporation were, at the time of the shift to Louisville, stockholders in a private company, Symbion, which has as its president Dr. Robert Jarvik, the inventor of the Jarvik 7. Symbion had an ambitious financial agenda. According to Jarvik, "What Genentech is doing with gene-splicing products, we want to do with artificial organs over the next decade" (Chase, 1984). Humana had also purchased the University of Louisville teaching hospital that is affiliated with Audubon. And Humana owns nearly ninety other hospitals, many of which could be prepared as centers for artificial heart implants, thereby guaranteeing a market and a demand for the device regardless of any views the public might have about the desirability of spending money on the device.

Historically, the artificial heart program has been buffeted by conflicts between those who favor totally implantable artificial hearts as the cure for cardiac failure and those who favor transplantation. The program has also been subject to powerful political pressure to move quickly to save many thousands who die each year of end-stage cardiac disease. The shift from Utah to Louisville introduces a new and more disturbing factor into the process of regulating and controlling technology development—profit.

By moving the artificial heart program to Louisville, DeVries perhaps hoped to avoid the strict application of the ethical and regulatory provisions that govern research involving human subjects at institutions that receive federal funding. While the Food and Drug regulations requiring institutional committee review prior to any implants of artificial hearts do apply to Humana Audubon, the composition of the committee at Audubon was quite different from that at Utah.

The Audubon committee consisted almost entirely of persons working directly for the institution, whereas the Utah institutional review board had members from a variety of departments outside the medical center. The Audubon committee had little prior experience with reviewing experimental protocols, whereas the Utah IRB had reviewed hundreds of research proposals in many different areas of medical research (Breo, 1984a).

Committee review at a for-profit hospital turned out to be far different than it had been at a publicly funded institution. After meeting only five times over the course of a few months, the Humana Audubon IRB gave its approval for a series of seven implants.

The potential for large profits inherent in the move was enormous. The fact that Humana owns a teaching hospital means that young surgeons could easily be trained in the techniques of artificial heart implantation, thereby creating a natural demand for the procedure.

It is unfortunate that, under private auspices, it is difficult to apply the traditional public methods of regulating the speed with which medical technology is developed and disseminated. The fact that the NIH has lost much of its enthusiasm for pneumatically driven, externally powered devices like the Jarvik 7 means little when research on the device can proceed with private funding. The fact that the institution where research on the artificial heart was done received publicity of the type that has surrounded the artificial heart program means that it is possible to use public opinion to overwhelm the skepticism of much of the medical community concerning the feasibility and desirability of the device. And the fact that it is much more difficult for existing review mechanisms (such as peer review and institutional review boards) to work effectively in private as opposed to public settings means that the traditional avenues for allowing professional and societal concerns to govern the pace of development of new technologies are of limited utility in an age of for-profit health care.

If the history of the artificial heart's evolution is taken as a representative example of how expensive new technologies evolve within our health care system, there would appear to be a strong case to be made for the inadequacy of the existing system of technology assessment in regulating the costs and direction of technological development in health care. Moreover, as the case of the artificial heart illustrates, it is difficult to say that the current system of technology development in health care produces those technologies that either the health care profession or the public would agree are those that are most needed or most cost-efficient.

Waste, inefficiency, and medical technology

As the case history of the artificial heart reveals, the existing system for regulating technological development in health care is not adequate. It can neither control the pace of development of expensive new devices nor allow sufficient public criticism of the development of commercially attractive, privately financed technology. The inadequacy of the existing system for regulating new technology at least casts doubts on those who advance the view that there is no fat in the system that can be cut prior to instituting rationing or restricting access to medical technology.

Usage patterns

There are also sound empirical reasons to doubt whether already existing technologies are being used effectively. While the state of epidemiological knowledge concerning the efficacy of existing medical technology is rudimentary, a number of studies have shown variations in the use of medical technology that would seem to disprove the view that all medical technology is to be viewed as effective and necessary merely because it exists and is widely used in medical practice.

A 1983 examination (Schroeder, 1984b) of five forms of medical technology at five similar hospitals in Belgium, West Germany, the Netherlands, the United Kingdom, and the United States revealed startling differences in the degree to which physicians in these countries utilize the same form of technology on roughly the same sort of patients. The study showed that the percentage of days in a typical hospital devoted to the provision of neonatal care varied from less than 1 percent of all hospital admissions in the United Kingdom to nearly 4 percent in a similar U.S. hospital. Open-heart surgery accounted for 0.5 percent of all the inpatient hospital days in a large Belgian tertiary care facility, while they accounted for over 1 percent of the days in an analogous institution in the United States. These variations may appear small, but differences in utilization rates of only a few tenths of a percentage point regarding a particular procedure can produce cost differences in the billions of dollars when extrapolated to entire hospital systems.

Even more disturbing variations in the utilization of technology were revealed in a study published in 1982 by Wennberg and Gittelsohn (see also Gleicher, 1984). These epidemiologists found that the amount and cost of hospital care in a particular community have more to do with the number of physicians present in the community and their specialities than with the health care needs of the residents of the community. They examined rates of surgery in matched populations within six New England states and found that the number of procedures done per 10,000 people for such common surgical interventions as tonsillectomies, hysterectomies, and prostatectomies varied enormously between similar communities. One hospital area in Rhode Island showed a rate of ten tonsillectomies per 10,000 residents while a similar area in Maine had a rate of over sixty per 10,000 residents. Within-state variations for hysterectomies in Vermont varied from a low of 25 per 10,000 residents to a high of 65 per 10,000.

Such studies cast severe doubt on the adequacy of the no-fat thesis concerning medical technology. It is evident that there are tremendous variations in the utilization of existing and well-accepted surgical procedures that can be attributed only to habit, custom, or financial incentive. The usage rates for particular technologies appear to bear little relationship to the medical needs of a particular community or population. These studies and the history of the evolution of new technologies such as the artificial heart should make it plain that there is much to do in the way of rooting waste and inefficiency out of the health care system before governmental decisions are made to begin restricting access to medical technology.

Conclusion

There is simply too little known by health care providers and regulators about what works and what doesn't in medical technology to support any claims about the need for rationing. The moral lesson of the history of medical technology in the post–World War II era is that adequate systems for assessing and controlling existing and evolving medical technologies do not exist. Policy makers would be well-advised to take steps to address this problem before decisions are made as to who may or may not receive certain kinds of health care.

References

Altman, L. 1984. "Surgeon's Move Highlights Controversial Trend." *New York Times* (Aug. 7):C-3.

Berenson, C., and B. Grosser. 1984. "Total Artificial Heart Implantation." *Archives of General Psychiatry* (41) (Sept.):910–16.

Bernstein, B. 1984a. "Is Technology Overemphasized?" *IEEE Engineering in Biology and Medicine* 3(2) (June):36–38.

———. 1984b. "The Misguided Quest for the Artificial Heart." *Technology Review* 87(8) (Dec.):13.

Breo, D.L. 1984a. "Ethical Issues Debated after Successful Implant of Second Artificial Heart." *American Medical News* 27(45) (Dec. 7):10, 54.

———. 1984b. "Barney Clark's M.D.-Son: I'm Ambivalent." *American Medical News* (April 22):9–10.

Budetti, P., et al. 1981. "The Costs and Effectiveness of Neonatal Intensive Care." Washington, DC: OTA (Aug.):PB82-101-411.

Caplan, Arthur L. 1982. "The Artificial Heart." *Hastings Center Report* (Feb.):22–24.

Chase, M. 1984. "Firm That Developed Artificial Heart Seeks to Build Bionic Market." *Wall Street Journal* (July 24):1.

Collen, M.F., ed. 1977. *Multiphasic Health Testing Services.* New York: John Wiley & Sons.

Comroe, J., and R. Dripps, 1976. "Scientific Basis for the Support of Biomedical Science." *Science* 192 (April 9):105–08.

DeVries, W., et al. 1984. "Clinical Use of the Total Artificial Heart." *New England Journal of Medicine* 310(5) (Feb. 2):278.

Fineberg, H. 1979. "Clinical Chemistries: The High Cost of Low-Cost Diagnostic Tests." In S. Altman and R. Blendon, eds., *Medical Technology: The Culprit behind Health Care Costs?*, 144–65. Hyattsville, MD, DHEW, PHS79-3216.

Fox, R., and J. Swazey. 1978. *The Courage to Fail.* 2d ed. Chicago: University of Chicago Press.

Ginsberg, E. 1984. "The Monetarization of Medical Care." *New England Journal of Medicine* 310(18):1162–65.

Gleicher, N. 1984. "Cesarean Section Rates in the United States." *Journal of the American Medical Association* 252(23) (Dec. 21):3273–3276.

Johnson, D. 1984. "Life, Death, and the Dollar Sign." *Journal of the American Medical Association* 252(2) (July 13):223–24.

Life Magazine. 1981. (Sept.):36.

Massachusetts Task Force on Organ Transplantation Report. 1984. Boston: Department of Public Health, Commonwealth of Massachusetts (Oct.): 39–71.

Melton, L.J., et al., 1982. "Rates of Total Hip Arthroplasty." *New England Journal of Medicine,* 307 (Nov. 11):1242–1245.

Moloney, T., and D. Rogers. 1979. "Medical Technology—A Different View of the Contentious Debate over Costs." *New England Journal of Medicine* 301:1413–19.

Office of Technology Assessment. 1982. "Strategies for Medical Technology Assessment." Washington, DC: GPO, 052-003-0087-4.

_____. 1984. "Abstracts of Case Studies in the Health Technology Case Study Series." Washington, DC: OTA (Nov.): OTA-P-225.

Schroeder, S., et al. 1984a. "The Failure of Physician Education as a Cost Containment Strategy." *Journal of the American Medical Association* 252 (July 13):225–30.

_____. 1984b. "A Comparison of Western European and U.S. University Hospitals." *Journal of the American Medical Association* 252(2): (July 13):240–46.

Schwartz, William, and Henry Aaron. 1984. *The Painful Prescription.* Washington, DC: Brookings Institute.

Shaw, M., ed. 1984. *After Barney Clark.* Austin: University of Texas Press.

Wennberg, J., and A. Gittelsohn. 1982. "Variations in Medical Care among Small Areas." *Scientific American* (April):120–26.

Wooley, S.R. 1984. "Ethical Issues in the Implantation of the Total Artificial Heart." *New England Journal of Medicine* 310(5) (Feb. 2):292–96.

18.

Hard data is the only answer to hard choices in health care

Let me begin with two stories about the way things are in health care today. I give many talks about the ethical issues which arise with respect to professional autonomy and the role physicians and other health care professionals play as patient advocates under the new economic constraints imposed in the name of cost-containment. Not infrequently my talk is followed by one given by a person who carries a big case full of software. This person gives a talk about how to beat the system of prospective payment instituted in Medicare and some state Medicaid programs. Health care providers are concerned about medical ethics, but they are even more concerned about the battering their bottom line is taking in many institutions. And concern about the costs of health care is not confined to the lecture hall.

Recently, a chief resident at the University of Minnesota Hospital told me about a case that was troubling the housestaff. A young woman who had a long history of intravenous drug abuse and prostitution had recently been admitted to the hospital. She was suffering from endocarditis, a bacterial infection that was damaging the valves of her heart. She had already undergone one heart valve replacement in Texas as a result of this disease. The cost for that procedure was over $75,000. When she appeared at the same hospital in Texas with the same condition a few years later, the hospital told her that they would not perform another operation.

Despondent, she came back to her home state, Minnesota, to seek a valve replacement. Some of the housestaff saw things exactly as had the doctors in Texas. She had clearly gotten reinfected because she was still sharing needles. Why should they perform an expensive operation on a woman who, in the words of one resident, "would just go out and do it all over again"?

Experiences such as these have left me with some sympathy for the view that it is nice to talk about ethics, but it is more important to understand how things actually are in our hospitals, nursing homes, and emergency rooms today. In some areas of the nation, harm is being done because doctors and administrators are overly concerned with costs. In other places hospitals and physicians seem to be more concerned with administering morality tests to their patients than they are in helping them.

There are three points I would like to make to show that bioethics does have something to say about the practical world. I want to make a specific recommendation about cost containment and equity. I also want to draw a philosophical distinction between allocation and rationing. I will also argue that we all ought to be willing to pay for the medical care of others, even when such payment is not for our own benefit and when those needing care may have contributed to their being sick or disabled through their own behavior.

The concept of obligation

Why should we care what happens to poor people or those who might in another era have been described as sinners? One response, which has gained numerous adherents in recent years, to those who engage in unsafe sex, fail to wear helmets while operating motorcycles, or drink to excess is "to hell with them." Some believe that the ethically responsible public policy response to the health care plight of the imprudent or the unfortunate can be formulated along something like the following lines: "Too bad, you probably deserve your problems. It's not my problem. Get out of my way, I'm coming into Mount Sinai to get a facelift or a tummy-tuck."

The response to the medically indigent and morally fallible in our society is not always one of empathy or sympathy for the plight of others. Perhaps morality can be used to generate a feeling of obligation to help which might not be present when we confine our response to a close examination of the contents of our wallets. Unfortunately, talk of obligations is not much in evidence in our current political policy debates about health care.

When can the concept of rationing be invoked?

Let me begin the examination of the concept of obligation with an examination of a crucial concept in health policy today: rationing.

One of the ways in which we allow rhetoric or ideology to overwhelm us is by being incautious about what the concept of rationing really means. Rationing, to the economist, simply describes any situation in which one has to divide a supply of resources amongst people who all want access to the resources. But this somewhat sterile description does not capture what rationing really entails, at least in the sense in which it is invoked in health policy rhetoric these days.

The rhetoric of health care cost containment these days is more akin to the ethic of the lifeboat, not discussions of marginal utility or whether we can ethically take away incremental benefits from someone. What people are talking about in academic circles, in Congress, in the Office of Management and Budget, in state legislatures, and in popular books such as those written by former governor of Colorado Richard Lamm and former Health and Human Services secretary Joseph Califano is withholding access to life-saving or life-extending medical care.[1-4]

There is a growing school of thought which runs, "Our nation is in a tough situation. We've got to gird up our emotional loins and be prepared to eject some of our fellow citizens from the health-care lifeboat. They are draining us of resources that we need to continue our economically sound voyage in competing in the world marketplace."

According to many analysts, the United States is currently facing a dire emergency. We are in a situation of lifeboat ethics with respect to health care. The moral question, and the only important moral question, is, What rules can we agree upon to guide us in answering the question of whom to toss over the side?

Answering this question is, by the way, highly lucrative labor for bioethicists. People feel much better about doing what they have to do if they can defend their triage policies in moral terms.

Rationing as a subset of allocation issues: the lifeboat

Rationing should be seen, from a moral point of view, as a very special and distinct subset of allocation issues. It is a particular and dire instance of what is permitted in responding to scarcity. Rationing should be used only to describe choices, not about marginal utilities or incremental benefits, but rather choices that require excluding some persons from life-saving benefits. Rationing applies in very particular circumstances. The clearest paradigm is the lifeboat.

On a lifeboat when scarcity exists there is nothing anyone can do to get more resources. In a lifeboat one simply cannot get any more food or water.

Furthermore, those on a lifeboat know, and there is no dispute about the fact, that the resource they need is required in order for them to live. You know that you must have food and water, not to feel better, but to live. You know that if you don't get food, or water, you will die.

On a lifeboat everyone wants the food and water that are available. There is no lifeboat ethics scenario if some passengers voluntarily decide to forgo access to food and water and die. The agony of rationing arises when all aboard want access to the resources that are available.

It is also true, if one is stuck in real lifeboat dilemmas, that there is not enough food and water to go around. This is a special, an extreme, form of scarcity. Resources cannot be shared below a minimal portion, since to go below the minimum will do no one any good. Unlike bubblegum or sunshine, no one can make do with a small portion.

These conditions are prerequisites for rationing to exist on a lifeboat. There is a shortage of a life-supporting, life-sustaining resource. Everybody would want it if they could have access to it.

There's nothing anyone can do to get any more of the resource. There's not enough of it to go around; the resource is nondivisible.

Admittedly rationing is sometimes needed. Some people, for instance William Schwartz and Henry Aaron in their widely hailed book, *The Painful Prescription*,[5] think you have to go to England to find real cases of rationing in health care. But there is no need to travel so far.

Rationing policies must be instituted in many areas of health care in the United States and have been for many, many years. Large American transplant centers must allocate organs and tissues among more recipients than there are organs and tissue available. And, in many American rehabilitation departments, there are many more people with spinal cord injuries and head trauma who want access to rehabilitation than there are facilities that can provide these services.

Rationing of organ transplants

What has been the American response when confronted with scarcity of such dimensions with respect to a life-sustaining resource that rationing is required? Consider the policies that have evolved in the field of organ transplants.

Ability to pay and age

The American response has been to use the ability to pay to ration access. There is not a major transplant center in the United States which does not require a means test for those seeking liver, pancreas, bone marrow, heart-lung, or lung transplants.

Our policy has also been to look very carefully at age. Age is used as a criterion every day. Transplant centers and transplant surgeons who say that 55 is too old for a liver transplant, or 65 is the age at which we will not give access to a heart transplant, are doing so on more than purely medical grounds. They are simply saying they have to adapt to a situation in which a life-saving resource is scarce and many people want it. Their response is to consider money. They think about age. What else do they do?

Efficacy and selection criteria

What doctors also think about in making rationing choices is the degree to which a procedure is known to work. There's a tendency to want to discourage access to some transplants in situations in which they have a poor chance of succeeding in preserving life.

Consider the notorious Baby Jesse case in California. A little girl was born with a heart defect. It was alleged that she was refused a transplant because she was the product of unmarried bliss.

But that is not all that happened. What was going on was that the physicians and social workers looked at the baby's family and decided they might not be competent to care for the baby if the surgery was done. So they did not admit the baby to the program. This kind of psychosocial judgment is based upon the need to ration. Provide more organs and more transplant centers capable of transplanting newborns, and psychosocial evaluations would be far more generous.

For new forms of transplantation, other values emerge. In rationing access in a new transplant program or for a new form of transplantation such as pancreas or lung transplants, doctors keep an eye over their shoulder to insure that their procedures have some degree of efficacy. They are also concerned to show that they are not going to kill patients at higher rates than other programs.

Those rationing access to the total artificial heart in Utah and Louisville kept upgrading the level of people in whom the hearts were inserted. Originally total artificial hearts were to go to those who could not be resuscitated during open-heart surgery. Later the criteria for admission were extended to include those with cardiomyopathy. Later still, additional criteria were added having to do with the psychological, social, and familial attributes of potential recipients.

The researchers argued (and continue to argue) that they needed people who were not quite so sick because the less ill would do better on the device. The same pattern of selectivity is in evidence in all other forms of transplantation. The health of patients is a factor much in evidence in rationing access to new medical treatments. There is a real need to show that new technologies work and that they are safe. Researchers triage access knowing that safety and efficacy must be demonstrated.

A slew of values come into play to govern rationing in the "real" world. Those trying to replace damaged organs look at the ability to pay, age, the health of potential recipients, and psychosocial factors in making their choices.

Access to dialysis in America and the United Kingdom

These same values are evident in the access patterns for hemodialysis in the United States and the United Kingdom during the past thirty years. It is particularly interesting to note the similarities in access patterns, given all the ballyhoo about the lessons on rationing we ought to learn from the British.

The availability of payment for dialysis in England made little difference to who got dialysis in the 1960s. Prior to our decision to create the End-Stage Renal Dialysis program and thus guarantee financial coverage for dialysis for those in end-stage renal failure, our distribution patterns were about the same as the United Kingdom's. The decision to pay for dialysis in 1972 was followed by a rapid expansion in the use of dialysis in the United States. But access to dialysis in the United Kingdom also underwent a rapid increase in the years following the American financing decision.

These similarities occurred because the other values just mentioned in the analysis of transplantation overwhelmed the fiscal incentives to provide or not provide the treatment. The primary value for the British nephrology community in the mid to late 1960s was making sure that the dialysis machine worked. They wanted to make sure that hemodialysis did not kill people faster than would happen by doing nothing. They were also trying to show that hemodialysis was better than doing kidney transplants.

These concerns determined the selection criteria that produced a dialysis population in England of people roughly 30 to 45 years old, who had a job, were psychologically stable, had few other diseases, and had a stable family. These early rationing criteria penalized the usual suspects. The poor, minorities, the drug addicted, the mentally ill, the elderly, the chronically ill, people who did not speak English, all dropped by the wayside because they were much tougher to work with in terms of obtaining good outcomes with a new technology.

American nephrologists also had a population of patients in the early and mid 1960s who were young or middle-aged, relatively healthy, middle and upper class, and in good mental health. Money was not the driving force in determining access to scarce hemodialysis machines, although it too played a role. The need to prove that the technology could work was the overriding moral norm that governed rationing during this period.

Specifically American values at work in selection and rationing

The same thing is true in other relatively new areas of health care. Decisions about who to admit to a rehabilitation unit for head injury or stroke victims frequently depend on who, in the attending physician's judgment, is likely to benefit the most from access to rehabilitation. Rationing has relatively little to do with need, because nearly all stroke and head injury patients need rehabilitation. Rationing has to do with who is seen as most likely to show the greatest improvement relative to other people the physician could admit. Decisions are oftentimes influenced by judgments about the degree to which a patient is motivated to strive for rehabilitation, his or her residual capacity to go back to independent living, and to go back to work.

The emphasis on work and independent living is interesting in the rehabilitation setting, since these are quintessentially American values. Other societies do not assign them the same weight that our physicians and third-party payors do.

Independence is the dominant value that we seem to care about, but we would have a hard time persuading many others in the world to care all that much about it. Work has an even more peculiar status. We are so enamored of the value of work in rehabilitation that we try to convince people to work who did not do so before they had their head trauma or stroke!

Many years ago I interviewed a man in a small acute-care rehabilitation facility. The staff complained bitterly that this fellow was noncompliant, he would not follow his rehabilitation regimen. He was particularly indifferent to his occupational and vocational therapy.

I was asked to go talk with him because no one else could figure out what to do with him. I asked him why he seemed uninterested in his rehabilitation. He said, "Well, I like to stare out the window and look at the construction going on across the street. That's what I like to do. And I don't want to do all these sorting tasks and licking envelopes and stuff that they're trying to make me do." I said, "Oh, what did you do before your accident?" He said, "Well, I hated working. I used to lie at home, stare out the window and watch construction." I am not quite sure how this fellow got past the triage screen for rehabilitation which placed so much weight on work, but I was sure he would not become a success if the only standard used to evaluate him was whether or not he returned to work.

Now whether our medical professionals should try to make people like this into something else as a result of the moral weight we put on work, I do not claim to know. But the values governing rationing in American health care are there for all to see if anyone really wants to see them. You do not have to travel to other places, other cultures, other societies.

My analysis of transplants, artificial organs, and rehabilitation leads me to claim that we have been rationing for quite some time in our society. And my analysis of the lifeboat case leads me to suggest that doctors, administrators, legislators, ethicists, nurses, bureaucrats, ex-governors, and Secretaries of Health and Human Services ought limit their use of the term "rationing" to those situations in which life-saving resources are scarce, and in which we know that resources cannot be stretched any further, that the resources will indeed save lives, and that people want access to them. If these conditions are not met, moral justification for rationing does not exist.

The case for inclusion, not exclusion, in health care

If this analysis is sound, then I do not believe a case can be made for instituting rationing throughout our health care system. There surely are areas of the health care system, such as organ transplantation or rehabilitation, in which rationing will be required now and for some time to come. But in large areas of health care we simply do not know whether access to resources is life-saving, much less beneficial in any way. And in too many cases we are giving care to people who have said they do not want it, or who would have said so had we instituted a public policy that would allow their voices to be heard when they cannot tell us what they want to do—in senility, coma, or mental illness.

If this is so, then we are under some obligation not to exclude people, but rather to include people in our health care system. Surely all ethical and religious traditions hold that minimal beneficence is required to save lives when it is possible to do so without risking one's own health or fiscal solvency.

When is the duty to help invoked?

Without going through a lot of technical argument, let me sketch an argument that would impose a duty of beneficence on anyone, provider or payor. If the following conditions are met, I think an obligation to help exists. To do this I will again use a paradigmatic case—that of rescuing a drowning victim.

Suppose you are a competent swimmer on your way to your favorite swimming hole. It is a hot summer day so you are already attired in your swimming suit. As you saunter down the road you pass a small, shallow pond. A little girl is thrashing about in the pond calling for help. You glance around, and there is no one else in sight. Are you obligated to help her?

The only possible answer is that you are. Why? Well, it is true that you do not know the girl. And it is true that you are not in any way responsible for her plight. Moreover, she may have fallen into the pond because of her own imprudent or negligent behavior. Nonetheless, you have an obligation to rescue her.

First, it is clear that she really is in need of help. And this is a standard requirement for any obligation to help; those seeking help must need it. Second, you know how to swim. You are even in your bathing trunks! The fact that she is shrieking things like, "Help, please help me," indicates not only a need but a desire for help. So a third condition for generating an obligation is met when the person in need wants help. And lastly, you can render aid without significant harm or peril to your own well-being. You are in your trunks, the pond is shallow, and you are on your way to go swimming anyway.

When benefits can be given to those in need who want help with a minimum of inconvenience, benefits ought be given.

In health care settings there are many people who have failing heart valves, premature babies, a need for rehabilitation after head injury or organ failure. We are obligated to help them if competent diagnosis reveals real needs and the person wants our help.

A third condition must also be met. We must know, just as the man in his swimming trunks, that if we do attempt to help there is a reasonable chance of doing so. It does not do much good for would-be rescuers to jump into ponds when they cannot swim, and it does no good to provide medical care if it is not known that the care will do any good.

Hard data on efficacy is necessary for any decision on rationing and moral obligation

Efficacy is at the heart of rationing and, as this argument makes clear, it is at the heart of obligations to assist as well. Yet our society spends more than $600 billion on health care while spending almost nothing to figure out whether any of it does any good. In discussions about whether our society should spend more or less on transplants or artificial hearts or prenatal care, or valve operations for addicts, or rehabilitation, or a thousand other things, no one can possibly decide because the data necessary for answering the question do not exist.

Unless hard data on efficacy exist, there is no way to derive a moral obligation to pay for providing medical care to others. All doctors, nurses, allied health professionals, social workers, third-party payors, trustees, and administrators can say is, we need a couple more billion for this or that, and it might help save lives. Or they can try to appeal to politicians through the deft use of the media by having photogenic patients beg, plead, and grovel in creative ways to elicit not a sense of obligation but a sense of charity.

What the medical professions, hospitals, nursing homes, institutions for the mentally ill, hospices, and health maintenance organizations should all be resolutely committed to is efficacy assessment, backwards and forwards, every day, all the time, for every procedure, be it diagnostic, palliative, therapeutic, preventive, rehabilitative, or cosmetic. Efficacy holds the key to the proper understanding of rationing. It is also the basis for generating a sense of obligation to help or pay for helping others. Unless the health care field can prove that there is a need for its services, that people want them, that they have a good chance of meeting those needs and that the needs can be met without demanding total sacrifice from society, it will have an extremely hard time persuading anybody to spend money for health care goods and services.

There is one last condition that needs to be mentioned in the context of the moral obligation to rescue or provide help to others. The degree of help being rendered does count.

To go back to my swimming case, if you are in your bathing suit not because you want to refresh yourself at the old swimming hole but because you are on your way to save many people who have had a boating accident, and happen to encounter our poor young girl in a swimming pond, then matters may be different. It does not make much sense to try to save the little girl if in doing so you forfeit the ability to save more people. If the odds of helping one are the same as helping more than one, then the weight of lives saved must be entered into the equation, other things being equal.

Few people would dispute the fact that we should not let the very real needs of a few overwhelm the ability of our health care system to provide for the very real needs of the many. But again, if there is no hard information about what does and does not work in health care, if doctors and nurses and allied health professionals are not certain whether an intervention has a high or a low probability of bringing about a benefit, then it will be very difficult to figure out what to do when conflicting demands for help exist. What is worse, without hard data every conflicting demand for help, for scarce health care dollars, looks insoluble.

If we allow ten new lung transplant programs to be created each year, if we make a commitment to provide access to rehabilitation for all who have suffered a stroke, what will the impact be on the overall health of the nation? The current structure of our health care system, with no systematic requirement for data to be quickly reported, makes it impossible to know. It is not that we lack the moral gumption to decide whether to help those who need transplants or rehabilitation, we simply do not have the numbers, the data, the analysis that would allow us to say anything constructive in attempting an answer.

The Institute of Medicine of the National Academy of Sciences and the Congressional Office of Technology Assessment have both issued reports[6,7] noting that less than 10 percent of all medical interventions have been subjected to any form of clinical trial. How can the American public be asked to spend money, be it retrospectively or prospectively, and feel happy about it if they lack the proof that their money buys results? If we had information on efficacy, we would know both where rationing is and is not necessary and where we are and are not obligated to help those in need. This seems a small price to pay for what is required in order to assure that our policies at the bedside and in the legislature are as ethical as we all agree they ought to be.

References

1. Churchill L. *Rationing health care in America.* South Bend, IN: University of Notre Dame Press, 1987.

2. Callahan D. *Setting limits.* New York: Simon and Schuster, 1987.

3. Califano J. *America's health care revolution.* New York: Random House, 1986.

4. Blank R. *Rationing medicine.* New York: Columbia University Press, 1988.

5. Schwartz W, Aaron H. *The painful prescription.* Washington, DC: The Brookings Institution, 1984.

6. Office of Technology Assessment. *Strategies for medical technology assessment.* Washington, DC: GPO, 1982.

7. Institute of Medicine. *Assessing medical technologies.* Washington, DC: NAS Press, 1985.

19.
Ethics, cost-containment, and the allocation of scarce resources

Our health care system is outstripping our ability—and, perhaps more importantly, the public's willingness—to pay for it. This crisis stems not so much from the existence of an absolute limit on health care resources[1] as from a growing realization that increasing expenditures will, if allowed to grow at the same rates of increase that have been present during the past two decades, inevitably interfere with spending for other national priorities, including education, housing, national defense, and with our nation's ability to compete in world markets.

The failure of cost containment

A number of cost containment strategies have been instituted by the federal government during the past two decades, including the encouragement of the creation of health maintenance organizations, the shift to prospective reimbursement based on diagnosis (DRGs),

TABLE 1

National health expenditures by year
(in billions of dollars)

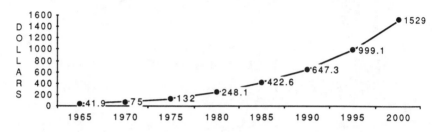

Source: Health Care Financing Administration

and the creation of both peer review organizations (PROs) to monitor procedures paid for by Medicare, and their forerunners, professional standards review organizations (PSROs), which monitored expenditures and treatment patterns in both Medicare and Medicaid.

None of these efforts has produced any significant reduction in costs.[2,3] In fact, health care expenditures have increased dramatically (both the total amount of money spent and as a percentage of the gross national product [see Tables 1–2]). The increases have, for many years, been at a rate higher than inflation. The medical care component of the consumer price index rose at an average compounded rate of 8.5 percent as against 4.8 percent for other items in 1980–1985. The rate was 6.9 percent versus 4.4 percent for 1988.

Equally disturbing is the fact that, despite the hundreds of billions of dollars spent, our health care system often fails to meet people's basic needs. About 37 million Americans are without health insurance, and thus are frequently without access to necessary care.

We spend a larger portion of our gross domestic product* (GDP) on health care than any other industrialized country (Table 3). Yet, the United States ranks 15th in male life expectancy, 7th in female life expectancy, and 19th in infant mortality compared to other industrialized nations. There is a growing public perception not only that health care costs are too high, but that health care resources are unwisely and inequitably distributed.

---

*The GDP—equal to the GNP less foreign earnings of international corporations—is more commonly used for international comparisons.

TABLE 2

National health expenditures as percent of GNP

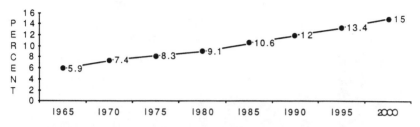

Source: Health Care Financing Administration

Factors underlying increases in health care cost

Many factors account for the steady (and projected) rise in health care expenditures. General increases in inflation and in the amount paid in wages to all workers have brought increases in expenditures for health care. In addition, a number of important factors specific to the health care sector are responsible for the continuing escalation in expenditures, including:

(1) Continued advances in medical technology

It is estimated that technological advances and increased intensity in the use of medical technologies account for 30–40 percent of health care cost increases.[4] New technologies often are less invasive and thus tend to be used more frequently than the older, more invasive ones they replace. For example, physicians are much more likely to use and patients to desire non-invasive techniques for diagnosis such as CAT and MRI scanning or ultrasound as opposed to invasive procedures such as contrast arteriography or exploratory surgery. Many new technologies also require more and better trained (and, thus, better paid) technicians.

Existing ethical standards in most areas of health care obligate health care professionals to employ interventions until they yield no additional benefits to patients. Concerns about legal liability reinforce decisions to provide all possible benefits with respect to diagno-

TABLE 3

Total health care expenditures as a share of Gross Domestic
Product: selected countries, 1986

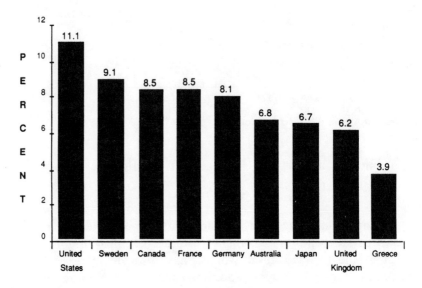

COUNTRY

Source: Organization for Economic Cooperation and Development

sis and treatment even when the chance of providing benefits is small.
The prevailing ethic of our health care system encourages, while the
legal system requires and existing economic incentives reward, maximal levels of intervention. Although each of the hundreds, perhaps
thousands, of new technologies that enter the medical care system
each year could, by itself, be absorbed into the system, not all can be
under present norms of utilization.

(2) The aging of the population

The U.S. median age, at an all-time high of 32.8, is projected to
be 38.4 in 2010 and 40.8 in 2030. The primary reason is the tremendous increase in the number of Americans 65 and over, which is
projected to rise from about 30 million in 1988 (12.5 percent of the
total population) to 39.2 million in 2010 (13.8 percent) and to 64.6 in
2030 (21.2 percent).[5]

Health costs are proportionately higher among the elderly, who require more ambulatory, hospital, surgical, and long-term care. These costs accelerate dramatically at the oldest ages and are particularly high in the final year of life. Although the elderly constitute only 12.5 percent of the population, they account for nearly 33 percent of all health care expenditures.[6] Per capita spending among those 65 and older is more than 3.5 times that of the total population.

(3) Increased prevalence of chronic diseases and disabilities

The prevalence of cardiovascular, degenerative, malignant, and other chronic diseases increases sharply with age. An aging population thus increases the need for long-term, non-curative care. The more successful medicine is in prolonging life, the more opportunities it creates for expensive care.[7]

Many patients—frequently the elderly but also those suffering devastating traumatic injuries as well as newborns born prematurely or with severe disabilities—can now be rescued by aggressive medical interventions. Some of those who are rescued survive with permanent disabilities or impairments which then require ongoing medical, nursing, and social expenditures to assist their rehabilitation and to enhance the quality of their lives.[8]

(4) AIDS

The number of people with AIDS has and will continue to increase relentlessly. During the first eight years of the AIDS epidemic, about 86,000 people in the U.S. developed the disease. The Center for Disease Control estimates between 390,000 and 480,000 cumulative cases will occur in the U.S. by 1993, with more than 75,000 new cases diagnosed in 1991 alone. Health care costs for AIDS (personal medical care costs and non-personal costs for research, education, screening, and general support services) are projected to increase from $1.6 billion (0.3 percent of total health care expenditures) in 1986 to about $10.3 billion (1.5 percent) in 1991.[9] In addition, productivity losses and other non-medical costs will be an estimated four times the medical costs.

(5) The partial success of efforts to increase access

Ironically, at a time when tens of millions of Americans still have no health insurance, a key factor which has fueled increases in health care costs has been the creation of programs to guarantee access to the health care system. The creation of Medicare and Medicaid has allowed millions of Americans to avail themselves of services they might not have received otherwise.

Limited health care resources

There can be little doubt that the factors described above have led to and will continue to fuel increases in the cost of health care. According to the health economist Victor Fuchs, "We can not have all the health or all the medical care that we would like to have. 'Highest quality care for all is pie in the sky.' We have to choose."[10]

Although there is still room for debate as to how much our society should pay for its health care, a consensus has developed—at least among government officials, corporate leaders, third-party payors, health policy analysts, some ethicists, and some union leaders—that we are reaching the limit of the percent of our resources that our nation is willing to devote to health care. Thus, many argue, universal access to all desired health care is an unrealizable ideal. Rationing, they argue, is the only viable public policy option. Some proponents of rationing argue that we have already instituted this policy, if not overtly then tacitly, since our country already is rationing health care, not only by the ability to pay but also by disease and by age.[11,12] Unfortunately, despite all the talk of the need to initiate or extend rationing as the only policy option capable of controlling escalating costs, those who use the term have not always been clear about what they mean.

What is rationing?

In order to understand the ethical criteria and principles that ought to govern rationing it is necessary to understand both the different types of distributional problems that arise in health care and the meaning of rationing itself. Rationing can take place at many different levels of decision-making.[13] And when rationing is the strategy used to respond to scarcity in health care settings, it carries consequences of tremendous moral importance.

The distribution of health care resources occurs at three distinct levels: (1) between health care and other social expenditures; (2) within the health care sector; and (3) among individual patients.[14] It might be useful to refer to the first two levels of distributional problems as "macroallocation" and to refer to the third level of distribution as "microallocation."

At the first level, health care competes with education, defense, and other industries to satisfy the myriad of human wants and needs. Even if our nation were to dramatically increase the amount spent on health care, it would be insufficient to provide universal access to all desired health care. The appetite for health care is infinitely expandable since it is almost always possible to secure some marginal increase in benefit by fulfilling wants or desires for more treatment.

Significantly increasing health care's share of the GNP, even if politically and economically feasible, thus will not solve the dilemma of limited health care resources: Spending more money is not by itself the answer to solving distributional problems at this level of macroallocation. Equity in macroallocation will still require drawing lines between what is needed and what is wanted in health care.

At the second level, in the words of the President's Commission on Ethical Problems in Medicine, "patients, health care professionals and institutions, and society at large must face an ethical problem. They must choose the uses to which limited—in some cases very scarce—resources must be put. The choices require comparing health care expenditures . . . within the health care budget: choices between treatment and research, between restorative steps for those already ill and preventive steps for those who may be at risk; choices among different age-groups, diseases, treatment settings, and so forth."[15] If the level of expenditure is held constant or allowed to increase only in small increments, the competing demands for the health care dollar will force hard choices among the various ways in which our society could spend monies earmarked for health care.

Decisions about how to spend dollars earmarked for health care are made in many different settings by many different people. Whether or not a hospital will buy a CAT scanning device or a group practice purchases an MRI machine are decisions influenced by many factors. But such decisions are pivotal in determining what choices will be faced at the level of microallocation.

The third level of distribution sometimes of necessity involves rationing. If there are fewer intensive care unit beds than patients who need them, fewer organs available for transplants than people dying of end-stage organ failure, or not enough crash carts and resuscitation teams available when more than one patient suffers a cardiac arrest, rationing would seem to be the only distributional option available to those who must make microallocation decisions.[16]

These examples are illustrative of exactly what is meant by rationing. In the health care setting, rationing can be defined as a conscious, reasoned decision by a health care provider faced with irremediable scarcity to deny access to life-extending medical interventions or to interventions that can help restore or ameliorate serious dysfunction for some patient or for a group of patients. Rationing presumes that health care interventions are both desired and known to be effective.

The term rationing is frequently used by economists and ethicists to describe any allocation decision or policy used to determine the distribution of scarce resources. But a narrower definition of rationing is to be preferred: rationing refers to the distribution of scarce resources that either save lives or significantly enhance the quality of life. The paradigmatic case of rationing in health care is triage on the battlefield, where doctors decide to focus their efforts only on those patients who are most likely to benefit from receiving care. Triage means denying care to some knowing that they will in all likelihood die.[17] Thus, in health care, rationing refers to a very well-defined subset of allocation policies—those which require a conscious decision or the adoption of an explicit policy wherein certain persons with known medical need are excluded from treatment that might save, prolong, or significantly enhance the quality of their lives.

The stakes are high where rationing is concerned in health care. Thus, the overriding moral imperative with respect to rationing in the health care system is not to determine what criteria or rules are fair. It is to make sure that, in the face of apparent scarcity, there is no distributional policy which is a viable alternative to rationing. Rationing, contrary to the more common use of the term, does not permit of any solution whereby resources can be expanded or stretched to meet the needs of those who seek the resource.

In most cases of scarcity, health care resources are rationed at the level of microallocation, and allocated at the level of macroallocation. For example, choosing Barney Clark from the pool of those dying of cardiac failure to receive the first artificial heart was a rationing decision. The decision by the University of Utah to devote resources to the development of an artificial heart program, rather than to any one of dozens of alternative programs, was an allocation decision.

Rationing can and does take place at both the macro and micro levels of allocation. But not all decisions to allocate resources in a particular way are instances of rationing. A decision to fund a particular research program rather than another, in and of itself, does not represent an instance of rationing since there is no conscious choice to allow someone or some group to die while others receive care that will allow them to live.

Caution is in order where the terms rationing and allocation are used. The ethics of allocation differs in important ways from the ethics of rationing. It may be that society will tolerate the use of criteria to accomplish the fair allocation of health care resources at the level of macroallocation (e.g., setting an explicit eligibility criterion based on age for access to health care, such as Medicare's use of age 65) which it will not accept as fair with respect to microallocation decisions (e.g., refusing access to dialysis to a patient because he or she is age 66). Conversely, the principles and rules used to make rationing decisions at the microallocation level may not be suitable for assuring equity at the level of macroallocation.[18]

Responses to the problem of limited health care resources

The intertwined issues of costs and access underlie America's health care crisis. Strategies to address this crisis generally are premised on two principles: (1) health care resources ought be used efficiently, and (2) resources ought be distributed equitably. There is no consensus, as yet, on whether our health policies should focus on cost and access simultaneously, or give cost containment top priority, or first make sure all Americans have access to health care and only then worry about cost containment.

Various options are available when confronting scarcity at either the macro or micro levels. It is possible to institute overt or tacit policies of rationing. It is also possible to pursue policies that attempt to avoid or delay the need for rationing. Perhaps the easiest "solution" would be to increase the percentage of the GNP devoted to health care; but this is unlikely and, furthermore, would only forestall, not eliminate, the need for rationing. The major payers for health care are bound by severe budget constraints—the federal government by the overriding budget deficit and corporations by growing pressure to remain competitive in the world market—and thus will redouble their cost containment efforts rather than significantly increase health care expenditures. And the factors underlying health care cost increases, particularly advances in medical technology and the aging of the population, would in any event soon outstrip our ability and willingness to pay for a health care system that would obviate rationing decisions.

Still, while some writers on cost containment and ethics have dismissed the importance or practicality of finding short-term solutions aimed at avoiding rationing by promoting efficiency,[3,6,12,14,19] it is ethically imperative to try and discover policy options that allow for rationing decisions to be delayed or avoided rather than to follow policies which call for explicit or tacit rationing. The stakes where rationing is involved in health care are so high—life and death, permanent disability or the restoration of function—that every effort must be made to resist or at least delay the implementation of rationing policies.

(1) Efficiency in the use of health care resources

In order to avoid the need for rationing at either the macro or micro levels of health care resource allocation, some argue that it is necessary to eliminate unnecessary care or waste. Unnecessary care can be defined in two ways—as care which has no demonstrated value to those who receive it or as care which has only a remote chance of producing marginal benefit.

Advocates of efficiency sometimes blur these two strategies.[20] And it might be argued that denying benefits, even marginal ones, to those in need is still a form of rationing. But, if the benefits being denied are not life-saving or significantly enhancing of the quality of life and if withholding or withdrawing them will not lead with certainty to adverse outcomes for some while others benefit, then it would seem inaccurate to describe policies which seek the elimination of marginal benefits as rationing.

Paradigms of unnecessary or wasteful care are laboratory screening and diagnostic tests performed without medically valid indications, various mental health interventions which appear to have no greater efficacy than that associated with the naturally occurring rates of disease remission,[21] the use of vitamins to supplement the diet of healthy persons, costly surgical operations and procedures performed without benefit to the patient (such as some Caesarean sections or the one out of seven coronary artery bypass surgeries performed for inappropriate reasons[22]) and "aggressive treatment of the terminally ill for whom treatment other than palliative care is no longer appropriate"[20] or desired. Wasteful and unnecessary care also includes care provided by incompetent and impaired health care providers. Not only is such care wasteful, it often causes iatrogenic problems that increase the overall costs of health care.

Some suggest that curtailing unnecessary care would permit the U.S. health care system to cover the cost of all truly beneficial care and thereby obviate the need for rationing.[18,20] Others argue that eliminating waste, which undoubtedly exists in the system, would not yield significant savings and would result only in a one-time reduction in expenditures.[3,19] Significantly improving the efficiency of the health care system requires (a) making providers more efficient and (b) systematically assessing the effectiveness of medical technologies. Other strategies to improve efficiency include (c) increasing market competition,[23,24] (d) emphasizing prevention,[25,26] and (e) providing more information about outcomes to consumers and purchasers of health care.[27]

(a) Making providers more efficient

Numerous studies have shown sharp differences from region to region in the use of medical resources (and, correspondingly, in per capita expenditures). These differences are not related to any obvious illness factors or the population's health care needs. Instead, they result primarily from variations in physician practice styles.[28,29]

There is wide disagreement within the medical and health professions over what constitutes appropriate diagnosis, treatment, rehabilitation, and palliation of many common conditions. Consequently, wide variations exist among physicians, nurses, and hospitals in the use of resources in the care of such conditions—from very conservative use to very elaborate use.[29,30]

These variations appear unrelated, in most cases, to health outcomes. If all health care providers adopted a more conservative style of practice—a style empirically established as consistently capable of producing good health outcomes—enormous savings could be realized.

Efficiency could also be improved by designing reimbursement policies which restrict access to certain procedures to institutional or private providers of demonstrated effectiveness. For example payment for some forms of organ transplants (lung, heart, bone marrow) is restricted by some third-party insurers (Prudential, John Hancock, Aetna) to transplant centers selected for the large number of transplants performed, high success rates and relatively low complication rates—in short on the basis of the center's proven efficiency. In 1987 the Medicare program took its first tentative steps in this direction by restricting coverage for heart transplants to those performed at designated transplant centers which had achieved demonstrable levels of success. Subsequently it has restricted payment for liver transplants to centers that qualify as "centers of excellence" by meeting certain standards for volume of procedures done and success rates.

(b) Assessing the effectiveness of medical technologies

Technology in health policy circles has a broad definition. It refers not just to the hardware of medicine but to all procedures carried out by health care providers as well as the organizational and support systems within which care is delivered.[31]

Using technology in this broad sense, it is evident that the United States has no coherent system for assessing the effectiveness or the efficacy of health care technologies. Although numerous federal agencies (e.g., National Institutes of Health, Office of Technology Assessment) and private organizations (e.g., medical device manufacturers, American Medical Association, health insurers) support or conduct medical technology assessment, the U.S. has no centralized, uniform, and readily accessible system for assessing all types of medical technology. FDA authority for assuring safety and efficacy extends only to drugs and some medical devices. There is no provision for the vast majority of diagnostic, rehabilitative, palliative, surgical, nursing, mental health, or non-pharmacological medical technologies to insure either their safety or effectiveness before their widespread dissemination and use.[31,32]

Moreover, existing assessment activities are voluntary. They concentrate almost exclusively on new technologies—not on those that are widely accepted and possibly outmoded. Thus, there are many expensive older technologies with questionable outcomes that remain eligible for reimbursement despite the fact that their effectiveness has not been established.

To improve efficiency, and to avoid or delay rationing at the micro and macro levels, emerging and existing medical technologies could be rigorously assessed to identify those that are safe and effective. Coverage and reimbursement policies could then be structured to promote the use of only those technologies which have established their safety and efficacy and of those providers who can demonstrate their ability to safely and effectively use them.

(c) Market competition

During the past decade there has been a profound shift from regulation toward a more competitive health care market. Some suggest that health care is not significantly different from other consumer goods and that, accordingly, the invisible hand of the marketplace will most efficiently distribute health care resources.[24,33] In a true competitive market, health care would be allocated or rationed principally according to the ability to pay.

However, health care differs in important respects from other kinds of products that consumers buy and sell in free markets. It is not clear that it is ethical to allow health care resources to be distributed by market forces alone. A large proportion of those in need of health care lack either the economic or the intellectual resources (e.g., the very young, the severely demented, the severely retarded, the illiterate) to make prudent choices in an open market. Providers have the ability not only to sell services but also to generate demand for them.

And it seems immoral simply to leave some portions of the population to fend for themselves in a free market if they lack the resources—for want of prudence, initiative, capacity, or for whatever reason—to obtain life-saving medical care for themselves and their dependents.

(d) Emphasizing prevention

Health care resources can be used to protect life and health by treating patients once they have become ill or injured, on the one hand, or to prevent death and disease by keeping people healthy on the other. Currently, private prevention programs make up less than 2 percent of total health care expenditures, and public health programs less than 2.5 percent.

More resources could be allocated for prevention as a way to increase efficiency and delay the need for rationing. Immunizations, prenatal care, access to contraception and other prevention programs are effective and relatively inexpensive ways to improve health status and control costs. But it is important to note that the evidence for the efficacy of prevention in many areas of health care is poor or non-existent.[34]

(e) Providing more information about outcomes to consumers and purchasers

Another strategy for promoting efficiency in the health care system is to assure that those who pay for health care have sufficient information regarding outcomes so as to make prudent choices.[27] The recent efforts of the Health Care Financing Administration (HCFA) to release hospital data on mortality and morbidity for Medicare recipients—and of states such as Iowa and Pennsylvania to compel the collection of data from all hospitals in these areas—represent early efforts to give those who purchase health care more information. But the availability of useful data for guiding consumer purchases, either by patients or by third parties, is still extremely limited. And, as was noted above, it is not clear that the consumers have the requisite expertise and capacities to always make proper use of information on outcomes in purchasing health care.

(f) Make greater use of technology

While technology is often cited as the prime culprit behind escalating health care costs there are many areas within health care where technology could be used to increase efficiency and lower costs. For example, hospital record keeping has far more in common with the 19th century than the 21st. Many institutions still keep their charts on paper and maintain huge storage rooms with large specialized staffs to access information. The inefficiency of this form of information storage and retrieval is obvious in an age of computers, modems and electronic mail. Significant cost reductions can be obtained simply by automating the handling of information in our health care institutions. The benefits of automation in information retrieval are not confined to hospital costs. Automating the collection, storage and retrieval of information would decrease the number of mistakes and iatrogenic incidents leading to adverse outcomes for patients thereby further decreasing the overall cost of care. More automation should also mean more informed patients, which should enhance compliance with medical recommendations thereby also allowing gains in efficiency.

(2) Equity in the allocation of health care resources

Equity in the distribution of health care resources at the level of macroallocation has alternatively been said to require (a) strict egalitarianism, (b) access based solely on medical necessity, (c) access to an adequate or minimal level of care, or (d) equal opportunity. Others have suggested that our nation can achieve equity in macroallocation by instituting rationing policies which utilize (e) age or (f) personal responsibility to limit access to health care.

(a) Strict egalitarianism

Equity as egalitarianism means everyone would receive the exact same level of resources to spend on health care. If health care resources are limited, then it is not possible to provide an optimal level of care to everyone. However, if access is to a standard of care that is lower than optimal, then equity as egalitarianism would deny an individual access to more or higher quality services than those available to everyone else, even if he or she were able to pay for those services or had special medical needs. To put this strategy bluntly, each person might get a government voucher good for a certain amount of health care, but no more. Those with compelling medical needs, such as newborns with severe congenital impairments, would have to cope with their medical needs with the same share of resources available to anyone else, impaired or not.

(b) Access based solely on medical necessity

Equity framed in terms of equal access to care according to "medical necessity" requires that all Americans be guaranteed "access to the health services which can reasonably be considered appropriate for meeting their medical needs."[35] The task is to articulate what constitutes reasonable need. No expenditure would be permitted for health care beyond this minimum, but everyone would have access, not to the same share of care, but to necessary care. Those with severe needs would have them met even if the cost of doing so were high.

(c) Access to an adequate level of care

Some suggest that only by defining equity as equal access to an adequate level of health care is an impossible commitment of resources to be avoided "without falling into the opposite error of abandoning the enterprise of seeking to ensure that health care is in fact available for everyone."[36] So defined, equity would mean that each member of society, regardless of ability to pay, would have equal access to an adequate level of health care. Services beyond this level, such as luxury hospital rooms, optional dental work, and cosmetic surgery, would be available for purchase in the health care market.

Precisely what constitutes an adequate level of care, or, alternatively, what comprises medically necessary care, has not yet been articulated. However, although disagreements exist at the margins, especially in cases of new and expensive technologies, sufficient consensus exists to make either standard useful.[35] The definition will change; specifying an adequate level of health care, or what is medically necessary, requires the creation of a mechanism capable of incorporating changing information on technology, consumer preferences, and resource availability.

(d) Equal opportunity

The distribution of health care can be guided by the principle of "fair equality of opportunity," such that all individuals have a fair chance of enjoying, at each stage of life, the "normal range of opportunities," i.e., "the array of life plans reasonable persons in (a given society) are likely to construct for themselves."[37] To achieve the goal of normal functioning, health care resources should be distributed to counter the opportunity disadvantages induced by impairment or disease. The problem with this position is that the needs of some persons are so great that providing them with care to allow them to have a level of opportunity equal with others would leave almost no resources for anyone else.

(e) Age as a standard

Many writers have suggested that age—not as a medical criterion (i.e., as a proxy for a person's physical condition) but as a "patient-centered criterion" (i.e., in reference to a person's history and biography)—could be used as a standard for allocating health care resources.[6,38] They see no hope for achieving cost control by any means other than the creation of explicit rationing policies at the level of macroallocation.

In typical age-based schemes, all people should have the opportunity to live a "natural life span"—to achieve a "full biographical life." Accordingly, the goal of medical care for people who have not yet achieved this is to avoid premature death and relieve pain and suffering. The goal of health care shifts for people who have lived a natural life span only to the relief of pain and suffering, not to extending life or resisting death.

(f) Personal responsibility

It is increasingly clear that many illnesses and injuries can be avoided by changes in lifestyle or personal habits. People who smoke, fail to exercise, do not use seatbelts or motorcycle helmets, or engage in other risky activities are more likely to need medical care. They are thus, to a degree, responsible for their illness or injury.

Some suggest the notion of personal responsibility for health (or illness) be used "for singling out for special treatment those who engage in unhealthy habits."[39] Such people should be encouraged, persuaded, or even coerced to change their behavior.[40] For example, healthful living habits could be promoted through education, the government could prohibit certain activities such as riding motorcycles without a helmet, or people who engage in risky behavior could be required to pay more for their health care insurance or for medical care when they become ill or injured. Finally, some suggest excluding from access to care persons who through their own choices increase the cost of care—unless they pay for it.[41,42]

(3) Equity in the rationing of health care resources

Even if it is possible to institute distributional policies which delay or avoid the need to ration at the level of macroallocation, it is still true that situations arise in the area of microallocation for which rationing is the only possible response.[16] For example, a finite and scarce supply of hearts limits the number of persons who can receive transplants. A shortage of beds in rehabilitation facilities limits the number of persons who can receive treatment for injuries, accidents, and disabling diseases. Limits on the number of MRI and PET scanners in the United States limit the number of diagnoses of life-threatening conditions that can be made using these machines. The shortage of nurses limits the number available to staff various units within hospitals and nursing homes.

There are many possible policies for rationing in response to scarcity. Rationing by age, social worth, prognosis, ability to pay, the absence of a disabling condition, patient motivation, and personal responsibility are all possible.[43] For the most part, physicians have relied on the level of medical urgency and of need as the most equitable criteria for rationing access to health care resources.

If rationing refers only to those situations in which valuable health care resources must knowingly be denied to one or more individuals while others receive them, it would appear that certain criteria would not be acceptable for guiding rationing decisions. Our society has agreed that race, gender, ethnic background, religious belief, and disability are all morally irrelevant when evaluating the worthiness of an individual or of a group to have access to social resources.

From the point of view of health care, it would appear that the primary goal of medical care should be to provide benefits to those in need. So rationing should be guided by the principle that health care providers should minimize the role of extraneous factors such as race or gender and strive to pursue distributional policies that have the greatest chance of providing the greatest benefit for the greatest number.

If maximizing benefit—or, to use older but more familiar terminology, avoiding harm and doing good—is the goal of health care, then factors such as the ability to pay are entirely irrelevant and inappropriate for those involved in microallocation decisions requiring rationing. Similarly, considerations of age, disability, motivation, or other patient characteristics are relevant only to the extent to which they are known to impact the chances of obtaining the benefits associated with particular medical interventions.

What society will accept as fair at the level of microallocation is closely tied to efforts to avoid comparative evaluations of the worthiness of saving one life instead of another. This is not to say that society views quality of life considerations as irrelevant. Rather, they are relevant only to the extent to which each individual believes quality of life is relevant in determining the desirability or worth of an intervention.

What is fair in microallocation need not be seen as fair in macroallocation. And what is obvious is that rationing is a distributional policy to be earnestly avoided at any level of allocation.

References

1. Reinhardt U. "We've Got a Health-cost Crisis? Bunk!." *Medical Economics* 1984;61:28–42.

2. Ginzberg E. "A Hard Look at Cost Containment." *N Engl J Med* 1987;316(18):1151–4.

3. Schwartz WB. "The Inevitable Failure of Current Cost-containment Strategies." *JAMA* 1987;257(2):220–24.

4. Jennett B. *High Technology Medicine.* Oxford: Oxford University Press, 1986.

5. U.S. Bureau of the Census. Projections of the Population of the United States, by Age, Sex, and Race: 1983 to 2080. In *Current Population Reports.* Series P-25, May 1984.

6. Callahan D. *Setting Limits: Medical Care in an Aging Society.* New York: Simon & Schuster, 1987.

7. Jennings B, Callahan D, Caplan A. "Ethical Challenges of Chronic Illness." *Hastings Cent Rep* 1988;18(1):1–16.

8. Caplan A. "Imperiled Newborns." *Hastings Cent Rep* 1987;17(6):5–32.

9. Scitovsky AA, Rice DP. "Estimates of the Direct and Indirect Costs of Acquired Immunodeficiency Syndrome in the United States, 1985, 1986, and 1991." *Public Health Rep* 1987;102(1):5–17.

10. Fuchs V. *Who Shall Live.* New York: Basic Books, 1974:7.

11. Cooper M. *Rationing Health Care.* New York: John Wiley, 1975.

12. Churchill L. *Rationing Health Care in America.* South Bend, IN: University of Notre Dame Press, 1987:14.

13. Childress J. "Who Shall Live When Not All Can Live?" *Soundings* 1970;53:339–355.

14. Evans R. "Health Care Technology and the Inevitability of Resource Allocation and Rationing Decisions." *JAMA* 1983;249(15):2047–53.

15. President's Commission for the Study of Ethical Problems in Medicine and Biomedical and Behavioral Research. *Summing Up.* Washington, DC: Government Printing Office, 1983:72.

16. Singer D, Carr P, Mulley A, Thibault G. "Rationing Intensive Care—Physician Responses to a Resource Shortage." *N Engl J Med* 1983; 309(19):1155–60.

17. Winslow, GR. *Triage and Justice.* Berkeley: University of California Press, 1982.

18. Caplan A. "A New Dilemma: Quality, Ethics and Expensive Medical Technologies." *New York Medical Quarterly* 1986;6(1):23–27.

19. Aaron HJ, Schwartz WB. *The Painful Prescription: Rationing Hospital Care.* Washington, DC: The Brookings Institution, 1984.

20. Angell M. "Cost Containment and the Physician." *JAMA* 1985;254(9):1203–07.

21. Fingarette H. *Heavy Drinking.* Berkeley: University of California Press, 1988.

22. Winslow CM, Kosecoff JB, et al. "The Appropriateness of Performing Coronary Artery Bypass Surgery." *JAMA* 1988;260(4):505–09.

23. Comptroller General of the United States. *Constraining National Health Care Expenditures.* Washington: GAO, 1985:GAO/HRD:85–105.

24. Lewin M, Meyer J. *Charting the Future of Health Care.* Washington: American Enterprise Institute, 1987.

25. Somers AR. "Why Not Try Preventing Illness As a Way of Controlling Medicare Costs?" *N Engl J Med* 1984;311:14.

26. Califano J. *America's Health Care Revolution.* New York: Random House, 1986.

27. Caplan A. "Hard Data on Efficacy: The Prerequisite for Hard Choices in Health Care." *Mt Sinai J Med* 1989. Reprinted in the present volume.

28. Wennberg J, Gittlesohn A. "Variations in Medical Care Among Small Areas." *Sci Am* 1982;246(4):120–34.

29. Wennberg J, Freeman JL, Culp WJ. "Are Hospital Services Rationed in New Haven or Over-Utilized in Boston?" *Lancet* 1987;1:1185–88.

30. Kane R, Caplan A. (eds.) *Everyday Ethics: Resolving Dilemmas in Nursing Home Life.* New York: Springer, 1990.

31. Office of Technology Assessment. *Strategies for Medical Technology Assessment.* Washington:GPO, September 1982.

32. Institute of Medicine. *Assessing Medical Technologies.* Washington: National Academy Press, 1985.

33. Olson M. *A New Approach to the Economics of Health Care.* Washington: American Enterprise Institute, 1981.

34. Russell LB. *Is Prevention Better Than Cure?* Washington, DC: Brookings Institution, 1986.

35. Bayer R, Callahan D, Caplan A, Jennings B. "Toward Justice in Health Care." *Am J Public Health* 1988;78(5):583–88.

36. President's Commission for the Study of Ethical Problems in Medicine and Biomedical and Behavioral Research. *Securing Access to Health Care.* Washington, DC: Government Printing Office, 1983:20.

37. Daniels N. *Just Health Care.* Cambridge: Cambridge University Press, 1985:33.

38. Kilner J. "Age as a Basis for Allocating Lifesaving Medical Resources: An Ethical Analysis." *J Health Polit Policy Law* 1988;13(3):405–23.

39. Wikler D. "Personal Responsibility for Illness." In D. Van De Veer (ed.), *Health Care Ethics.* Philadelphia: Temple Univ. Press, 1987.

40. Blank R. *Rationing Medicine.* New York: Columbia University Press, 1988.

41. Veatch R. "Voluntary Risks to Health: The Ethical Issues." *JAMA* 1980;243:50–55.

42. Englehardt HT. "Allocating Scarce Medical Resources and the Viability of Organ Transplantation." *N Engl J Med* 1984;311(1):66–71.

43. Rescher N. "The Allocation of Exotic Medical Lifesaving Therapy." *Ethics* 1969;79(3)173–86.

Index

Aaron, Henry: cost of medical technology, 288; rationing of health care, 306

Abernathy, V.: definition of competency, 212

Access: genetic counseling programs, 132; organ transplant referrals, 171; causes of rising health-care costs, 285, 289, 320; failure to meet basic needs, 316; equity in allocation and medical necessity, 330; equity in allocation and adequate level of care, 330–31

Accidents: present methods of organ procurement, 148, 181

Acute illness: relationship to chronic illness, 222–25; professional authority and individual autonomy, 225–26; moral obligation of public, 226–29; bioethic literature on provider/patient relationship, 241

Admissions: standards for organ transplant programs, 168–69

Age: chronological as distinct from aging, 198; rationing of organ transplants, 306; demographic causes of rising health-care costs, 318–19; equity in allocation of health-care resources, 331

Aging: normality, naturalness, and disease, 195–96; medical intervention, 197; description of process, 197–99; naturalness, design, and function, 199–200; concept of biological function, 200–201; religious and evolutionary explanations of function, 201–203; theories of and concept of disease, 203–205; ethical arguments against treating as disease, 206–208. See also Elderly

AIDS: public health and genetic screening and testing, 137; causes of rising health-care costs, 319

Allocation: example of moral efficacy in, 4–5; exclusion of philosophers from decision-making, 10; inadequacies of present methods of organ procurement, 147; public trust and fairness of organ distribution system, 157, 160–62; data needed to assess fairness of organ distribution system, 162–63; identifying pool of potential organ recipients, 164–67; admission to transplant center waiting lists, 168–69; transplant centers and distribution rules, 169–70; policies, principles, and values in organ distribution, 170–75; rehabilitation and termination of treatment, 250; equity and health care resources, 329–32. See also Rationing

Altruism: subject participation in biomedical research, 90; public willingness to serve as organ donors, 153; required-request approach to organ donation, 155; fairness of organ-distribution system, 160; nationality and organ transplants, 171

American Fertility Society: IVF success rates, 109–10; right to privacy and reproduction, 112

American Medical Association: moral requirements of medical profession, 243

Analogical reasoning: role in scientific theorizing, 35

Animal-breeding industry: influence on animal experimentation, 47

Animal experimentation: legitimacy of means and ends, 43–45; areas of contention concerning moral legitimacy, 45–53; sentience and purposiveness as criteria of moral worth, 54–57; conclusions on legitimacy, 57–58; reasons for current interest, 59–60; question of animal rights, 60–61; scientists and critics, 61–62; intuition and common sense in ethics, 63–64; democracy, moral uncertainty, and controversy, 64–65; scientists and morally relevant issues, 65–69. See also Xenografts

Animal-welfare movement: contemporary concerns, 59–60; responsibilities of scientists in a democracy, 64

Antigen matching: inequities in organ-distribution system, 161, 172–73

Antivivisectionism: moral legitimacy of animal experimentation, 47–49

Applied ethics: moral efficacy in medicine, 3–5; reasons for mixed record of success, 10–12; inadequacies of engineering model, 12–14; when failure is not failure, 14–16; art of moral engineering, 16–17. *See also* Ethics; Philosophers

Arteries: naturalness, design, and function, 199–200

Authority: social role of moral experts, 29, 37; acute and chronic illness and autonomy, 225–26

Autoimmune theory: genetic mutations and aging process, 204

Automation: record keeping and technology, 329

Autonomy: privacy as part of, 75; privacy as basic human need, 77; desire to respect and conflicts with professional judgments, 216–17; medical treatment of elderly, 217–20; acute and chronic illness and authority, 225–26; societal emphasis on and chronically ill and disabled, 229; demedicalizing of chronic illness and disability, 237; bioethic literature on provider/patient relationship, 241–42: competency and rehabilitation, 247–50; decisions to end rehabilitative care, 250–51; educational model of rehabilitation, 253; preeminence of in bioethics and legal studies of patient/provider interactions, 256–58; elderly and protection and enhancement of, 258–60; failures to adequately protect, 260–62; failure of donor cards in organ procurement, 262–63; inadequate scope of living wills, 265–67; supplementing living wills, 267–72; advance directives and locus of responsibility, 273–75; information needed for values baseline, 276–77; problems with values baseline for elderly, 278–79

Axiomatic-deductive model: logical relationship of facts to theories, 35

Ayer, A. J.: rejection of moral expertise, 22

Baby Jesse case: rationing of health care, 307

Bailey, Leonard: early attempts at xenografts, 178, 179

Behavior: modification and prevention of irreversible organ failure, 185

Belgium: usage patterns of medical technology, 299

Beneficence: health care and moral foundations of in American society, 227–28; demedicalizing of chronic illness and disability, 237; specific circumstances and moral obligation, 311–12

Benevolence: competency and autonomy, 216–17

Bennett, William: political activism and applied ethics, 21; political criticism of moral expertise, 23–24

Best interest: competency and medical judgments, 216, 219

Bioethics: foundationalism and moral theory, xvi–xvii; literature on provider/patient relationship, 241–42; elderly and discussions of autonomy, 257–58. *See also* Applied ethics; Ethics; Philosophers

Biotechnology: commercialization and human genome mapping project, 123–24

Boruch, Robert: privacy and need for identifiable health information, 79, 80–83

Brown, Louise: ethical debate on IVF, 105, 108

Cadavers: demand for organs and tissues from, 146

California: availability of genetic screening and counseling, 135–36; living-will legislation, 263

Catholic Church: Vatican pronouncement on assisted reproduction and IVF, 105

Cells: biological process of aging, 198, 203

Ceremony: moral engineering as, 16

Children: genetic disorders and genome-mapping project, 121; genetic engineering and human growth hormone, 139–40; pool of potential kidney-transplant recipients, 180; scientific status of xenografts, 184

Chromosomes: genetic mutations and aging, 203, 204. *See also* Genetics

Chronic illness: economic issues raised by increase in, 211–22; relationship to acute illness, 222–25; professional authority and individual autonomy, 225–26; moral obligation of public, 226–29; medical model, 230–33; disease and reclassification of, 233–34; conceptualization and policy dilemma, 234–35; demedicalizing and policy, 235–37; causes of rising health-care costs, 319

Clark, Barney: development of artificial heart, 290, 294, 295, 323

Class: skepticism about moral expertise, 26; research subjects and skewed pools, 87; access to genetic services, 131; organ-transplant allocation, 171, 172

Clinical practice: moral principles and meaning of competency, 215–17. *See also* Diagnosis

Collagen: cross–linkages and aging, 203

Commerce: development of artificial heart, 296–98

Commercialization: ethical issues of genome mapping project, 124

Commissions: growth in utilization of moral experts, 19

Common sense: engineering model, 13–14; intuition in ethics and animal experimentation, 62–64

Competency: determining care of elderly patients, 210–11; elderly and vulnerability, 211–12; problem of definition, 212–14; clinical standards and determinations of, 214–15; moral principles and meaning of in clinical settings, 215–17; ethical issues in medical treatment of elderly, 217–20; bioethic literature on provider/patient relationship, 241–42; autonomy in rehabilitation, 247–50. *See also* Incompetency

Competition: pervasiveness in medical research and ethics, 107; heart transplants and medical centers, 161–62

Compliance: chronically ill and disabled patients, 232

Conceptual analysis: philosophical skills, 6

Confidentiality: contractual model of medical relationships, 245; problems with values baseline, 278

Congress: genome-mapping project, 118; living-will legislation, 258; evolution of artificial heart, 293–94

Congressional Office of Technology Assessment: data on efficacy, 313–14

Consent: possible reforms to existing policies of organ donation, 151, 152; required-request policy for organ procurement, 152–53. *See also* Informed consent

Conservators: appointment and court-reviewed demonstration of incompetency, 259

Consumer, medical: benefits of biomedical research, 96; provision of information to, 328

Consumer price index: medical costs as component of, 316

Contractual model: provider/patient relationships, 244–46

Conversation: collection of information on autonomy, 275

Cooley, Denton: evolution of artificial heart, 290–92, 293

Cooperatives: obligations of members, 91–92; teaching hospital as, 93–94; research institutions, 94–95

Cosmetics: animal experimentation, 48

Costs: third-party payors and IVF, 107–108; efficacy of IVF, 110; genome-mapping project, 118; societal support for organ transplantation, 159; physicians and allocation of organ transplants, 167; admission to transplant-center waiting lists, 168, 172; social and economic costs of treating aging as disease, 207; third-party payors and chronic illness, 224–25; causes of rising costs, 285–87, 317–20; medical technology and, 288–89; development of artificial heart, 294–95; health-care providers and ethical issues, 302–303; rationing of organ transplants, 306; failure of containment strategies, 315–16; efficiency in use of health-care resources, 324–29. *See also* Economics

Counseling: value neutrality as moral foundation of genetic, 128–37

Courts: growth in utilization of moral experts, 19; reproductive rights, 112; brain death, 159; attempts at definition of competency, 213; right of competent adults to refuse medical treatment, 242; protection of right to autonomy, 259, 260

Cross-linkages: protein and nucleic-acid molecules and aging process, 203, 204

Culture, American: response to experts and expertise, 29; concept of expertise and view of knowledge, 30; definition of privacy, 74; universality of provisions of privacy, 76–77

Cyclosporine: history of organ transplantation, 158–59

Cytotoxic drugs: pharmacology and human experimentation, 183–84

Davis, Frederick: concept of privacy, 72, 73

Death and dying: reservations and fears about as barrier to organ donation, 149, 263; laws and court decisions recognizing brain death, 159; public acceptance of brain death, 159–60; aging and question of naturalness, 197

DeBakey, Michael: evolution of artificial heart, 290

Democracy: incompatibility with moral expertise, 24–25, 31; animal experimentation and responsibilities of scientists in, 64; moral uncertainty and controversy in animal experimentation, 64–65

Demographics: causes of rising health-care costs, 286

Department of Energy: genome-mapping project, 118, 119

Design: aging and function, 199–200

Deviance: genome-mapping project and concept of normality, 138

DeVries, William: evolution of artificial heart, 292, 293, 296, 297

Diagnosis: benefits of genome-mapping project, 121; potential pool of organ transplant recipients, 166–67

Dialysis: pool of potential kidney-transplant recipients, 179; end-stage renal disease program, 224–25; rationing in U.S. and U.K., 308–309

Disabilities and disabled: diagnosis and genome-mapping project, 121; organ-transplant allocation system, 171; economic issues raised by increase in, 221–22; medical model, 230–33; conceptualization and public policy, 234–35; demedicalizing and public policy, 235–37; causes of rising health-care costs, 319. *See also* Rehabilitation

Discrimination: ethical issues in genetic research, 126, 127, 137; inequities in organ-distribution system, 161, 171, 172; ethical arguments against treating aging as disease, 206–207

Disease: diagnosis and genome-mapping project, 121; normality and naturalness of aging process, 195–96; theories of aging and concept of, 203–205; ethical arguments against treating aging as, 206–208; relationship between acute and chronic illness, 222–25; uncertainty about categorization of chronic medical problems, 229; definition under medical model, 230; chronic illness, disability, and medical model, 231–33; reclassification of chronic illness, 233–34

DNA: human-genome mapping project, 119

DNI (do not intubate), DNR (resuscitate), DNT (treat) orders: failures to protect autonomy, 261

Donor cards: failure of existing policies for organ donation, 148–50, 262–63

Driver's licenses: organ procurement and encouraged voluntarism, 148

Drugs: cyclosporine, 158–59; cytotoxic, 183–84; government regulation of testing, 188. *See also* Pharmacology

Duty. *See* Obligation

Economics: issues raised by increase in chronic illness and disability, 221–22. *See also* Costs

Educational model: provider/patient relationship and rehabilitation, 251–54

Egalitarianism: equity in allocation of health-care resources, 329–30

Eisenberg, Leon: participation in research as public good, 89

Eisenstadt vs. Baird: reproductive rights, 112

Elderly: organ transplant allocation, 171; competency and determination of care, 210–11; vulnerability and competency, 211–12; membership approach to determination of competency, 215; conflict between benevolence and respect for autonomy, 217; ethical issues and medical treatment, 217–20; bioethical discussions of autonomy, 257–58; protection and enhancement of autonomy, 258–60, 266; causes of rising health-care costs, 318–19. *See also* Aging

Elephant Man (story): moral equality, 50

Embryos: research on and respect, 114–16

Emmanuel, Ezekiel and Linda: living wills and medical directives, 267–68

Employment: philosophical qualifications for medical, 6–7

Ends: legitimacy of in animal experimentation, 43–45

End-stage renal-disease program: costs of chronic illness, 224–25; access to dialysis, 308

Engineering model: description of in applied ethics, 7–8; effectiveness of philosophers using, 8–10; mixed record of success of applied ethics in medicine, 10–12; inadequacies of in applied ethics, 12–14; art of moral engineering, 16–17; moral expertise, 33–36, 36–38

Enzymes: biological changes of aging, 198

Epidemiology: justification for violation of privacy, 78–80

Equality: democracy and moral expertise, 31; moral legitimacy of animal research, 46, 48–49, 49–53

Equal opportunity: allocation of health-care resources, 331

Equity: exclusion of philosophers from decision-making, 10; public trust and fairness of organ distribution system, 160–62; allocation of health-care resources, 329–33

Ethics: universal foundationalism, xii–xvi; question of existence of moral expertise, 27–28; definition of moral expertise, 28–32; moral equality and recent history of discipline, 50; pervasiveness of competition in medical research, 107. *See also* Applied ethics; Bioethics; Medical ethics; Philosophers

Eugenics: ethical issues in genetic research, 125, 127

Evolution: function of aging, 200, 201–202, 208

Facts: application of moral expertise, 33–36

Fair play: moral duty and participation in research, 91–93; teaching hospital as social cooperative, 93–94; research institutions and obligations of patients, 95

Family: required-request approach to organ donation, 154; articulation of values and competency, 219; societal obligations to chronically ill and disabled, 229; rehabilitation and provider/patient relationship, 247, 252–53; veto power over autonomy of deceased, 264–65; values-history as supplement to living will, 270, 271; autonomy and collection of information for values baseline, 276

Fertility. *See In vitro* fertilization (IVF)

Florida: public policy and organ donation, 150

Food and Drug Administration: regulation and xenograft research, 188; evolution of artificial heart, 291–92; lack of system for assessing effectiveness of technology, 326–27

Foundationalism: universal and moral theory, xii–xvi; moral expertise and reexamination, 37

Free choice: societal emphasis on and chronically ill and disabled, 229

Free riders: concept of fair play, 92

Fried, Charles: participation in research as public good, 89

Fuchs, Victor: limited health-care resources, 320

Function: aging and design, 199–200; aging and concept of biological, 200–201; approach to competency determination, 215

Funding: genome-mapping project, 120; chronic illness and disability, 224–25

Gametes: research on and respect, 114–16

Genetics: diagnostic benefits of genome-mapping project, 121, 126; microsurgery and benefits of genome-mapping

project, 122; history of abuses in reproductive research, 124–25; expanding knowledge of and understanding of human nature and self-perception, 125; value neutrality and clinical, 128–30; value neutrality in screening, counseling, and information disclosure, 130–37; normalcy, deviance, and perfection and prospect of new knowledge, 137–41; mutations and aging process, 203, 204. *See also* Chromosomes; DNA; Genome-mapping project

Genome-mapping project: description, 118–20; goals, 120–23; ethically distinct issues raised by, 123–25; ethical issues in reproduction, 126–28

Germany: clinical genetics and eugenic goals of state, 127. *See also* Nazis

Gibson, Joan: values-history form, 271

Gifts: language of and organ donation, 155

Goffman, Erving: role of privacy in self-identity and personhood, 76

Government: reproductive rights and regulation of IVF, 111–13; funding of genome-mapping project, 120; definition of competency, 212–13; failure of cost-containment strategies, 315–16. *See also* Courts; Legislation

Grannum v. Berard: definition of competency, 213

Gross domestic product (GDP): proportion of U.S. spent on health care, 316

Guardians: appointment and court-reviewed demonstration of incompetency, 259

Hare, R. M.: on existence of moral expertise, 28

Hart, H. L. A.: moral duty and participation in research, 91

Health Care Financing Administration (HCFA): provision of information to consumers and purchasers, 328

Health maintenance organizations (HMOs): chronic illness and disability, 224

Heart transplants: transformation of interventions from experimentation to therapy, 106; age restrictions on, 146; survival rates of cadaver grafts, 151; history of, 158, 159; competition between medical centers, 161–62; need for transplantable solid organs, 180–81; present supply of transplantable solid organs, 181, 182; scientific status of xenografts, 182; evolution of artificial heart, 290–95; rationing policies, 307

Hegel, Georg Wilhelm Friedrich: moral experts, 26

Height: societal preferences and human-growth hormone, 140

Hippocratic Oath: moral requirements of medical profession, 243

Hospitals: policies and efficacy of philosophers in medicine, 10; diversionary and co-optative uses of applied ethics, 15–16; teaching as social cooperative, 93–94; responsibility for failure of present methods of organ procurement, 149, 160, 264, 265; required-request approach to organ donation, 153–54; regulations on DNR and DNI orders, 259; commerce and medical research, 296, 297

Humana Audubon: evolution of artificial heart, 293, 296

Human experimentation: moral scandals and prevention of abuses, 86–87; regulation of xenograft research, 188–89; evolution of artificial heart, 290–93. *See also* Subjects, research

Human growth hormone: genetic engineering and supply of, 139–40

Humans: mental properties and moral worth, 50–51. *See also* Human experimentation; Subjects, research

Hypoplastic left-heart syndrome: infants and congenital heart disease, 181

Identity: privacy as basic human need, 77

Ideology: skepticism about moral expertise, 26; human equality and moral expertise, 31

Illinois: definition of competency, 213

Immune deficiency syndrome: technology and health-care costs, 287. *See also* AIDS

Impartiality: philosophical qualifications for medical employment, 7

Incompetency: protection of patient autonomy, 259. *See also* Competency

Independence: values and rationing, 309

Independent committee review: human reproductive materials, 115. *See also* Institutional review boards; Peer review

India: genetic research and procreation, 126

Inevitability: criteria for defining naturalness, 199

Infants: numbers with congenital heart disease, 181; scientific status of xenografts, 184; premature and costs of technology, 287

Information: value neutrality and disclosure of genetic, 130–37; providers and responsibility for autonomy, 274; collection of for values baseline, 276–77; timeliness of values baseline, 278–79; provision to consumers and purchasers, 328; record keeping and technology, 329

Informed consent: research institutions and obligation of patients as subjects, 94–95; objections to use of IVF, 105; human reproductive materials, 115; competency as essential element of patient care, 210; in acute or emergency treatment and in rehabilitation, 242; contractual model of physician/patient relationships, 244–45, 246

Institute of Medicine of the National Academy of Sciences: data on efficacy, 313–14

Institutionalization: adverse impact on competency, 212

Institutional review boards: commerce and medical research, 297. *See also* Independent committee review; Peer review

Institutions: totalitarianism and invasion of privacy, 76

Insurance industry: lack of fairness in organ-transplant allocation, 172; reluctance to pay costs of chronic illness and disability, 224; organ transplants and restrictions of reimbursement policies, 326

Intelligence: value neutrality in genetic counseling, 132

Intuition: common sense in ethics and animal experimentation, 62–64

In utero fetal surgery: genetic research and reproductive rights, 126

In vitro fertilization (IVF): standard and non-standard forms of procedure, 103–104; harm and ethical debate, 104–105; nature and ethical debate, 105–106; transformation of from experimentation to therapy, 106–108; as technology or technique, 108–109; success rates and efficacy of, 109–11; reproductive rights and liberties, 111–13; respect and research on efficacy, 113–16

Jarvik, Robert: commerce and medical research, 296

Jarvik 7: limitations of artificial heart, 295

Jonas, Hans: participation in research as public good, 89, 90

Journals, professional: allocation of organs for transplantation, 161

Justice: participants and free riders in medical research, 88; theories of and organ-distribution system, 163

Kass, Leon: critics of IVF, 104, 105
Kelman, Herbert C.: risks of social harms, 81
Kidneys: early transplant surgery and dialysis, 146; survival rates of cadaver grafts, 151; history of organ transplantation, 158, 159; tissue typing and organ allocation decisions, 173; need for solid transplantable organs, 179–80; present supply of transplantable solid organs, 181, 182; scientific status of xenografts, 182; artificial organ replacement as permanent therapeutic option, 186. *See also* Dialysis
Koop, C. Everett: criticism of genetic testing, 129

The Lancet (journal): gene therapy and human self-improvement, 138
Lasagna, Louis: participation in research as public good, 89
Left, political: skepticism about moral expertise, 26
Legislation: advances in organ transplantation, 159; protection and enhancement of autonomy of elderly, 258–59; model language for living-will statutes, 266. *See also* Government
Lifestyles: autonomy and collection of information on, 276; personal responsibility and allocation of health-care resources, 331–32
Liver: transplants as experimentation or therapy, 107; history of organ transplantation, 158, 159; need for transplantable solid organs, 180; present supply of transplantable solid organs, 181, 182; scientific status of xenografts, 182
Living wills: legislation recognizing, 258; failures to protect autonomy, 261, 263–65; physicians and protection of autonomy, 261–62; inadequate scope of, 265–67; methods of supplementing, 267–72
Logical positivism: foundationalism in twentieth–century ethics, xiii
Logicians: definition of moral expertise, 32–33
Lundin, K.: definition of competency, 212

McCloskey, H. J.: derivative nature of privacy, 72–73

McDermott, Walsh: participation in research as public good, 89
Maine: rates of surgery in matched populations, 299
Market: possible reforms to existing policy of organ procurement, 151–52; competition and cost-containment strategy, 327–28
Means: overemphasis on by engineering model, 13; legitimacy of in animal experimentation, 43–45
Media: public trust and inequities in organ distribution system, 161
Medicaid/Medicare: air conditioners and respiratory patients, 5; advances in organ transplantation, 159; end-stage renal-disease program, 224–25; failure of cost-containment strategies, 316; improvement of access, 320; organ transplants and rationing, 326
Medical directives: supplements to living wills, 267–69
Medical ethics: effectiveness of philosophers using engineering model, 8–10. *See also* Applied ethics; Bioethics; Ethics
Medical model: chronic illness and disability, 230–33
Mehinacu Indians: cultural practices for attaining privacy, 76
Membership approach: determination of competency, 214–15
Memory: aging process and psychological change, 198
Metabolic disorders: value neutrality in genetic counseling, 132
Methodology: moral concerns and advances in scientific, 81
Meuffels, Willebrodus: development of artificial heart, 290
Mills, John Stuart: incompatibility of moral expertise with democracy, 24–25; paternalism and moral expertise, 29
Minorities: inequities in organ distribution system, 161, 171, 172, 173
Missouri: court decisions on competency and autonomy, 260
Moral agency: moral equality of humans and animals, 53
Moral experts and expertise: growth in utilization of, 18–20; response of philosophers to claims of, 20–22; philosophers on attempts to apply, 22–23; political correctness, 23–24; reasons for philosophical skepticism about, 24–27, 36–38; question of existence, 27–28;

definition, 28–33; facts and applications of, 33–36
Morality: changing interests and needs in real world, 11; effectiveness of philosophers using engineering model, 9–10; advances in scientific methodology, 81. *See also* Ethics
Moral theory: universal foundationalism, xii–xvi; bioethics, xvii; mixed record of success of applied ethics in medicine, 10–12; reasons for skepticism about moral expertise, 25–26; facts and application of moral expertise, 33–36
Mosaicism, genetic: value neutrality in genetic counseling, 132
Motivation: chronically ill and disabled patients, 232
Murphy, E. A.: normality and disease, 196

National health insurance: ethical debate, 289
National Heart Institute: evolution of artificial heart, 293–94
National Institutes of Health: genome-mapping project, 118, 119
Nationality: organ-transplant allocation system, 170–71
Naturalness: aging, normality, and disease, 195–96; death and dying, 197; aging, design, and function, 199–200
Nazis: abuse of research subjects in human experimentation, 86; abuses in reproductive research, 124
Need: moral legitimacy of animal experimentation, 46, 47–48; privacy as basic, 77; medical urgency and organ-transplant allocation, 173–74; existence of and societal obligation, 226; equity in allocation of health-care resources, 330
Neugarten, Bernice: category of old-old, 211
Newsletters: claims to moral expertise, 18
New York: court decisions on competency and autonomy, 260
Nielsen, Kai: applied ethics and moral theory, 25
Noble, Cheryl: political criticism of moral expertise, 23–24
Nomological-deductive model: compared to engineering model, 8
Normality: genome-mapping project and issue of human perfectability, 138; aging process and disease, 196
Nozick, Robert: concept of fair play, 92
Nuremberg trials: abuse of research subjects, 86. *See also* Nazis
Nurses: failure to make organ-donation requests, 160; collection of information for values baseline, 275. *See also* Professionals, health-care
Nursing homes: adverse impact on competency, 212; personal autonomy and professional authority, 226; elderly and autonomy in daily life, 266

Obligation: moral basis for participation in biomedical research, 89–93; teaching hospitals as social cooperatives, 93–94; research institutions and patients, 94–98; organ donation as charity or duty, 155–57; public policy and concept of, 303–304; rationing and public policy, 304–305; circumstances and imposition of duty, 311–12; data on efficacy and rationing, 312–14
Old-old: elderly and competency, 211
Organ procurement: inadequacy of present methods, 145–48, 181–82, 186; failure of encouraged voluntarism, 148–50, 262–63, 264, 265; possible reforms of existing policy, 150; required request as policy alternative, 152–55; donation as charity or obligation, 155–57; public distrust of medical establishment, 160; urgent need for transplantable solid organs, 179–81
Organ transplantation: fragility of societal support for, 158–62; data needed to assess fairness and equity of allocation system, 162–63, 163–64; identifying pool of potential recipients, 164–67; admission to transplant-center waiting lists, 168–69; transplant centers and distribution rules, 169–70; policies, principles, and values in allocation, 170–75; existing rationing policies, 306–308; insurance companies and rationing, 326. *See also* Xenografts
Outcome approach: determination of competency, 214–15

The Painful Prescription (Schwartz and Aaron): costs of medical technology, 288; rationing of health care, 306
Parsons, Talcott: cultural and social dimensions of disease, 231
Paternalism: traditional model of provider/patient relationship, 243–44; early stages of rehabilitation process, 248–50; educational model of rehabilitation, 252; autonomy and literature of health-care ethics, 259
Patients: teaching hospital as social cooperative, 93–94; research institutions and obligation to serve as subjects, 94–

95; current views on ethics of provider relationships, 240–43; traditional model of paternalism in provider relationships, 243–44; contractual model of provider relationships, 244–46; decisions to terminate rehabilitative treatment, 250–51; educational model in rehabilitation, 251–54

Patient Self Determination Act of 1989: living-will legislation, 258

Payments: as method for discharging obligation to serve as research subject, 97

Peer review: research protocols and obligation to serve as subject, 95

Perception: aging process and psychological change, 198

Perfectability: genetic research and issue of human, 138–41

Personality: physicians and allocation of organ transplants, 167

Pharmacology: introduction of drugs into human beings, 183–84. *See also* Drugs

Philosophers: activities of in medical settings, 5–6; qualifications for medical employment, 6–7; effectiveness of engineering model, 8–10. *See also* Applied ethics; Ethics; Moral experts and expertise

Physicians: inadequacies of engineering model, 14; failure of present methods of organ procurement, 149, 160; patient eligibility for organ transplantation, 167; ethical arguments against treating aging as disease, 206; traditional model of paternalism in patient relationships, 243–44; contractual model in patient relationships, 244–46; living wills and failure to protect autonomy, 261–62; diagnostic testing behavior and costs of medical technology, 288, 289; numbers in community and variations in use of technology, 299; efficiency and cost-containment strategies, 325–26. *See also* Professionals, health care

Pinkard, Terry: conceptual analysis of privacy, 71–72, 73–75

Plato: on moral expertise, 20

Policy, public: efficacy of philosophers in medicine, 9, 10; value neutrality in genetic counseling, 136–37; improvement, perfection, and genetic knowledge, 140–41; inadequacies of present method of organ procurement, 148–50, 186; possible reforms in organ procurement, 150; required request as organ-procurement policy alternative, 152–55; advances in organ transplanta-

tion, 159; organ allocation system, 170–75; moral foundations of beneficence in American society, 227–28; conceptualization of chronically ill and disabled, 234–35; demedicalizing chronic illness and disability, 235–37; evolution of artificial heart, 293; concept of obligation, 303–304; rationing and obligation, 304–305

Political prisoners: invasion of privacy, 76

Politics: correctness and moral experts and expertise, 23–24; skepticism about moral expertise, 26; potential pool of organ-transplant recipients, 166; relationship between chronic and acute illness, 223–25

Popper, Karl: Plato and moral expertise, 20

Power of attorney statutes: autonomy of elderly, 258–59

Preferred provider organizations (PPOs): chronic illness and disability, 224

President's Commission for the Study of Ethical Problems in Medicine and Biomedical and Behavioral Research: definition of competency, 212, 214

President's Commission on Ethical Problems in Medicine: health-care rationing, 321

Preventive health care: benefits of genome-mapping project, 122–23; as cost-containment strategy, 328

Principles of Medical Ethics (AMA): moral requirements of medical profession, 243

Priority: moral legitimacy of animal experimentation, 47, 49; claims of and desire to transmute experiments into therapy, 107

Prisons: organ procurement policies, 150

Privacy: importance to patient and moral efficacy of medical ethicists, 4; reasons for concern about in social sciences, 70–73; as essentially contested concept, 73–75; definition and importance, 76–78; buying power of in moral marketplace, 78–80; protection of and scientific health, 80–83; reproductive rights, 112; contractual model of medical relationships, 245; problems with values baseline, 278

Problem: selection and definition of moral problems, 12–13; individuation and identification of moral problems, 35–36

Procreation: religious objections to IVF

as morally illicit, 105–106. *See also In vitro* fertilization; Reproduction

Professionals, health-care: efficacy of philosophers in medical setting, 9–10; inadequacies of engineering model, 14. *See also* Nurses; Physicians

Progeria: genetic disease and aging process, 198

Provider/patient relationship: current views on ethics of, 240–43; traditional model of medical paternalism, 243–44; contractual model, 244–46; unique aspects of clinical care in rehabilitation, 246–47; competency and autonomy in rehabilitation, 247–50; decisions to terminate rehabilitation, 250–51; educational model in rehabilitation, 251–54

Provivisectionism: arguments on moral legitimacy of animal research, 46–47

Psychology: desire to transmute experiments into therapy, 107; changes in aging process, 198

Public good: moral basis for participation in biomedical research, 89–90

Public health: justification for invasion of privacy, 78–80; value neutrality in genetic counseling, 136–37

Publicity: public distrust of organ-distribution system, 160–61

Public opinion: willingness to serve as organ donor, 152–53, 263

Purposiveness: moral worth of animals and humans, 52–53, 56–57

Quality of life: values history, 270

Ramsey, Paul: critics of IVF, 104

Randomized clinical trials: bad science and skewed subject pools, 88–89

Rationing: technology and escalation in health-care costs, 289; public policy and obligation, 304–305; as subset of allocation, 305–306; organ transplants, 306–308; dialysis in U.S. and U.K., 308–309; American values, 309–10; case for inclusion in health care, 310–11; efficacy and moral obligation, 312–14; definition, 320–23; equity and health-care resources, 332–33. *See also* Allocation

Rawls, John: concept of fair play, 91–92

Record keeping: technology and efficiency, 329

Referrals: physicians and allocation of organ transplants, 167; organ transplants and set of norms governing, 171–72

Regan, Tom: animal rights, 60–61, 67

Regulation: xenograft research involving human subjects, 188–89; circumvention in technological development, 292; technology and adequacy of existing methods, 293–95; commerce and medical research, 297. *See also* Food and Drug Administration

Rehabilitation: provider/patient relationships and informed consent, 242–43; contractual model of provider/patient relationships, 245–46; unique aspects of clinical care and provider/patient relationships, 246–47; competency and autonomy, 247–50; decisions to terminate treatment, 250–51; educational model of, 251–54; existing rationing policies, 306; American values and rationing, 309–10

Religion: objections of IVF, 105–106; function of aging, 200, 201

Reproduction: rights, liberties, and IVF, 111–13; ethical issues in applicability of genetic knowledge to human, 124–25, 126–28; naturalness and disease, 196; evolutionary function of aging, 202. *See also In vitro* fertilization; Procreation

Research: institutions and subjects as patients, 94–98; efficacy of IVF, 113–16; clinical studies of xenografts, 182; ethics of further xenograft studies, 185–87; killing of animals for xenograft studies, 187–88; regulation of xenografts involving humans, 188–89; evolution of artificial heart, 290–93; adequacy of existing methods of regulation, 293–95; commerce and development of artificial heart, 296–98. *See also* Statistical research; Subjects, research

Resources: moral efficacy of medical ethicists, 4–5; limitations of health care, 320. *See also* Allocation

Respect: privacy as derivable from principle of, 75; for reproduction materials in IVF research, 113–16

Responsibility: personal and allocation of health-care resources, 331–32

Rhode Island: rates of surgery in matched populations, 299

Right, political: skepticism about moral expertise, 26

Rights: utilitarian analysis of moral worth, 56; question of animal, 60–61; informed consent and obligations of research subjects, 95; reproductive and IVF, 111–13; procreation and genetic research, 126

Roth, L.: definition of competency, 212

Ryle, Gilbert: definition of expertise, 30

Schiller: definition of competency, 213

Schroeder, William J.: artificial heart, 290, 293, 294

Schwartz, William: costs of medical technology, 288; rationing of health care, 306

Science: moral philosophy, xiii, xiv–xvi; theory and philosophy of, 33–36; skewed subject pools, 88–89. *See also* Research

Scientists: involvement in animal experimentation and critics, 61–62; responsibilities of in democracy, 64; arrogance and animal experimentation, 65; morally relevant issues in animal experimentation, 65–69

Selection: evolutionary function of aging, 202

Self-improvement: genetic research and issue of human perfectability, 138–41

Sentience: moral worth of humans and animals, 52–53, 54–56, 57

Sex: fetal and value neutrality in genetic counseling, 132

Sickle cell anemia: genetic research and reproductive rights, 126

Sick role: cultural and social dimensions of disease, 231

Singapore: genetic research and procreation, 126

Singer, Peter: definition of moral expertise, 32–33, 35, 36; sentience and moral worth, 54–56; question of animal rights, 60–61; moral equality and animal experimentation, 66

Slavery: intuition and common sense in ethics, 63, 64

Social contract: duty to participate in research, 90–91

Social science: reasons for concern about privacy, 70–73; protection of privacy and scientific health, 80–83

Socrates: moral expertise, 20, 24, 28

Soviet Union: clinical genetics and eugenic goals of state, 127

Space seclusion: importance of in animal and human behavior, 77

Standardization: information on values, 277

Stanford Heart Transplantation program: age restrictions on heart transplants, 146

State Department: politics and organ transplant allocation, 166

States: definition of competency, 212–13; living wills, 258. *See also* Legislation

Statistical research: protection of privacy and scientific health, 80–83

Subjects, research: privacy and social sciences, 82; information available on participants in biomedical research, 87–88; skewed pools and bad science, 88–89; moral basis for participation in biomedical research, 89–93; teaching hospital as social cooperative, 93–94; research institutions and obligations of patients, 94–98; regulation of xenograft research, 188–89. *See also* Human experimentation

Substituted judgment: competency and medical judgments, 216, 218–19

Suicide: intuition and common sense in ethics, 63, 64

Supreme Court: reproductive rights, 112

Surgery: rates of in matched populations, 299

Symbion Corp.: commerce and development of artificial heart, 296

Teaching: moral efficacy of applied ethics in medicine, 3–4; disinterest in medical ethics, 9, 10; claims of moral expertise, 21–22; hospitals as social cooperatives, 93–94; hospitals and commerce in medical research, 297

Technology: efficacy of IVF, 110; causes of rising health-care costs, 285, 286–87, 317–18; evolution of artificial heart, 290–93; adequacy of existing methods of regulation, 293–95; waste and inefficiency, 298–300; effectiveness assessment as cost-containment strategy, 326–27; greater use of as cost containment strategy, 329

Territoriality: importance of in animal and human behavior, 77

Theory: foundationalism and science, xv–xvi; philosophy, history, and sociology of science, 34. *See also* Moral theory

Therapy: efficacy of IVF, 110–11; benefits of genome-mapping project, 122–23

Thomson, Judith: right to privacy, 72, 73

Triage: as example of rationing, 322

Trust, public: barriers to organ donation, 149, 263; equity in organ-allocation system, 175; living wills, 264; values history, 271, 279; health-care providers and patient autonomy, 275

Truth: paternalism and contractual models of provider/patient relationships, 244–45

Uniform Anatomical Gift Acts: inadequacies of present methods of organ procurement, 148; reforms of organ-procurement policies, 150–51

United Kingdom: usage patterns of medical technology, 299; rationing of dialysis, 308–309

United Nations: reproductive rights, 112

United Network for Organ Sharing (UNOS): antigen-matching and inequities in organ-distribution system, 161, 173; organ-distribution rules, 169–70

United States: numbers of medical centers doing heart transplants, 161–62; citizenship and potential recipients of organ transplants, 164–65, 171; usage patterns of medical technology compared to other countries, 299; rationing policies, 306, 308–309; values and rationing, 309–10; lack of system for assessing effectiveness of technology, 326–27

Universality: criteria for defining naturalness, 199

University of Arizona: evolution of artificial heart, 293

University of Utah: evolution of artificial heart, 296, 323

Usage patterns: waste and inefficiency in medical technology, 298–300

Utilitarianism: sentience and moral worth, 54–55; Singer's and Regan's positions on animal rights, 61; justification of invasion of privacy, 79–80

Values: neutrality and clinical genetics, 128–30; neutrality in genetic screening, counseling, and information disclosure, 130–37; organ-transplant allocation system, 170–75; competency and medical treatment of elderly, 217–20; capacity of elderly for autonomy, 258; supplementation of living wills, 269–72; advance directives and locus of responsibility, 273-75; autonomy and collection of information, 276–77; problem of measurement, 277–78; problems with baseline, 278–79; American and rationing, 309–10

Vasoconstriction: aging and natural arterial function, 200

Vatican: pronouncement on assisted reproduction and IVF, 105

Vermont: rates of surgery in matched populations, 299

Voluntarism, encouraged: reasons for failure of policy, 148–50

Vulnerability: elderly and competency, 211–12

Waiting lists: inadequacies of present methods of procuring organs, 146; admission to transplant center, 168–69

Wallace, R. J.: justification for violation of privacy, 78–80

Washington: definition of incompetence, 213

Weismann, August: evolutionary function of aging, 200

Wells, Diane: definition of moral expertise, 32–33, 35, 36

Width: as essentially contestable concept, 74

Wisdom: elderly and articulation of personal values about health care, 218, 220; capacity of elderly for autonomy, 258

Women: as research subjects, 87

Work: values and rationing, 309–10

Xenografts: ethical issues raised by first attempts, 178–79; scientific status of, 182–84; ethics of further human experimentation, 185–87; killing animals for research involving, 187–88; regulation of research involving human subjects, 188–89. *See also* Animal experimentation

XYY syndrome: value neutrality in genetic counseling, 132

Zafra, Victor: evolution of artificial heart, 291–92